D0122586

Series Editors:
Steven F. Warren, Ph.D.
Joe Reichle, Ph.D.

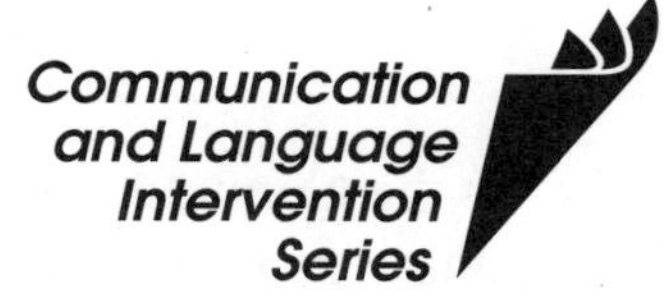

Volume 9

Autism Spectrum Disorders

Also in the Communication and Language Intervention Series:

Volume 5
Language Intervention:
Preschool Through the Elementary Years
edited by Marc E. Fey, Ph.D.
Jennifer Windsor, Ph.D.
and Steven F. Warren, Ph.D.

Volume 6
Assessment of
Communication and Language
edited by Kevin N. Cole, Ph.D.
Philip S. Dale, Ph.D.
and Donna J. Thal, Ph.D.

Volume 7
Transitions in
Prelinguistic Communication
edited by Amy M. Wetherby, Ph.D.
Steven F. Warren, Ph.D.
and Joe Reichle, Ph.D.

Volume 8
Exploring the
Speech–Language Connection
edited by Rhea Paul, Ph.D.

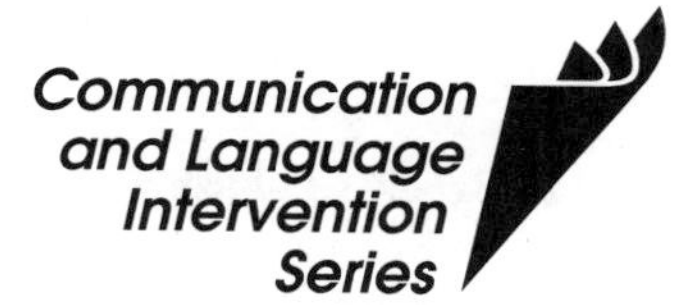

Volume 9

Autism Spectrum Disorders

A Transactional Developmental Perspective

edited by

Amy M. Wetherby, Ph.D., CCC-SLP
Professor
Department of Communication Disorders
Regional Rehabilitation Center
Florida State University
Tallahassee

and

Barry M. Prizant, Ph.D., CCC-SLP
Director
Childhood Communication Services
Cranston, Rhode Island

Adjunct Professor
Center for the Study of Human Development
Brown University
Providence, Rhode Island

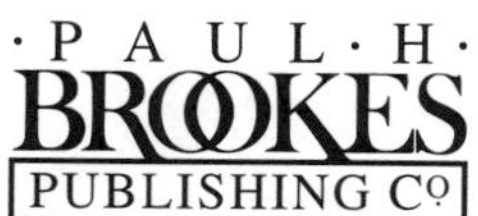

Baltimore • London • Toronto • Sydney

Paul H. Brookes Publishing Co.
Post Office Box 10624
Baltimore, Maryland 21285-0624

www.brookespublishing.com

Typeset by Eastern Composition, Binghamton, New York.
Manufactured in the United States of America by
The Maple Press Co., York, Pennsylvania.

The vignettes in Chapters 11 and 13 are based on the authors' actual experiences. All names have been changed; some identifying details have been altered to protect confidentiality.

This book is printed on recycled paper. 

Second Printing, January 2001.

Library of Congress Cataloging-in-Publication Data

Autism spectrum disorders: a transactional developmental perspective / edited by Amy M. Wetherby and Barry M. Prizant.

p. cm.—(Communication and language intervention series; 9)
Includes bibliographical references and index.
ISBN 1-55766-445-5
1. Autism in children. 2. Autistic children—Rehabilitation. I. Wetherby, Amy M. II. Prizant, Barry M. III. Series.
RJ506.A9 A9238 2000
618.92'8982—dc21 99-053060

British Library Cataloguing in Publication data are available from the British Library.

Contents

Part II Assessment and Intervention Issues

Series Preface

The purpose of the *Communication and Language Intervention Series* is to provide meaningful foundations for the application of sound intervention designs to enhance the development of communication skills across the life span. We are endeavoring to achieve this purpose by providing readers with presentations of state-of-the-art theory, research, and practice.

In selecting topics, editors, and authors, we are not attempting to limit the contents of this series to those viewpoints with which we agree or that we find most promising. We are assisted in our efforts to develop the series by an editorial advisory board consisting of prominent scholars representative of the range of issues and perspectives to be incorporated in the series.

We trust that the careful reader will find much that is provocative and controversial in this and other volumes. This will be necessarily so to the extent that the work reported is truly on the so-called cutting edge, a mythical place where no sacred cows exist. This point is demonstrated time and again throughout this volume as the conventional wisdom is challenged (and occasionally confirmed) by various authors.

Readers of this and other volumes are encouraged to proceed with healthy skepticism. In order to achieve our purpose, we take on some difficult and controversial issues. Errors and misinterpretations inevitably are made. This is normal in the development of any field and should be welcomed as evidence that the field is moving toward and tackling difficult and weighty issues.

Well-conceived theory and research on development of both children with and children without disabilities are vitally important for researchers, educators, and clinicians committed to the development of optimal approaches to communication and language intervention. For this reason, each volume in this series includes chapters pertaining to both development and intervention.

The content of each volume reflects our view of the symbiotic relationship between intervention and research: Demonstrations of what may work in intervention should lead to analyses of promising discoveries and insights from developmental work that may in turn fuel further refinement by intervention researchers.

An inherent goal of this series is to enhance the long-term development of the field by systematically furthering the dissemination of theoretically and empirically based scholarship and research. We promise the reader an opportunity to participate in the development of this field through the debates and discussions that occur throughout the pages of the *Communication and Language Intervention Series*.

Editorial Advisory Board

Contributors

The Editors

Amy M. Wetherby, Ph.D., CCC-SLP, Professor, Department of Communication Disorders, 107 Regional Rehabilitation Center, Florida State University, Tallahassee, FL 32306.

Dr. Wetherby is Professor and former Chair of the Department of Communication Disorders at Florida State University. She received her doctorate from the University of California–San Francisco/Santa Barbara in 1982. She has had more than 20 years of clinical experience in the design and implementation of communication programs for children with autism and severe communication impairments and is an American Speech-Language-Hearing Association fellow. Dr. Wetherby's research has focused on communicative and social-cognitive aspects of language difficulties in children with autism and, more recently, on the early identification of children with communicative impairments. She has published extensively on these topics and presents regularly at national conventions. She is a co-author of the *Communication and Symbolic Behavior Scales* (with Barry M. Prizant [Applied Symbolix, 1993]). She is the Executive Director of the Florida State University Center for Autism and Related Disabilities and is Project Director of U.S. Department of Education Model Demonstration Grant No. H324M980173 on early identification of communication disorders in infants and toddlers and Personnel Preparation Training Grant No. H029A10066 specializing in autism.

Barry M. Prizant, Ph.D., CCC-SLP, Director, Childhood Communication Services, 2024 Broad Street, Cranston, RI 02905; Adjunct Professor, Center for the Study of Human Development, Brown University, Providence, RI 02912.

Dr. Prizant has more than 25 years experience as a clinical scholar, researcher, and consultant to young children with autism spectrum disorders (ASD) and related communication disabilities and their families. He is an American Speech-Language-Hearing Association fellow and is a member of the Interdisciplinary Council on Developmental and Learning Disabilities. Formerly, he was Associate Professor of Psychiatry in the Brown University Program in Medicine, Professor in the School of Communication Sciences and Disorders at Emerson College, and Advanced Post-Doctoral Fellow in Early Intervention at University of North Carolina at Chapel Hill. He has developed family-centered programs for newly diagnosed toddlers with ASD and their families in hospital and university clinic environments. He has been an invited presenter at two State of the Science Conferences on ASD at the National Institutes of Health (NIH) and has contributed to the NIH Clinical Practice Guidelines for early identification and diagnosis of ASD. Dr. Prizant's current research and clinical interests include identification and family-centered treatment of infants, toddlers, and young children who have or are at risk for sociocommunicative difficulties, including ASD.

The Chapter Authors

Natacha Akshoomoff, Ph.D., Research Clinical Neuropsychologist, Laboratory for Research on the Neuroscience of Autism Laboratory, Children's Hospital Research Center, 8110 La Jolla Shores Drive, La Jolla, CA 92037. Dr. Akshoomoff received a doctorate in clinical psychology (neuropsychology specialization) in 1992 from the University of California–San Diego/San Diego State University Joint Doctoral Program in Clinical Psychology and also completed a clinical psychology predoctoral internship (neuropsychology track) at the University of Florida. From 1992 to 1995 she was a postdoctoral fellow in developmental cognitive neuroscience at the University of California–San Diego. Her research focuses on developmental neuropsychology, with an emphasis on the development of attention, using behavioral, cognitive electrophysiological, and functional magnetic resonance imaging methods. Dr. Akshoomoff wrote the chapter she contributed to this volume while she was Assistant Professor in the Psychology Department at Georgia State University.

Marie E. Anzalone, Sc.D., O.T.R., Assistant Professor of Clinical Occupational Therapy, Programs in Occupational Therapy, Neurological Institute, Columbia University, 710 West 168th Street, Eighth Floor, New York, NY 10032. Dr. Anzalone has extensive experience in pediatric occupational therapy specializing in sensory integration with young children, neonatology, and self- and mutual regulation during mother–infant play. Her current research focuses on mother–child interaction during play and the efficacy of sensory integration intervention.

Loisa Bennetto, Ph.D., Assistant Professor, Department of Clinical and Social Sciences in Psychology and Department of Pediatrics, University of Rochester, Meliora Hall, Box 270266, Rochester, NY 14627. Dr. Bennetto's research focuses on neurocognitive functioning in autism and other developmental disorders. Specifically, she studies how executive functioning, memory, and imitation relate to the development of social cognition and relatedness.

Pamelazita Buschbacher, Ed.D., Assistant Professor, Department of Child and Family Studies, Louis de la Parte Florida Mental Health Institute, University of South Florida, 13301 Bruce B. Downs Boulevard, Tampa, FL 33612. Dr. Buschbacher has more than 20 years of experience as a speech-language pathologist and holds a doctorate in early childhood and special education. Her research, publication, and presentation interests include supporting young children with autism and related disabilities in developmentally appropriate ways, communication development/intervention, early childhood development, and inclusion.

Malinda Carpenter, Ph.D., Postdoctoral Researcher, Max Planck Institute for Evolutionary Anthropology, Inselstrasse 22, D-04103 Leipzig, Germany. Dr. Carpenter's research interests include the development of joint attention, imitation, theory of mind, and other social-cognitive skills in children with autism, typically developing children, and apes.

Barbara Cutler, Ed.D., Educational Consultant, New Autism Consultants, 7 Teresa Circle, Arlington, MA 02474. Dr. Cutler, who has degrees from Harvard University and Boston University, has worked for more than 25 years as an educational consultant in autism. Her son, who has autism, is President of the Autism National Committee.

Barbara Domingue, M.Ed., Project Director, Community Autism Resources, Adsum, Inc., Post Office Box 1511, Fall River, MA 02722. Ms. Domingue is Project Director of Community Autism Resources of Adsum, Inc., which provides information, technical assistance, educational consultation, and advocacy to individuals with ASD and their families. She received her master's degree in special education with a specialization in autism from Lesley College in Cambridge, Massachusetts. She and her husband have three children, one of whom has autism.

Glen Dunlap, Ph.D., Professor, Department of Child and Family Studies and Department of Special Education, and Director, Division of Applied Research and Educational Support, University of South Florida, 13301 Bruce B. Downs Boulevard, Tampa, FL 33612. Dr. Dunlap is Director of the Research and Training Center on Positive Behavioral Support and Executive Director of the Center for Autism and Related Disabilities at the University of South Florida. He has worked for more than 25 years with children with autism and their families.

Karen A. Erickson, Ph.D., Professor, University of New Hampshire, 105C Morrill Hall, Durham, NH 03824. Dr. Erickson is a professor of early childhood and special education in the Department of Education at the University of New Hampshire and formerly was the Education Coordinator at the Center for Literacy and Disability Studies in North Carolina. The focus of Dr. Erickson's work is literacy assessment and instruction as it relates to students with significant disabilities. Her current work includes the development of a web-based reading and writing curriculum for adolescents with severe speech and physical impairments who read at the beginning level, development of a standardized reading assessment for people with severe speech and physical impairments, and school-based research of a technical assistance project aimed at providing inclusive education to young children with autism.

Lise Fox, Ph.D., Associate Professor, Department of Child and Family Studies, Louis de la Parte Florida Mental Health Institute, University of South Florida, 13301 Bruce B. Downs Boulevard, Tampa, FL 33612. Dr. Fox is Director of the Individualized Support Project, a model demonstration and outreach program that provides early intervention for young children with autism and serious challenging behavior and their families. She also serves as an administrative team member of the Center for Autism and Related Disabilities at the University of South Florida.

Stanley I. Greenspan, M.D., Clinical Professor, Department of Psychiatry, Behavioral Sciences, and Pediatrics, George Washington University Medical Center, 7201 Glenbrook Road, Bethesda, MD 20814. Dr. Greenspan is Supervising Child Psychoanalyst at the Washington Psychoanalytic Institute; Chairman of the Interdisciplinary Council on Developmental and Learning Disorders; founder and former President of ZERO TO THREE: National Center for Infants, Toddlers, and Families; and former Director of the National Institute of Mental Health's Clinical Infant Development Program and Mental Health Study Center. Dr. Greenspan is author or editor of numerous books and articles and has received several national awards, including the American Psychiatric Association's highest award for child psychiatry research. His work has been the subject of a PBS *Nova* documentary, "Life's First Feelings."

Catherine Lord, Ph.D., Clinical Psychologist, Professor of Psychiatry, and Director, Developmental Disorders Clinic, University of Chicago, 5841 South Maryland Avenue, Chicago, IL 60637. Dr. Lord is the director of an interdisciplinary clinic that provides diagnosis, assessment, consultation, and treatment for individuals of all ages with ASD and their families. The clinic's research group is actively involved in longitudinal studies of children referred for autism at age 2 and younger, studies of attention and communication, and studies of the genetics of autism. The clinic also provides training in research and clinical diagnoses using the Autism Diagnostic Interview–Revised (ADI–R; *Journal of Autism and Developmental Disorders,* 1994) and the Autism Diagnostic Observation Schedule–WPS Edition (ADOS–WPS; Western Psychological Services, 1999).

Janet McTarnaghan, M.Ed., Educational Consultant, Community Autism Resources, Adsum, Inc., Post Office Box 1511, Fall River, MA 02722. Ms. McTarnaghan consults with families and educators to support individual children with ASD in school environments. Her responsibilities also include the provision of in-service training on ASDs in schools and other agencies and the development and facilitation of peer support programs. She has worked for a number of years to provide support services to families of children with disabilities and has been an elementary school teacher and special education teacher in both private and public schools.

Pat Mirenda, Ph.D., Associate Professor, Department of Educational and Counselling Psychology and Special Education, University of British Columbia, 2125 Main Mall, Vancouver, British Columbia V6T 1Z4, Canada. Dr. Mirenda's primary areas of expertise include augmentative and alternative communication, positive behavioral support, and inclusion of students with severe disabilities in schools.

Peter Mundy, Ph.D., Professor of Psychology and Executive Director, Florida State Center for Autism and Related Disabilities, University of Miami, 212 Merrick Building, Coral Gables, FL 33146. Dr. Mundy is Director of the Child Division within the Department of Psychology. He has published numerous empirical and theoretical articles on the nature of early social deficits of children with autism. His research continues to explore the importance of early joint attention skill development for children with atypical or typical development.

Susan Risi, M.A., Research Associate, Department of Child and Adolescent Psychiatry, University of Chicago Hospitals, 5841 South Maryland Avenue, MC 3077, Chicago, IL 60637. Ms. Risi is completing her doctorate in clinical psychology at Florida State University. Currently, she is a research associate in the Department of Child and Adolescent Psychiatry at the University of Chicago Hospitals focusing on the diagnosis and treatment of autism.

Sally J. Rogers, Ph.D., Professor of Psychiatry, University of Colorado Health Sciences Center, 4200 East Ninth Avenue, Box B-148, Denver, CO 80262. Dr. Rogers is the principal investigator of a research program that is exploring the development of core symptoms of autism. She is also Director of Clinical Services at JFK Partners, a university affiliated program for individuals with developmental disabilities that provides training, research, and clinical care across the life span. She has been involved in treating children with autism for more than two decades and is the author of many papers and chapters on characteristics of autism and approaches to treatment.

Patrick J. Rydell, Ed.D., Director, Rocky Mountain Autism Services, 6520 South Oak Court, Littleton, CO 80127. Dr. Rydell is the director of Rocky Mountain Autism Services, a private practice dedicated to individuals who have autism and their families. He has contributed numerous peer-reviewed articles and book chapters pertaining to sociocommunicative disorders and interventions specific to individuals with ASD. Dr. Rydell speaks frequently at national and international conferences on issues related to ASDs.

Adriana L. Schuler, Ph.D., Professor, Department of Special Education, San Francisco State University, 1600 Holloway Avenue, San Francisco, CA 94132. Dr. Schuler's primary research interest is the interrelations between thinking and language. She has lectured extensively in the United States as well as abroad on the communicative, cognitive, and social dimensions of autism. Her work on emerging language in autism, thought without language, and prelanguage intervention approaches has been published in a number of different languages.

Jennifer Stella, M.S., Doctoral Candidate in Psychology, Center for Autism and Related Disabilities, University of Miami, 212 Merrick Building, Coral Gables, FL 33146. Ms. Stella is a full-time clinical staff member of the Center for Autism and Related Disabilities at the University of Miami. Her research has focused on improving the methods available for the assessment of autism and related disabilities, as well as on better understanding the possible fundamental features of this disorder, such as social-orienting disturbance.

Michael Tomasello, Ph.D., Co-Director, Max Planck Institute for Evolutional Anthropology, Inselstrasse 22, D-04103, Leipzig, Germany. Dr. Tomasello's research interests focus on processes of social cognition, social learning, and communication in human children and great apes. He is editor of *The New Psychology of Language: Cognitive and Functional Approaches to Language Structure* (Lawrence Erlbaum Associates, 1998), co-author of *Primate Cognition* (with J. Call [Oxford University Press, 1997]), and author of *First Verbs* (Cambridge University Press, 1992).

Diane Twachtman-Cullen, Ph.D., CCC-SLP, Autism Consultant, Autism and Developmental Disabilities Consultation Center, Post Office Box 13, Cromwell, CT 06413. Dr. Twachtman-Cullen is a communication disorders specialist and practicing speech-language pathologist specializing in autism, Asperger syndrome, and related conditions. She provides consultation services and training seminars internationally on the behalf of individuals with autism and Asperger syndrome. Dr. Twachtman-Cullen holds a Sixth Year Diploma in early childhood education and a doctorate in special education, has published numerous books and chapters, and serves on several professional advisory boards, including the panel of Professional Advisors of the Autism Society of America as well as the Asperger Syndrome Education Network of America, Inc.

Serena Wieder, Ph.D., Clinical Psychologist, 1315 Woodside Parkway, Silver Spring, MD 20910. Dr. Wieder specializes in the assessment and treatment of developmental disorders of relating and communicating in young children. She publishes widely and is co-author with Dr. Stanley I. Greenspan of *The Child with Special Needs: Encouraging Intellectual and Emotional Growth* (Addison Wesley Longman, 1998). Dr. Wieder is Associate Director of the Interdisciplinary Council on Developmental and Learning Disorders and is a member of the Board of Directors of ZERO TO THREE: National Center for Infants, Toddlers, and Families.

G. Gordon Williamson, Ph.D., Associate Clinical Professor, Rehabilitation Medicine Department, Columbia University, 710 West 168th Street, Eighth Floor, New York, NY 10032. Dr. Williamson directs Project BEAM at the John F. Kennedy Medical Center in

Edison, New Jersey, which provides outreach training to promote the social and adaptive competence of young children and families living in urban poverty. Dr. Williamson is a member of the Board of Directors of ZERO TO THREE: National Center for Infants, Toddlers, and Families and serves as Vice President of the New York ZERO TO THREE Network. He is a member of the Board of Directors and the Academy of Research of the American Occupational Therapy Foundation and has lectured widely throughout the United States, South America, and the Middle East.

Pamela J. Wolfberg, Ph.D., Consultant and Researcher, 1882 22nd Avenue, San Francisco, CA 94122. Dr. Wolfberg is in private practice and specializes in the peer socialization and play development of children with ASD. As originator of Integrated Play Groups, she leads efforts to develop peer play programs within the United States and abroad. She is author of *Play and Imagination in Children with Autism* (Teachers College Press, 1999), which is based on an award-winning ethnographic study.

Acknowledgments

I wish to acknowledge my family for their enduring support of my career. To my parents, Sue and Mel Miller, and my brother, Walter Miller, I am grateful for their unwavering love and support and for teaching me the importance of education and hard work. To my children, Rebecca and Shane Wetherby, and my husband, Dean Gioia, I am thankful for their willingness to share my time and for their ongoing love and support.

I also wish to acknowledge four individuals who have served as mentors, colleagues, and friends and have each contributed in unique and invaluable ways to my career—Drs. Carol Prutting, Robert Koegel, Adriana L. Schuler, and last but not least, my co-editor, Dr. Barry M. Prizant.

Finally, I wish to acknowledge the children with autism and their families, whom I have gotten to know over the years, for allowing me to learn so much from them.

Amy M. Wetherby

This book is dedicated to my father, Sam Prizant, who passed away after a long and fulfilling life only a few months prior to the publication of this book. The path I chose in my professional career was due in part to his unwavering support. This book is also dedicated to my son, Noah, whose journey through the toddler years during the writing of this book constantly reinforced the absolute necessity of understanding and supporting the development of all children from a developmental and transactional perspective. I also wish to acknowledge my wife, Dr. Elaine Meyer, for her understanding, love, and support during the completion of this volume.

I wish to acknowledge my co-editor, Dr. Amy M. Wetherby, for her friendship and professional partnership over the past three decades, and three personal mentors: Dr. Judy Duchan, my dissertation director and long-time friend, whose pioneering work in pragmatics demonstrated how essential it is for professionals to dig deep to understand how children make sense of their experience; Dr. David Yoder, for his personal support and friendship over the years and for his contributions in child language disabilities and augmentative and alternative communication, which have had a profound impact on professionals working with children with disabilities; and Dr. David Luterman, my professional colleague and dear friend over the past decade, whose wisdom, insight, and professional contributions regarding the family context of childhood disability have deepened challenges and rewards for countless professionals.

Finally, this book is dedicated to children and their families who live with the daily challenges of ASDs. They continue to provide the most profound lessons to professionals about how we can be helpful in our work, if only we are willing and able to listen.

Barry M. Prizant

Autism Spectrum Disorders

1

Introduction to Autism Spectrum Disorders

Amy M. Wetherby and Barry M. Prizant

The terms *autism spectrum disorders (ASDs)* and *pervasive developmental disorders (PDDs)* currently are used synonymously to refer to a wide spectrum of neurodevelopmental disorders that have three core features: impairments in social interaction, impairments in verbal and nonverbal communication, and restricted and repetitive patterns of behavior (American Psychiatric Association, 1994). Major advances have been made since the 1980s in understanding the social and communication difficulties of children with ASD or PDD. This progress has resulted in a greater emphasis on early sociocommunicative patterns in the diagnostic criteria for the generic category of PDDs, which includes the subcategory of autistic disorder (American Psychiatric Association, 1994). More specifically, the following essential features for autistic disorder compose the diagnostic criteria in the *Diagnostic and Statistical Manual of Mental Disorders, Fourth Edition:*

1. Impairment in social interaction, manifested by impairment in the use of nonverbal behavior, lack of spontaneous sharing, lack of socioemotional reciprocity, and/or failure to develop peer relationships
2. Impairment in communication, manifested by delay in or lack of development of spoken language and gestures, impairment in the ability to initiate or maintain conversation, repetitive and idiosyncratic use of language, and/or lack of pretend play
3. Restricted repertoire of activities and interests, manifested in preoccupation with restricted patterns of interest, inflexible adherence to routines, repetitive movements, and/or preoccupation with parts of objects

Because language and communication difficulties are essential features of this syndrome, educators and practitioners need to have current understanding of these characteristics and issues pertaining both to assessment and to intervention programs for children with ASD.

Autism is now understood to be of neurogenic origin and can have a dramatic impact on the family members of individuals with ASD. New treatment strategies are frequently introduced and discussed in the media and the professional literature; however, there is great variability regarding the extent to which treatments address the core characteristics of ASDs. In fact, much disagreement remains as to the nature of the core characteristics as opposed to secondary or frequently observed associated characteristics. Furthermore, most published intervention studies fail to employ meaningful outcome measures that document changes in barriers to learning that are characteristic of ASDs or meaningful lifestyle changes for the individual or family.

This volume provides a theoretical and research foundation for understanding the nature of the communication and language problems experienced by children with ASD and for guiding decision making in educational programming and, in particular, communication assessment and intervention. The first part (Chapters 2 through 8) examines the developmental context of children and their families and explores the underpinnings of ASDs and how these relate to communication and language problems. The second part (Chapters 9 through 15) examines issues pertaining to education and treatment for children with ASD. Because the topic of autism is so broad across the life span, this volume focuses on the first decade of life, spanning infancy, childhood, and elementary school age.

A DEVELOPMENTAL TRANSACTIONAL PERSPECTIVE

The theoretical and research framework underlying this book draws heavily from the transactional model of child development. That is, child development is viewed as a transactional process that involves a developmental interaction vis-à-vis the child and communicative partners (McLean, 1990; McLean & Snyder-McLean, 1978). Developmental outcomes at any point in time are seen as a result of a continuous dynamic interplay among child behavior (which is greatly influenced by neurophysiological variables), caregiver responses to the child's behavior, and environmental variables that may influence both the child and the caregiver (Sameroff, 1987; Sameroff & Chandler, 1975; Sameroff & Fiese, 1990). Over time, when a young child's social behavior can be accurately interpreted or read by a caregiver and the caregiver is able to respond in such a way as to meet the child's needs or to support social exchange, both caregiver and child develop a sense of efficacy (Dunst, Lowe, & Bartholomew, 1990; Goldberg, 1977). A cumulative effect of positive contingent responsiveness is that interactions become more predictable as expectancies and contingencies increase. This perspective emphasizes the reciprocal, bidirectional influence of the child's social environment, the responsiveness of communicative partners, and the child's own developing communicative competence.

A child's emotional and physiological regulation, which underlies the capacity to be "available" for learning and participating actively in a social context, is seen as an essential foundation within the transactional model. Development is therefore influenced by a child's ability to maintain some degree of emotional and physiological regulation and to produce increasingly readable and conventional signals, as well as by a caregiver's ability to respond effectively to the child's signals and to embed reciprocal and mutually satisfying transactions in everyday activities and routines. We believe that the nature of the social, communication, and language impairments in autism can best be understood by reflecting on the acquisition process from a transactional developmental perspective and have invited distinguished researchers and clinicians to contribute toward this end.

CURRENT ISSUES IN COMMUNICATION AND LANGUAGE OF CHILDREN WITH AUTISM

Dawson and Osterling (1997) reviewed eight early intervention programs for preschool children with autism, ranging from intensive, one-to-one discrete trial approaches to programs in inclusive environments using naturalistic procedures. They concluded that the level of success achieved across these programs was fairly similar; these programs generally were effective for about half of the children. Effectiveness was determined based on changes in measures such as IQ scores and classroom placement. They noted that few of these programs documented progress on goals addressing social and communicative aspects of development.

Their conclusions provide important implications for intervention programs and directions for future research. First, no evidence indicates that one program or approach works better than others, and, therefore, caution is warranted in drawing conclusions about intervention efficacy. Second, there is much to be learned about effective programs to enhance social and communication skills in children with autism because little empirical data are available. These findings underscore the need to better understand which specific intervention methods work best to accomplish which goals for which children. We contend that directions for future research, particularly intervention studies, should be rooted in theory and research about the nature of ASDs and of the developmental process.

OVERVIEW OF THIS VOLUME

We have invited authors who represent a range of orientations and perspectives (e.g., behavioral, neurobehavioral, developmental, family systems) to contribute to this volume. This volume will help clinicians and educators gain access to the most current theories and research to better understand children with ASD and be exposed to guidelines for developing innovative intervention approaches to enhance social, communication, and language skills in these children.

Part I of this volume examines the developmental context and explores the underpinnings of ASDs and how these relate to communication and language difficulties. Lord and Risi (Chapter 2) begin with an overview of the diagnostic features of ASDs and the differentiating characteristics of the subcategories. They discuss the importance of the diagnosis with a focus on diagnosis in young children. They compare and contrast research on diagnostic measures based on parent report and observational measures in 2- and 3-year-olds. Implications for earlier and more accurate diagnosis are provided, with an emphasis on changes in developmental characteristics during the preschool years.

Carpenter and Tomasello (Chapter 3) describe the social-pragmatic approach to language acquisition with a focus on the process of cultural learning. They review research on how children acquire language and examine the role of joint attention, the flow of social interaction, and social-cognitive foundational skills. They examine the process of language acquisition in children with autism from a social-pragmatic perspective and discuss how impairments in the foundational skills of joint attention, understanding others' communicative intentions, and role-reversal imitation can explain many other impairments in the language of children with autism.

Mundy and Stella (Chapter 4) examine three prominent models to account for the social communication impairments of autism, the theory of mind (ToM) model, the executive function model, and the social orientation model. They conclude that the social orientation model has the best explanatory power for the developmental progression of autism in that it accounts for the earliest-emerging features of the disorder. They hypothesize that the early social-orienting disturbance may have a negative impact on postnatal brain development and on executive function and ToM development. In discussing implications they highlight the importance of measures of joint attention.

Rogers and Bennetto (Chapter 5) examine the roles of imitation and executive function to account for the deficits in social relatedness; communication; and restricted, repetitive behaviors in autism on the basis of empirical research published since the late 1980s. In reviewing findings on imitation, motor impairments, and dyspraxia in autism, they conclude that there is support for autism-specific impairments on imitative and nonimitative motor tasks. In reviewing findings on executive function, they conclude that there is consistent evidence of impairments on global tasks of executive functions in older and higher-functioning individuals but not in preschoolers. On the basis of Stern's (1985) model of emotional development, they hypothesize that a severe and early deficit in imitation/praxis could impair the physical coordination of social exchanges but argue that the affective system holds clues about the primary impairment of autism.

Wetherby, Prizant, and Schuler (Chapter 6) review research on the nature of communication and language impairments in autism, focusing on the capacities for joint attention and symbol use. They examine research on developmental patterns that reveals how strengths and weaknesses in communication, social-affective, and symbolic abilities cluster in distinct profiles in children with autism. They explore how developmental theory can contribute to a better understanding of the communication patterns in autism and provide implications for earlier diagnosis, meaningful measures of abilities and outcomes, and decisions about intervention efficacy.

Anzalone and Williamson (Chapter 7) present an overview of theories on motor planning and sensory processing in ASDs. They also examine issues of sensory integration dysfunction relative to the variety of ways it may be manifest in children with ASD and its impact on adaptive functioning. Implications for infusing treatment principles into educational programs for children with ASD are discussed, with particular emphasis on changing the environment and incorporating a daily sensory diet to prevent sensory defensiveness and promote self-regulation.

Akshoomoff (Chapter 8) explores the neurological underpinnings of autism. She reviews neuroimaging and autopsy studies and examines two neurodevelopmental models of autism: a complex model involving multiple neural systems and the cerebellum and an attention model. She discusses how early damage to specific neurological sites can lead to the behavioral symptoms of autism and suggests the importance of addressing the speed of shifting attention and the size of the attentional "spotlight" in early intervention programs.

Part II of this volume examines issues pertaining to communication and language in the education and intervention for children with ASD. Prizant, Wetherby, and Rydell (Chapter 9) begin with a historical perspective on approaches to enhancing language and communication abilities of children with ASD. They provide a critical analysis of a continuum of approaches ranging from traditional behavioral to developmental, social-pragmatic approaches, including middle-ground "hybrid" approaches that draw from both behavioral and developmental research and educational traditions. They conclude by describing an evolving model for establishing therapeutic priorities that focuses on capacities in communication and emotional regulation and for developing the requisite transactional supports (i.e., family members, peers, environmental supports) necessary to optimally enhance children's development.

Twachtman-Cullen (Chapter 10) describes the specific sociocommunicative challenges faced by higher functioning children with ASD, including children with a diagnosis of Asperger syndrome. She explores these challenges in reference to theories on information processing and social-cognitive constructs such as ToM. Guidelines for enhancing abilities also are addressed with attention given to the complex and often subtle nature of the problems experienced by these children and the related challenges in education and communication enhancement.

Schuler and Wolfberg (Chapter 11) provide an overview of theories and research on patterns of play development in children with ASD. Particular attention is given to aspects of social play and how such impairments affect social and language development. The authors present guidelines for promoting play development within a social inclusionary context based on their extensive clinical and research experience on "integrated play groups" for children with ASD.

Greenspan and Wieder (Chapter 12) discuss their functional approach, in which a child's developmental profile is examined to capture the unique features of processing strengths and weaknesses, which orients the clinician toward the proper intervention plan. An emphasis is placed on understanding core emotional functional capacities as they relate to and support many aspects of a child's development. They then describe the underpinnings of their Developmental, Individualized, Relationship-Based Intervention (DIR) model to enhancing social and emotional development of children with ASD, with practical suggestions and examples for implementing the "floor time" approach.

Fox, Dunlap, and Buschbacher (Chapter 13) offer a way to understand the challenging behavior of children with autism and recognize the critical role of the family context. They describe positive behavioral support, which is a process for understanding the purposes of challenging behavior and developing a plan of support that promotes the development of new skills while reducing the need for and occurrence of the behavior. This approach is rooted in research and theory on the communicative purpose of challenging behavior, which is reviewed in this chapter. They offer a lucid description of the functional assessment process, including gathering information, formulating hypotheses about the function of the behavior, and developing a behavioral support plan.

Mirenda and Erickson (Chapter 14) provide a comprehensive review of the current research literature pertaining to augmentative and alternative communication (AAC) and literacy issues for children with ASD. Implementation of AAC and literacy strategies is discussed in relation to the often-observed visual processing strengths as well as sociocommunicative impairments of children with ASD. Guidelines for decision making in selecting communication systems and fostering literacy skills are presented.

Domingue, Cutler, and McTarnaghan (Chapter 15) consider the process of coping and adapting among families of children with ASD, giving particular emphasis to the experience of families from the family's perspective. The first two authors share their unique insights from the perspective of being both professionals and parents. Suggestions for incorporating family-centered practices of support, assessment, and intervention are presented, with specific justification why working within a family-centered model is essential for children with ASD and their families.

The common bond shared by all of the authors is the understanding that children with ASD and their families are uniquely individual and that there is no single explanation that accounts for the developmental profiles and challenges of all of the children. Thus, there is no single intervention approach or treatment modality that can address the varied needs of all children and their families.

CONCLUSIONS

Clinicians, educators, and parents will find a wealth of information in this volume that will enhance their understanding of children with ASD. This information can then be applied to supporting the development of specific children using individualized approaches, which are so essential to addressing the unique needs of each child. Our hope is that this volume also provides direction for researchers as well as practitioners to further explore specific topics and offers decision-making guidelines and innovative strategies that can be used in developing comprehensive approaches for children with ASD. The clinician/educator as "scientist" will need to explore and document the effectiveness of specific intervention procedures with particular children.

REFERENCES

American Psychiatric Association. (1994). *Diagnostic and statistical manual of mental disorders* (4th ed.). Washington, DC: Author.

Dawson, G., & Osterling, J. (1997). Early intervention in autism. In M. Guralnick (Ed.), *The effectiveness of early intervention* (pp. 307–326). Baltimore: Paul H. Brookes Publishing Co.

Dunst, C.J., Lowe, L.W., & Bartholomew, P.C. (1990). Contingent social responsiveness, family ecology, and infant communicative competence. *National Student Speech Language Hearing Association Journal, 17,* 39–49.

Goldberg, S. (1977). Social competence in infancy: A model of parent–infant interaction. *Merrill-Palmer Quarterly, 23,* 163–177.

McLean, J.E., & Snyder-McLean, L.K. (1978). *A transactional approach to early language training.* Columbus, OH: Charles E. Merrill.

McLean, L.K. (1990). Communication development in the first two years of life: A transactional process. *ZERO TO THREE Bulletin, 11,* 13–19.

Sameroff, A. (1987). The social context of development. In N. Eisenburg (Ed.), *Contemporary topics in development* (pp. 273–291). New York: John Wiley & Sons.

Sameroff, A., & Chandler, M. (1975). Reproductive risk and the continuum of caretaking causality. In F. Horowitz (Ed.), *Review of child development research* (Vol. 4, pp. 187–244). Chicago: University of Chicago Press.

Sameroff, A., & Fiese, B. (1990). Transactional regulation and early intervention. In S. Meisels & J. Shonkoff (Eds.), *Early intervention: A handbook of theory, practice, and analysis* (pp. 119–149). New York: Cambridge University Press.

Stern, D. (1985). *The interpersonal world of the human infant.* New York: Basic Books.

Part I

Theoretical and Research Foundations

Understanding the Developmental Context of Autism

2

Diagnosis of Autism Spectrum Disorders in Young Children

Catherine Lord and Susan Risi

Autism is a developmental disorder that originates prior to birth or in early infancy. Although there are many reasons to believe that autism is a neurobiological disorder with a strong genetic component, a biological marker has not yet been found. Therefore, the syndrome must be defined on the basis of observed or described behaviors. The behaviors, as depicted in the formal diagnostic systems of the American Psychiatric Association (APA; 1994) and the World Health Organization (WHO; 1993), are described in terms of a pattern of deficits in social behavior and communication accompanied by restricted and repetitive behaviors or interests as well as an age of onset prior to 36 months.

AUTISM AS A SPECTRUM DISORDER

Since the late 1970s, not only has the description of autism been increasingly refined, but the concept also has been extended to that of a spectrum disorder (Gillberg, 1990; Wing & Gould, 1979). Autism is defined by a triad of deficits in social reciprocity, communication, and repetitive behaviors or interests, each of which can occur at different levels of severity. Although deficits in these three areas often co-occur in individuals without autism (Bolton et al., 1994), children affected by similar difficulties in social reciprocity and either communication or restricted behaviors often need the same services and follow the same course as those with autism. Even among people with deficits in all three areas, individuals can vary significantly in the degree to which they are affected by behaviors associated with autistic disorder. Incomplete manifestations of the syndrome may be observed, such as in people with marked social and communication deficits but without repetitive behaviors. These deficits may still cause significant and lifelong impairment, even though they do not meet the three-domain definition of autism.

The term *pervasive developmental disorders* (PDDs) was first adopted to provide a formal diagnosis for individuals who shared critical deficits similar to those associated with autism but who did not meet the full criteria of a diagnosis of autism. The intention was to emphasize the pervasiveness of the impairments in many aspects of life while still differentiating autism from general cognitive disabilities such as mental retardation. As shown in Figure 2.1, the notion of a spectrum assumes that, until biological markers are found, classical autism is the prototype of the disorder. Other disorders extend from this prototype in decreasing severity and in decreasing number of domains affected.

Exactly which disorders should be included in the spectrum and how broadly this spectrum extends is controversial (Mahoney et al., 1998; Tanguay, Robertson, & Derrick, 1998) and differs slightly across the American and international diagnostic systems: the *Diagnostic and Statistical Manual of Mental Disorders, Fourth Edition* (DSM-IV; APA, 1994), and the *International*

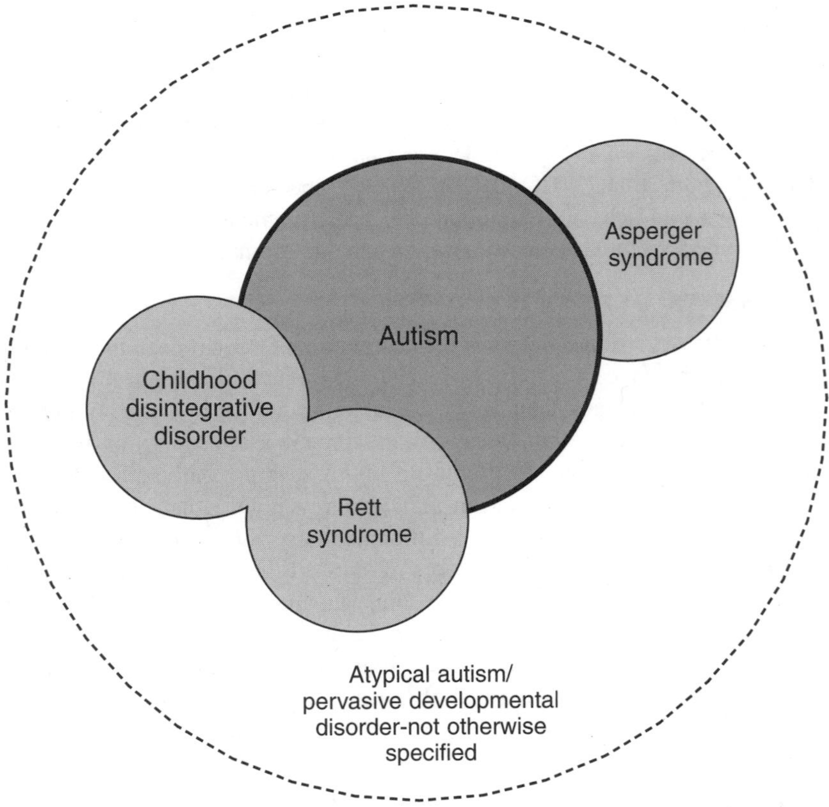

Figure 2.1. Relationship among autism spectrum disorders. Overlapping circles represent that symptoms overlap although the disorders do not. The prototypical disorder, autism, appears in the center; other disorders extend from this prototype in decreasing severity and in decreasing number of domains affected.

Classification of Diseases, Tenth Revision (ICD-10; WHO, 1993), respectively. There is little disagreement, however, that there is a spectrum. There is also an increasing call from researchers and clinicians to use the term *autism spectrum disorders* (ASDs) instead of *PDDs*. Such a shift in terminology recognizes that services are often appropriate for individuals with ASD, beyond autism, and acknowledges that there may be few absolute distinctions between broader (ASDs, PDDs) and narrower (autism) definitions. Although there is some variability in terminology (*atypical autism* versus *PDD*) among individual investigators and in how diagnostic distinctions are drawn (Miller & Ozonoff, 1997), there is virtual unanimity that individuals with lesser degrees of deficit should be considered as part of the autism spectrum.

Autism is also differentiated from other ASDs in ways other than severity and number of domains affected. As shown in Table 2.1, PDD-not otherwise specified (PDD-NOS) and atypical autism are distinguished from autism by age of onset, presence of language or cognitive delay, presence of co-morbid factors, and specific neurologic features. In some cases, these features are a necessary part of the other diagnoses. For example, childhood disintegrative disorder is defined by typical development until age 2, followed by a clear loss

Table 2.1. Factors that differentiate autism from other major *Diagnostic and Statistical Manual of Mental Disorders, Fourth Edition* (DSM-IV), and *International Classification of Diseases, Tenth Revision* (ICD-10), autism spectrum disorders

Disorder	Onset/Course	Delay	Severity	Domains affected
Autism	Prior to 3 years[a]	May or may not be associated with general delays[a]	Exceeds standard thresholds of number of features[a]	Social, communication, *and* repetitive[a] behaviors
Childhood disintegrative disorder	Typical development up to 2 years; loss of speech *and* at least one other skill[c]	Usually associated with mental retardation requiring extensive supports[b]	Thresholds not specified but appear same as autism	Abnormalities in two of three domains of autism
Asperger syndrome	Onset may be before or after 3 years[b]	No general delay in cognition or language[c]	Must exceed threshold in social area[b]	Social and circumscribed interests[b]
Atypical autism (ICD-10)/ pervasive developmental disorder-not otherwise specified (DSM-IV)	May fail to meet autism onset criteria[b]	May or may not be associated with developmental delays	May fall below threshold in one or more areas[b]	Social and either communication or repetitive behaviors or both[c]

[a]Autism criteria.

[b]May differ from autism.

[c]Always differs from autism.

of language and social skills. In other cases, differences in onset may or may not distinguish the disorders. For example, a child may receive a diagnosis of Asperger syndrome because he or she does not meet autism criteria for onset before age 3 years and has no cognitive or language delay. Another child might meet the criteria for Asperger syndrome because he or she has severe social deficits and circumscribed interests but may not have sufficient language impairments or repetitive behaviors to receive an autism diagnosis, even though he or she did show early onset.

AUTISM AS A DEVELOPMENTAL DISORDER

Autism is an important example of a childhood-onset disorder that reflects developmental interactions. The relationship between autism and development occurs in two directions. First, the manifestations of autism are affected by development. Younger children with autism differ from older children and adults with autism similar to the ways in which autism is distinct from other disorders. Developmental trends have been identified in a number of the characteristics that best define autism within particular age groups. For example, a lack of response to others' attempts to direct attention is one of the most consistent findings in younger preschool children with autism, but this trait becomes less of an effective differential feature as children grow older and more developmentally able (Mundy, Sigman, & Kasari, 1994). Similarly, simple theory of mind tasks tend to accurately differentiate children with autism from children without autism who have developmental disabilities and have sufficient language to participate in the tasks but not necessarily from those who have more sophisticated language or cognitive skills. The tasks are not particularly useful with nonverbal children (with or without autism) or with very high-functioning individuals (Happé, 1995).

In addition to autism being affected by development, it is highly likely that having autism affects the experiences of a child growing up and, in this way, affects development. Detailed observations of the behavior of children with autism in social environments suggest that they tend to have far less social interaction than other children in unstructured environments or even during unstructured times in a structured environment (e.g., at home when no one is actively working with them) (Lord & Magill-Evans, 1995). Children with autism are less likely to look at people's faces, a behavior that is very important in early language development. These differences in behavior affect differences in the information available to young children with autism and, thus, may affect rate or breadth of development (Sigman et al., 1999; Ungerer, 1989; see Chapter 4).

IMPORTANCE OF A DIAGNOSIS

Given the lack of clear association between autism and a specific neurobiological marker, one can ask why a diagnosis of autism in young children might be important. Identifying standard diagnoses is critical to investigating medical and scientific issues. Although there have been many exciting neurobiological findings in the field of autism since the 1990s (Bailey et al., 1995; Minshew, 1991; Sigman et al., 1999; Yeung-Courchesne & Courchesne, 1997; see Chapter 8), replication of neurobiological studies across sites has sometimes been very difficult. Establishing standard diagnostic criteria, particularly in young children, would allow the criteria to be well described and followed. The developmental patterns that emerge will be crucial to an understanding both of initial biological differences and of changes in these differences with time and experience.

Diagnosis should also yield important information about course of development and response to treatment. For families, a diagnosis often means access to services. This is particularly the case for a young child or a child older than school age who may not have a central agency or body that takes responsibility for designing an appropriate program. For parents, understanding that other families have children with similar difficulties may provide comfort as well as relief from the possibility that somehow the parents were responsible for this disorder.

Standard diagnosis also allows more efficient and accurate communication among professionals and less confusion for parents who are trying to understand what is occurring in their child's development and to identify where appropriate help can be sought. Often different diagnoses reflect a rational process in understanding a child's disabilities, but this process still is one that can be quite confusing for parents. A 2-year-old with autism first may be referred for a hearing test and speech-language therapy by a pediatrician. The speech-language pathologist may describe the child correctly as having a communication disorder. After working with the child for several months, the speech-language pathologist may become concerned that the child's behaviors cannot be accounted for by a language deficit and may suggest a referral to a psychologist or early education specialist. In the meantime, the pediatrician may also be concerned about the child's level of progress and refer him or her to a pediatric neurologist. One of these professionals may bring up the possibility of autism, but often the professional does this by saying that he or she believes a child does not have autism because, as discussed later in this chapter, many 2-year-olds who later meet criteria for autism do not show the full pattern of behavior at this young age. By the time parents meet an expert in autism, they have often accumulated an array of diagnoses and opinions. One very important issue is how best to work with parents and support them as a diagnosis is sought, without misleading them either by inappropriately ruling out autism or by providing an overly inclusive diagnosis too early.

DIAGNOSIS IN YOUNG CHILDREN

Most relevant to this discussion is the dramatic change since the 1980s in the age of recognition and referral for children with ASD. In the 1980s many children with autism had their first contact with professionals familiar with the disorder when they entered or became ready to enter school. With more media coverage; greater dissemination of information about the disorder; and increasing sophistication, particularly in the fields of communication disorders and pediatrics, ages for initial referral have dropped significantly from later preschool and early school age years to ages 2 and 3 and even younger.

Previous Studies of Early Diagnosis

In spite of this change in the age of initial referral, relatively little is known about the reliability and validity of diagnoses of ASD in young children. Earlier treatment studies using nonstandard diagnoses showed different results in outcome from each other (Lovaas, 1987; Rogers & Lewis, 1989). Very early follow-up studies of children with features of autism suggested that children with the most unusual motor behaviors had better outcomes than did children who were referred predominantly because of the absence of appropriate social behaviors; at older ages, the latter group frequently appeared to have significant mental disabilities but not necessarily autism (Knobloch & Pasamanick, 1975). Several early psychiatric follow-up studies, in which experienced investigators made diagnoses of children younger than 3 years and then followed these children, showed these examiners to be quite accurate in predicting stable diagnoses of autism (Gillberg et al., 1990; Lord, 1995). In these cases, however, the most effective diagnostic strategy was using overall clinical judgment; standard frameworks of diagnosis and methods were not particularly appropriate for these very young children. In a large-scale epidemiological study, initial results suggested that a screening instrument, the Checklist for Autism in Toddlers (CHAT; Baron-Cohen et al., 1996), was quite effective in identifying children with autism at 18 months old (Baron-Cohen, Allen, & Gillberg, 1992). Further results for the same sample, however, indicated that the instrument may have missed a substantial proportion of children diagnosed with ASD at 5 years (Charman, Baron-Cohen, Baird, Cox, Swettenham, & Wheelwright, 1999). Additional studies are underway to investigate these questions. Other research has shown clinical measures to be quite accurate in placing 2-year-olds within the autism spectrum but not in differentiating within the spectrum or in identifying children with mild ASD (Stone et al., 1999).

Similarly, another study (Lord, Pickles, DiLavore, & Shulman, 1996) found that an experienced clinician's diagnosis of autism at age 2 was associated with the same diagnosis in 72% of the children at age 3, with all but one of the children who had received an autism diagnosis at age 2 (94%) continuing to fall within the autism spectrum range (PDD-NOS) at age 3. Diagnoses of PDD-NOS at age 2 were less consistent over time, with only 42% of the children retaining the specific PDD-NOS diagnosis at age 3. Outcomes for children with PDD-NOS were equally split so that for half of the remaining children, symptoms had worsened to autism by age 5 and for half, symptoms lessened and were then considered to be outside the spectrum (Lord et al., 1996).

Empirical Studies of Autism in Young Children

In contrast to the variation in results of the follow-up studies, the cross-sectional, empirical research with preschool children with autism has been much more consistent across tasks and laboratories. Difficulties in joint attention, including response to others' attempts to direct attention and the child's initiation of attempts to obtain joint attention, have been found consistently to be associated with autism (McEvoy, Rogers, & Pennington, 1993; Mundy et al., 1994). A number of investigators have also found that reduced propensity to looking at faces, lack of response to name, and limited pretending (Hertzig, Snow, & Sherman, 1989; Osterling & Dawson, 1994) differentiate young children with autism from children with similar nonverbal profiles and, sometimes, from children with similar degrees of language impairment.

DIFFICULTIES IN DIAGNOSING VERY YOUNG CHILDREN

Clinical issues in diagnosing very young children remain. Discrepancies between areas of development that allow identification of specific social deficits as opposed to more generalized developmental delay are more difficult to document in very young children (Lord, 1997). For children whose nonverbal developmental skills fall at an early infant level, descriptions of dramatic differences between nonverbal skills and social skills become quite difficult (Lord, Shulman, Pickles, & DiLavore, 1997). For example, if a 2-year-old cannot stack blocks, place objects in containers, or carry out simple object permanence tasks, an examiner may feel uncomfortable saying that the child has *specific* social deficits, though the child's social behavior and communication may show even greater impairments than his or her nonverbal skills. In these cases, it is important to recognize that there are severe delays that include social and communicative deficits and possibly autism; diagnostic specification can follow.

Variability in typical young children also affects measurement; an examiner may question whether a child who does not seek out interaction during observation is acting like a "typical 2-year-old" who is hesitant with a stranger or who "has a mind of his or her own" or whether the child has specific social deficits. Standard scoring procedures for "refusals" on the major developmental tests for young children highlight this difficulty. Clinicians may feel uncertain that a child's failure on a particular item has to do with lack of ability rather than a lack of understanding the task or lack of motivation to complete a task that may have little interest or value to a young child. Measures of social behavior in young children can address this uncertainty, however, by creating activities in which the children clearly want to participate and by using tasks with scoring normed for the relevant age group.

In addition, diagnoses of autism in older children are helped by parental descriptions of relationships with other children and the clinician's opportunities to observe children interacting with peers. Many 2-year-olds do not interact with other children outside their families very often, or these opportunities are very much determined by the adults who are present and who make social arrangements for the children. Thus, interpreting the definition of *friendship* in a 2-year-old is difficult, and age-appropriate examples of "peer" interaction such as interest in other children of the same age or response to siblings' overtures need to be sought.

Furthermore, a substantial minority of children with autism experience plateaus or regressions in development in the second year of life. Obtaining information about a child during this time may be difficult because skills are changing during the period of observation.

PARENTS AS SOURCES OF INFORMATION

Parents of 2-year-olds have much greater knowledge about their children's behavior and history of development than do any other people. Research on acquiring information from parents of children with other disorders has indicated that parents are excellent sources of information but that they may not interpret what they see as would an expert in autism (Schopler & Reichler, 1972). One of the difficulties is that with autism, parents have to recognize as deficits behaviors that are "transparent" in everyday social interaction (Lord, 1995). That is, when a very young child does not look at a parent, the parent often simply moves over to be within the range of the child's vision without necessarily noticing that he or she has done so. When parents are asked about the child's eye contact, they may not report any difficulties or, more commonly, may report that they have not noticed anything but that others have commented about it.

Canadian Early Diagnosis Study

In a Canadian study of early diagnosis (Lord, 1995), researchers saw 30 children younger than 3 years referred for possible diagnoses of autism and administered a standardized parent interview, the Autism Diagnostic Interview–Revised (ADI–R; Lord, Rutter, & LeCouteur, 1994). The children also received a best-estimate clinical diagnosis from the same clinician who had administered the ADI and who had conducted psychological testing and informal observations. At age 3, the children saw a different clinician. The ADI–R and psychological tests as well as the standard observations were readministered. A second diagnosis was made by the original clinician who, in 29 of 30 cases, agreed with the judgment of the new clinician. Two items from the parent interview were the clearest discriminators of children at age 2 who continued to receive a diagnosis of autism at age 3. These items had to do with children's attention to neutral statements made by other people (not including their names) and the degree to which the children spontaneously directed other people's attention in any manner (e.g., pointing, vocalizing, gesturing in some other way).

Several aspects of these findings are important. First, both of these interview items had to do with social communication. At age 2, as shown in Table 2.2, there was not one example of a restricted and repetitive behavior that was universal or frequent enough to be considered a strong diagnostic feature of autism. Although there were children who engaged in behaviors such as hand and finger mannerisms or lining up objects, many of the 2-year-olds with later, stable diagnoses of autism did not do so at age 2.

Second, the nature of the questions that were most effective at predicting diagnosis in the parent interview was somewhat different than the findings from the direct observational studies on which they were based. That is, asking parents whether their child responded to his or her name was not a particularly helpful question, although differences have been found using ratings from videotapes showing whether children responded to their names (Osterling & Dawson, 1994). On the other hand, asking parents whether their child responded to a neutral statement, such as "Oh no! It's raining again!" *without specific prompting or calling* of the child's name, was quite effective.

The behaviors described and the contexts were similar, but the interview question needed to be different from those that researchers had coded from videotapes in the previous studies. It seems most likely that the videotape and interview studies are both correct but that there are differences between observational and interview methods of acquiring information. When parents were asked whether their children with autism responded when their names were called, parents almost uniformly said, "Yes." When they described the ways in which they called their children's names, however, it was clear that parents

Table 2.2. Parent interview questions that best predicted autism at age 3

Questions at age 2
Does your child usually respond to a neutral statement (e.g., "Oh, it's raining") when you don't call his or her name or go to him or her?
Does your child try to get you to look at things at a distance (e.g., stars, signs) even when he or she is not asking for them?
Does your child understand any words outside of the usual routine that he or she hears them in (e.g., understanding "Grandma" or "cookie" when neither is in sight or expected)?
Questions at age 3
Does your child usually respond to a neutral statement (e.g., "Oh, it's raining") when you don't call his or her name or go to him or her?
Does your child spontaneously point with his or her finger to get you to look at something just to "share" noticing it with you (not as a request)?
Does your child ever move his or her hands or fingers in unusual ways or hold them in unusual positions?
Does your child use your hand as a tool, such as by placing it right on a container that he or she wants opened or on a doorknob that he or she wants turned?
Does your child say any words (besides "mama" or "dada") spontaneously (not in imitation) that clearly have meaning to him or her and to you and that he or she uses consistently every day?

Source: Lord (1995).

were going right up to their children and saying their names in close proximity, in a very animated fashion. Parents who said that their children did not respond to their names often were referring to other contexts, such as calling a child from another room; this situation was actually more likely to occur for children without autism than children with autism and so made scoring of this question even more variable. Thus, although not responding to name is a good discriminator in direct observation, a question about response to neutral statements was a better discriminator in the parent interview.

By age 3 years, as shown in Table 2.2, five items were identified as the clearest discriminators of a current diagnosis of autism. One of these was the same item as discussed previously, attention to a neutral voice. Another item was a more precise description of directing attention, which involved the child's pointing to express interest. By age 3, hand and finger mannerisms had become sufficiently common that they contributed to stable diagnoses. Children's use of other people's bodies as tools was also an identifying feature. The second-to-last item dealt with whether children led parents by the hand and then placed the hand on an object, such as a doorknob or a container, to get help. Although at age 2, both predicting items had to do purely with social reciprocity, by age 3, restricted and repetitive behaviors (i.e., hand and finger mannerisms) and unusual modes of communication (e.g., use of others' bodies as a tool) contributed to the identification of autism.

This study was based on a clinic referral sample from a department of pediatrics. It included a substantial proportion of children with significant cognitive disabilities. Though very few of the children with or without autism in the sample could speak at age 2, language items were, in fact, useful in discriminating children with autism from children with cognitive delays without autism. At age 2, children who *understood no words out of context* had a high probability of having autism. It is important to note that children with moderate to severe hearing loss or other sensory difficulties, as well as children with multiple disabilities, were not included in this sample. By age 3, children who *did not use any meaningful words consistently* were also much more likely to have autism than was expected. A *meaningful word* was defined as a word that a child consistently said, with a specific intention, *not* in imitation or upon request, in an appropriate context, at least once a day over a period of at least a month. Words that sometimes "popped out" that the child did not use consistently in the same situation were excluded. Although these language questions were highly associated with autism, there were also children with autism who did not have such severe language problems. Thus, these factors indicate risk for autism but are not necessary for the diagnosis.

The same study (Lord, 1995) indicated that standard diagnostic criteria tended to overdiagnose children with significant cognitive delays as having autism at age 2, but underdiagnose a small proportion of children with autism who did not yet show clear, repetitive behaviors. This may have been in part because parents did not yet recognize the children's behaviors as unusually repetitious. For example, a 2-year-old's repeatedly throwing small objects or flipping through magazines is not extraordinary. The repetitious quality of these behaviors may be apparent only after the child continues them for a substantial period of time and fails to engage in other behaviors.

In the Canadian study (Lord, 1995), clinical diagnosis at age 2 was more accurate than were the standard diagnostic instruments. Yet, there was concern that these diagnoses were not based on a clear framework but on the clinician's rather undefined weighting of different factors. These results are similar to findings by Gillberg and colleagues (1990), who were also able to predict at age 2 children who would continue to have autism at age 3 or older, but who similarly found that the most stable diagnoses at age 2 were not necessarily equivalent to those yielded by formal ICD-10 criteria.

Two-year-olds who were misdiagnosed with autism by the instruments (i.e., ADI–R; Childhood Autism Rating Scale [CARS; Schopler, Reichler, & Renner, 1986]) in this study tended to have more significant cognitive delays than the rest of the children in the sample. Children who did not receive standard diagnoses of autism at age 2 but did at age 3 tended to be higher-functioning children. These children had some language at age 2 and had more socially directed behavior than most children with autism. By age 3, their language had often become more clearly stereotyped and their social behavior, although continuing to improve, was more obviously not as reciprocal as other children their age.

OBSERVATIONAL MEASURES FOR EARLY DIAGNOSIS

Because the Canadian study primarily relied on the parent interview and only informally on observation, the researchers' next goal was to follow a larger sample using a wider variety of measures. For this purpose, a standardized observation of social and communicative behavior and play was developed for young children. This was the Pre-Linguistic Autism Diagnostic Observation Schedule (PL-ADOS; DiLavore, Lord, & Rutter, 1995). This measure was modeled after a previously designed standardized observation of social behavior for older children, the Autism Diagnostic Observation Schedule (ADOS; Lord et al., 1989). The purpose of the ADOS and PL-ADOS was to standardize contexts for observation of behaviors associated with autism. This included standardization of content of the observation (in terms of specific behaviors coded), thresholds for abnormality in individual behaviors, and interpretation of observations in the form of providing an overall algorithm for diagnosis. For each task, a hierarchy of "presses" or social structures is provided so that during the first administration of a task a child is able to take as much initiative as possible. When this does not occur, the examiner gradually makes the tasks more specific and increasingly structured to observe the child's response.

For example, in observing how a child responds to his or her name, the procedure in the PL-ADOS is as follows. Initially, the examiner calls the child's name. If the child does not respond to several attempts, then a parent is asked to call the child's name several times. If the child still does not respond, then the parent is asked to say anything or make any sound that he or she thinks might elicit the child's attention. If this does not occur, then the parent is encouraged to go to the child and try to elicit a response. This approach means that a child may "succeed" on each task and not be presented with repeated failure. Both the child's behavior and the effort and structure required from the parent or examiner are included in the ratings. The PL-ADOS differed from the ADOS, the original observation schedule, in that parents were expected to be part of the assessment and were seen as part of the hierarchy of social presses.

The normative data from the PL-ADOS indicated that it very accurately distinguished 3- and 4-year-old children with autism from children with other disorders and from typically developing children (DiLavore et al., 1995). A diagnostic algorithm, intended to be a partial operationalization of DSM-IV/ICD-10 criteria (appropriate to the context of an office visit and interactions with a "friendly" stranger), was derived. The one major limitation to the PL-ADOS was that the algorithm underdiagnosed higher-functioning children who already used beginning phrases and sentences. The PL-ADOS has now been incorporated into a more comprehensive instrument, the Autism Diagnostic Observation Schedule–WPS Edition (ADOS–WPS; Lord, Rutter, DiLavore, & Risi, 1999), which provides different modules for children on the basis of developmental and language levels and so addresses this problem of underinclusion.

North Carolina Early Diagnosis Study

The PL-ADOS was next used in a second, larger study in North Carolina, in which 110 two-year-olds referred for possible autism to the TEACCH (Treatment and Education of Autistic and related Communications Handicapped Children) program and 21 children with developmental delays serving as comparisons were followed until age 5. When the children were 2 years old, clinicians made best-estimate diagnoses of probable autism or not autism. When the children were 5 years old, an independent clinical diagnosis, as well as an overall diagnosis, was made using the ADI–R and clinical impression. A preliminary analysis of the PL-ADOS used with children at age 2 to predict autism at age 5 (Lord, 1997) has yielded findings similar to earlier studies' findings. As with the previous sample, even at age 2, the highest-functioning children began to "fall out" of the algorithm (i.e., were underidentified). Otherwise, the PL-ADOS, if anything, was more specific and sensitive to autism than the parent report measure. In the second, larger study, contrary to findings in previous studies, clinical diagnosis was the least accurate predictor of children seen first at age 2 who would be diagnosed as having autism at age 5. Clinicians making overall judgments tended to consistently underdiagnose autism in 2-year-olds, in contrast to the overdiagnosis that occurred with the parent interview. Differences from previous findings may be attributed to differences in the samples or to differences in clinicians' willingness to formally label autism in very young children.

Generally, with the PL-ADOS, behaviors in specific contexts were not as effective in discriminating among children with different diagnoses as were judgments of behaviors across several contexts. Although there were very stable differences between diagnostic groups in response to the joint attention task, these differences were also strongly influenced by development (DiLavore & Lord, 1995). Overall, judgments of a child's social reciprocity made during these and other tasks were more consistently associated with diagnosis across development than with scoring of specific behaviors. For example, differences in requesting, which characterized the youngest and developmentally lowest-functioning children in this sample, were not necessarily still apparent at later ages; however, judgments about the quality of a child's social overtures when he or she was motivated to approach an adult were consistent across chronological age and developmental level. Thus, the value of the observation (i.e., the PL-ADOS) in discriminating children with autism from children with other diagnoses was that it standardized a number of the tasks and how clinicians rated them, but there were few simple "tests" for autism that were effective across age ranges.

Generally, the trajectories yielded by developmental tests at age 2 were remarkably straight (Taylor, Pickering, Lord, & Pickles, 1998). Growth curve analyses were able to project linear trends for individual children based on their receptive and expressive language scores on a variety of measures including the Mullen Scales of Early Learning (MSEL; Mullen, 1989) and the Vineland Adaptive Behavior Scales (Sparrow, Balla, & Cicchetti, 1984) as well as the Bayley Scales of Infant Development (Bayley, 1969). Even though the absolute scores on these tests varied somewhat depending on the content of the items, it was quite possible to predict trajectories from 2 years to 5 years for the children. Children with a diagnosis of autism at age 5 tended to show less variation in their scores and to have lower scores in receptive and expressive language at all time points than did children in any of the other diagnostic groups.

When diagnoses at age 2 were used, however, there was less homogeneity for the children with autism than when diagnoses at age 5 were employed. In no case in this study did a child change from a diagnosis of autism at 2 to a diagnosis outside the autism spectrum at 5. However, children with tentative diagnoses of autism who showed significant improvements in cognitive functioning between age 2 and 5 often received diagnoses of PDD-NOS at age 5.

This finding provides hope for improvements in the symptoms of autism in a subset of the population. The children most likely to follow this pattern were children who had higher language scores at age 2. Although most of the children in the study had minimal speech during the first assessment, the difference between a 2-year-old with a few words and some ability to follow directions out of context and a child with no words and no consistent comprehension of language was dramatic in terms of the likelihood of diagnostic changes from age 2 to 5.

These results are similar to the findings from the earlier parent interview study (Lord, 1995), which indicated that children who did not understand any words out of context at age 2 and who did not use any words had a high probability of having autism. The results reinforce the need for a careful skills assessment, not only of children's sociocommunicative functioning but also of their language levels, even at very young ages. Most communication and language therapists are able to generate such scores. Often, however, they are uncomfortable doing so because findings indicate very low levels of language skill (e.g., language levels below 1 year) and because of their concern that they cannot discriminate lack of ability from lack of cooperation. These findings, across a variety of tests, and now across two samples, suggest, however, that results of even relatively rudimentary scales measuring expressive and receptive language in very young children, such as the MSEL, the VABS, and the Sequenced Inventory of Communication Development–Revised (Hedrick, Prather, & Tobin, 1984), provide quite useful information about a child's expected rate of progress.

CLINICAL AND EDUCATIONAL IMPLICATIONS

Overall, it is likely that many children with autism can be identified at age 2, though not necessarily with standard diagnostic criteria. Diagnostic criteria for autism and the methods used to measure them are less meaningful at age 2 than at older preschool years for a number of reasons. First, the absence of specific social behaviors in children younger than age 3 occurs in disabilities (most typically mental retardation) other than ASDs. Thus, although not pointing to express interest is a reasonable discriminator of social behavior between a child with autism and a child with a mild language disorder at age 3, it may not necessarily discriminate a child with autism at age 2 from a 2-year-old with severe cognitive delay who does not have autism. Generally, however, such measures do allow for accurate discriminations once children have a mental age of 18 months and reach a chronological age of 3 years or older.

Second, fewer children with autism show clear repetitive or odd behaviors at age 2 than at age 3. This difference is exacerbated by the fact that parents or other individuals who are not experienced with autism may not recognize these behaviors as repetitive in young children, even when they do occur.

The behaviors may also be tied to specific contexts in very young children (e.g., a child who only flips swizzle sticks when he has his cup to flip them in). In addition, some children with autism may only develop these behaviors between ages 2 and 3 or even later.

Third, more children referred for possible autism change diagnoses between ages 2 and 3 than during any other year-long period in later development. At least in the groups of children we studied, these changes in diagnoses were predominantly between autism and atypical autism/PDD-NOS. They were represented by two pathways: 1) improvements in social behavior, generally for children who had less severe language delays, resulting in a shift from autism to PDD-NOS or from PDD-NOS to nonspectrum disorders or 2) increasingly apparent repetitive behaviors in children who had not met criteria for autism at age 2 because of absence of these behaviors, resulting in a shift from PDD-NOS to autism. In any case, children suspected of having autism at age 2 are rarely without difficulties later. In the sample in the North Carolina study (Lord, 1997), only 10 of 110 children *referred* for possible autism (not *diagnosed* with possible autism) at age 2 did not receive a diagnosis of either autism or PDD-NOS at age 5. Of these 10 children, 9 showed mental retardation or quite severe language delays, with only 1 child receiving a final diagnosis of oppositional behavior. The last child, although referred for possible autism at age 2, was never believed to have had an ASD diagnosis by the research team.

Children who received stable diagnoses of autism at age 5 did not necessarily appear to have prototypical autism at age 2. Generally, they were not aloof. Most of them were quite responsive to physical interaction, such as tickling. Most were quite attached and close to their mothers, at least in the sense of being upset by separations from them and being aware of their presence. Many children did not show odd behaviors or unusual mannerisms.

In contrast, most of the children later diagnosed with autism failed to respond when someone spoke to them in a neutral fashion, did not try to direct others' attention, and did not bring objects from another room on request (other than in a predictable context, such as going to get their shoes to go out). Information about these behaviors could be elicited during standardized observations and described in parent interviews. At age 2, social criteria on their own, as opposed to the three-domain pattern (limited social reciprocity; limited communication; restricted, repetitive behaviors) that defines autism at other ages, were most useful in recognizing autism. By age 3, the same children typically showed deficits in all three diagnostic areas—social reciprocity, communication, and restricted and repetitive behaviors—though they continued to seem less socially atypical than older children with autism.

"Small" differences in developmental level affected how autism was manifested in the preschool years. A child who had even a few consistent, meaningful, and spontaneous words at age 2 tended to be more able to respond to certain social tasks, such as following a pointed finger, than did a child with no consistent words. In general, trajectories made on the basis of very simple measurements of early language functioning were remarkably linear. These findings suggest the need to be certain that early screening includes measurements (and quantification) of cognitive and language functioning as well as areas specifically related to autism.

Overall, general judgments of social reciprocity and the ability to communicate, made on the basis of standardized observation, were the strongest and most stable predictors of autism. In earlier studies, such as in the DSM-IV field trial (Volkmar et al., 1994), however, these measures were also the items most difficult for nonexperts to complete reliably. This suggests that screening methods, to be carried out by primary practitioners, may need to be organized in quite a different fashion than do measures indicating a diagnosis. That is, screening measures should not rely on subtle judgments but need to be based on information from parents or a few discrete observations that serve as markers for risk. Screening and diagnosis have different purposes from each other and may need to be organized in different ways. In addition, in a clinical assessment, the process of working with parents to increase their understanding of their children and to provide access to appropriate services is as important, if not more important, than the resulting classification. Practitioners should consider which role (screening or diagnosis) they wish to fill and make sure parents have the opportunity for a full diagnosis from them or from others. Helping parents with the process of understanding their child's disabilities and how a particular professional fits into this process may avoid confusion and help prepare them to seek further information. A speech-language pathologist who describes a child as having sensory or motor planning difficulties may be accurately describing one aspect of a child's difficulties but may not be ruling out autism or cognitive delay. If the therapist can warn the parents that a very young child with severe difficulties in language comprehension or unusual behaviors is at risk for autism, this warning may help parents find information and other services but also leaves room, if the risk is not apparent as the child grows older, for other diagnoses later on. Focusing on specific behaviors, what they mean, and how they can be addressed (for example, teaching a child to point or to initiate a game or to play with a toy) allows the therapist to provide parents with hope and a way to actively help their child while they are beginning to understand the long-term implications of a diagnosis such as autism.

DIRECTIONS FOR FUTURE RESEARCH

Neurobiological research is the most likely source to help prevent or treat autism before symptoms arise. This research requires standard diagnostic methods and early identification and appropriate referrals. Better ways of describing and delineating children and adults within the broader spectrum of autistic disorders will also be critical. Research in clinical practice has provided insight into the effects of a number of specific approaches to early intervention that have been very valuable. Directly addressing even larger questions with young children who have received standardized diagnoses, such as how much and which therapies are most effective for which children, is of great importance. Because standard methods of diagnosis are available for children as young as 2 years, there is now no reason to study treatments carried out on poorly described samples when this limits replication and dissemination. Still, research must consider not only the implications for science but also the effects of various findings on families. For example, what is the effect on parents when they are told their child is "at risk for autism"? How can increased knowledge about the disorder result in increased support for children and families?

CONCLUSIONS

Much more is known about the diagnosis of young children with autism now than was known in the late 1980s. Methods are available that provide ways of acquiring structured information from parents and for observing children directly in diagnosis. Measurement of levels of language and nonverbal functioning have been shown to be reliable and valid and to have great importance in interacting with autism-specific factors to predict outcome. Conceptualization of how screening and diagnosis fit together is improving, with increased awareness of the need to consider consequences for children and families. There is much work to be done, but great progress has been made.

REFERENCES

American Psychiatric Association. (1994). *Diagnostic and statistical manual of mental disorders (DSM-IV)* (4th ed.). Washington, DC: Author.

Bailey, A., LeCouteur, A., Gottesman, I., Bolton, P., Simonoff, E., Yuzda, E., & Rutter, M. (1995). Autism as a strongly genetic disorder: Evidence from a British twin study. *Psychological Medicine, 25,* 63–77.

Baron-Cohen, S., Allen, J., & Gillberg, C. (1992). Can autism be detected at 18 months? The needle, the haystack, and the CHAT. *British Journal of Psychiatry, 161,* 839–843.

Baron-Cohen, S., Cox, A., Baird, G., Swettenham, J., Nightingale, N., Morgan, K., Auriol, D., & Charman, T. (1996). Psychological markers in the detection of autism in infancy in a large population. *British Journal of Psychiatry, 168,* 158–163.

Bayley, N. (1969). *Manual for the Bayley Scales of Infant Development.* San Antonio, TX: The Psychological Corporation.

Bolton, P., Macdonald, H., Pickles, A., Rios, P., Goode, S., Crowson, M., Bailey, A., & Rutter, M. (1994). A case-control family history study of autism. *Journal of Child Psychology and Psychiatry and Allied Disciplines, 35,* 877–900.

Charman, T., Baron-Cohen, S., Baird, G., Cox, A., Swettenham, J.G., & Wheelwright, S. (1999, April). *A six-year follow-up study of the CHAT (Checklist for Autism in*

Toddlers). Paper presented at a symposium at the biennial meeting of the Society for Research in Child Development, Albuquerque, New Mexico.

DiLavore, P., & Lord, C. (1995, April). *Do you see what I see? Requesting and joint attention in children with autism.* Poster presented at the biennial meeting of the Society for Research in Child Development, Indianapolis.

DiLavore, P., Lord, C., & Rutter, M. (1995). Pre-Linguistic Autism Diagnostic Observation Schedule (PL-ADOS). *Journal of Autism and Developmental Disorders, 25,* 355–379.

Gillberg, C. (1990). Autism and pervasive developmental disorders. *Journal of Child Psychology and Psychiatry and Allied Disciplines, 31,* 99–119.

Gillberg, C., Ehlers, S., Schaumann, H., Jakobsson, G., Dahlgren, S.O., Lindblom, R., Bagenholm, A., Tjuus, T., & Blidner, E. (1990). Autism under age 3 years: A clinical study of 28 cases referred for autistic symptoms in infancy. *Journal of Child Psychology and Psychiatry and Allied Disciplines, 31,* 921–934.

Happé, F.G.E (1995). The role of age and verbal ability in the theory of mind task performance of subjects with autism. *Child Development, 66,* 843–855.

Hedrick, D.L., Prather, E.M., & Tobin, A.R. (1984). *Sequenced Inventory of Communication Development–Revised* (SICD–R). Seattle: University of Washington Press.

Hertzig, M.E., Snow, M.E., & Sherman, M. (1989). Affect and cognition in autism. *Journal of the American Academy of Child and Adolescent Psychiatry, 28,* 195–199.

Knobloch, H., & Pasamanick, B. (1975). Some etiologic and prognostic factors in early infantile autism and psychosis. *Pediatrics, 55,* 182–191.

Lord, C. (1995). Follow-up of two year-olds referred for possible autism. *Journal of Child Psychology and Psychiatry and Allied Disciplines, 36,* 1365–1382.

Lord, C. (1997, August). Preschool diagnosis of autism spectrum disorders. In S. Campbell (Chair), *Developmental trajectories from infancy through school-age.* Symposium conducted at the meeting of the American Psychological Association, Chicago.

Lord, C., & Magill-Evans, J. (1995). Peer interaction of autistic children and adolescents: Developmental processes in peer relations and psychopathology [Special issue]. *Development and Psychopathology, 7,* 611–626.

Lord, C., Pickles, A., DiLavore, P.C., & Shulman, C. (1996). *Longitudinal studies of young children referred for possible autism.* Paper presented at the biannual meeting of the International Society for Research in Child and Adolescent Psychopathology, Los Angeles.

Lord, C., Rutter, M., DiLavore, P.C., & Risi, S. (1999). *Autism Diagnostic Observation Schedule–WPS Edition (ADOS–WPS).* Los Angeles: Western Psychological Services.

Lord, C., Rutter, M., Goode, S., Heemsbergen, J., Jordan, H., Mawhood, L., & Schopler, E. (1989). Autism Diagnostic Observation Schedule: A standardized observation of communicative and social behavior. *Journal of Autism and Developmental Disorders, 19,* 185–212.

Lord, C., Rutter, M., & LeCouteur, A. (1994). Autism Diagnostic Interview–Revised: A revised version of a diagnostic interview for caregivers of individuals with possible pervasive developmental disorders. *Journal of Autism and Developmental Disorders, 24,* 659–685.

Lord, C., Shulman, C., Pickles, A., & DiLavore, P. (1997, April). *Learning and not learning to speak: Examples from a longitudinal study of preschool children with autism spectrum disorders.* Paper presented at a symposium at the biennial meeting of the Society for Research in Child Development, Washington, DC.

Lovaas, O.I. (1987). Behavioral treatment and normal educational and intellectual functioning in young autistic children. *Journal of Consulting and Clinical Psychology, 55,* 3–9.

Mahoney, W., Szatmari, P., Maclean, J., Bryson, S., Bartolucci, G., Walter, S., Hoult, L., & Jones, M. (1998). Reliability and accuracy of differentiating pervasive developmental disorder subtypes. *Journal of the American Academy of Child and Adolescent Psychiatry, 37,* 278–285.

McEvoy, R.E., Rogers, S.J., & Pennington, B.F. (1993). Executive function and social communication deficits in young autistic children. *Journal of Child Psychology and Psychiatry and Allied Disciplines, 34,* 563–578.

Miller, J.N., & Ozonoff, S. (1997). Did Asperger's cases have Asperger disorder?: A research note. *Journal of Child Psychology and Psychiatry and Allied Disciplines, 38,* 247–251.

Minshew, N. (1991). Indices of neural function in autism: Clinical and biological implications. *Pediatrics, 87*(Suppl.), 774–780.

Mullen, E. (1989). *Mullen Scales of Early Learning.* Cranston, RI: T.O.T.A.L. Child, Inc.

Mundy, P., Sigman, M., & Kasari, C. (1994). Joint attention, developmental level, and symptom presentation in young children with autism. *Development and Psychopathology, 6,* 115–128.

Osterling, J., & Dawson, G. (1994). Early recognition of children with autism: A study of first birthday home videotapes. *Journal of Autism and Developmental Disorders, 24,* 247–257.

Rogers, S.J., & Lewis, H. (1989). An effective day treatment model for young children with pervasive developmental disorders. *Journal of the American Academy of Child and Adolescent Psychiatry, 28,* 207–214.

Schopler, E., & Reichler, R.J. (1972). How well do parents understand their own psychotic child? *Journal of Autism and Childhood Schizophrenia, 2,* 387–400.

Schopler, E., Reichler, R.J., & Renner, B.R. (1986). *The Childhood Autism Ratings Scale (CARS) for diagnostic screening and classification of autism.* New York: Irvington.

Sigman, M., Ruskin, E., Arbelle, S., Corona, R., Dissanayake, C., Espinosa, M., Kim, N., Littleford, C., & Lopez, A. (1999). Social competence in children with autism, Down syndrome, and other developmental delays: A longitudinal study. *Monographs of the Society for Research in Child Development, 64.*

Sparrow, S., Balla, D., & Cicchetti, D. (1984). *Vineland Adaptive Behavior Scales.* Circle Pines, MN: American Guidance Service.

Stone, W.L., Lee, E.B., Ashford, L., Brissie, J., Hepburn, S.L., Coonrod, E.E., & Weiss, B.H. (1999). Can autism be diagnosed accurately in children under three years? *Journal of Child Psychology and Psychiatry and Allied Disciplines.*

Taylor, A., Pickering, K., Lord, C., & Pickles, A. (1998). Mixed and multilevel models for longitudinal data: Growth curve models of language development. In B.S. Everitt & G. Dunn (Eds.), *Statistical analysis of medical data: New developments* (pp. 1–15). New York: Oxford University Press.

Tanguay, P.E., Robertson, J., & Derrick, A. (1998). A dimensional classification of autism spectrum disorder by social communication domains. *Journal of the American Academy of Child and Adolescent Psychiatry, 37,* 271–277.

Ungerer, J.A. (1989). The early development of autistic children: Implications for defining primary deficits. In G. Dawson (Ed.), *Autism: Nature, diagnosis, and treatment* (pp. 75–91). New York: Guilford Press.

Volkmar, F.R., Klin, A., Siegel, B., Szatmari, P., Lord, C., Campbell, M., Freeman, B.J., Cicchetti, D.V., Rutter, M., Kline, W., Buitelaar, J., Hattab, Y., Fombonne, E., Fuentes, J., Werry, J., Stone, W., Kerbeshian, J., Hoshino, Y., Bregman, J., Loveland, K., Szymanski, L., & Towbin, K. (1994). Field trial for autistic disorder in DSM-IV. *American Journal of Psychiatry, 151,* 1361–1367.

Wing, L., & Gould, J. (1979). Severe impairments of social interaction and associated abnormalities in children: Epidemiology and classification. *Journal of Autism and Developmental Disorders, 9,* 11–29.
World Health Organization. (1993). *ICD-10 classification of mental and behavioural disorders.* Geneva: Author.
Yeung-Courchesne, R., & Courchesne, E. (1997). From impasse to insight in autism research: From behavioral symptoms to biological explanations. *Development and Psychopathology, 9,* 389–419.

3

Joint Attention, Cultural Learning, and Language Acquisition

Implications for Children with Autism

Malinda Carpenter and Michael Tomasello

Many researchers look at language as a purely formal object. In this approach, the syntax of language is innate, and even the acquisition of individual words is underlain by innate word-learning constraints. Language is thought to be a cognitive module distinct from other cognitive and social capacities (Chomsky, 1986; Pinker, 1995). In contrast, the social-pragmatic approach to language and its acquisition views language very differently (Bruner, 1983; Nelson, 1985; Tomasello, 1992). In this view, each of the world's natural languages has its own set of communicative conventions, in the form of linguistic symbols created over thousands of years, by means of which its speakers attempt to influence the interest, attention, knowledge, and behavior of other members of their speech communities. This is not to deny that there are universals in the way symbols are created, learned, and used across languages. Instead of being innate and language-specific, however, these universals are universals both in the way human beings experience the world and in the ways they interact and communicate with one another socially.

In the social-pragmatic approach to language acquisition, the focus is on both the structured social world into which the child is born and the child's capacities for tuning into and participating in that structured social world (Tomasello, 1992). In this view, young children are not engaged in a reflective cognitive task in which they are attempting to make correct "mappings" of word to world based on adult "input"; rather, they are engaged in social interactions in which they are attempting to understand and interpret adult communicative intentions so as to make sense of the current situation (Nelson, 1985). When attempting to comprehend adult use of novel linguistic symbols, children use all kinds of interpretive strategies based on the pragmatic assumption that adult linguistic symbols are somehow *relevant* to the ongoing social interaction (Bloom, 1993; Bruner, 1983; Sperber & Wilson, 1986). The child who knows that his mother wishes him to eat his peas (because she is holding them up to his mouth and gesturing) assumes that her utterance is relevant to that intention, and this understanding of communicative intentions is what guides that child's interpretations of any novel language in the situation. The child may then learn to produce the same symbols when he wishes for others to experience a situation in the same way, thus entering into the world of bidirectionally (intersubjectively) understood linguistic symbols (Tomasello, 1996).

In the social-pragmatic view, then, children acquire linguistic symbols as an integral part of their social interactions with adults in much the same way that they learn many other cultural conventions. Tomasello, Kruger, and Ratner (1993) have called this process *cultural learning.* In this chapter we spell out this view of language acquisition in more detail, focusing first on how children "get off the ground" in language acquisition via processes of joint attentional interaction, then on how they progress in word learning in the second year of life, and then on the social-cognitive skills on which language acquisition depends. Finally, we apply this general theoretical approach to the acquisition of language by children with autism. The language difficulties of these children are well known, but we believe they may be better understood when they are seen in the light of other difficulties these children have with social and communicative activities in general.

JOINT ATTENTION AND EARLY LANGUAGE

The problem of how children learn linguistic symbols was first clearly articulated by Wittgenstein (1953): How can a child learn a word when no nonlinguistic procedures can unambiguously illustrate its reference? Wittgenstein noted that even an ostensive definition—the seemingly simplest case of language acquisition in which one person "shows" another what a word means—is problematic because it assumes that both teacher and learner know what "showing" is and precisely how it serves to pick out individual referents in some language-independent way. The point was crystallized by Quine (1960) in his parable of a native who utters the expression "Gavagai!" and "shows" a foreigner the intended referent by pointing out a salient event as it unfolds. Given the stipulation that native and foreigner have no way to establish a common view of the event nonlinguistically, however, there is basically no way that the foreigner can know whether the native's novel expression is being used to refer to the event, to some participant in the event, to some part of the participant's body, to the color of the participant's hair, or to any of an infinite number of aspects of the situation. This is the basic problem of referential indeterminacy.

Bruner (1975, 1983) addressed this problem and gave a basically Wittgensteinian answer: The child acquires the conventional use of a word by learning to participate in a form of life that he or she understands first nonlinguistically, so that adults' language can be grounded in shared experiences whose social significance he or she already appreciates. One key component of this process is a child who can understand adults as intentional beings well enough to share attention with them in some shared activity (we discuss this later). There is another component, however, when what is at issue are things cultural and conventional. To learn a conventional symbol the child must live in a world that has structured social activities in which he or she can participate and whose structure he or she understands. These structured social activities often involve the recurrence of the same general activity on a regular basis so that the child can come to comprehend how the activity works, how the various social roles in it function, and so forth. And, of course, it must be the case that the adult uses a novel linguistic symbol in a way that the child can comprehend within that shared activity.

The basic idea may be illustrated by imagining an adult attempting to learn a foreign language. In one scenario, one can imagine the adult trying to learn from interactions in which a native speaker simply approaches and starts talking in the foreign tongue—out of nowhere, so to speak. It is very unlikely that in such situations the learner would acquire the conventional use of any forms from the foreign language at all. In another scenario, we may imagine that the learner enters a store or a train station and begins interacting with the storekeeper or ticket-seller in some meaningful ways. In these situations it is highly likely that some new language will be learned because both interactants share an understanding of one another's interactive goals in terms of purchasing and selling items, and so it is very likely that in many cases the learner can infer the native's communicative intentions independently of language. As the two interact in searching for objects, exchanging objects, exchanging money, and so forth, the learner may actually acquire some new language if the native speaker uses that new language in some way that suggests to the learner some reason for making that utterance at that time. This may happen, for instance, when the native speaker utters a novel word while holding out his or her hand from behind the cash register after the learner has acquired an object from the shelf. In such cases the learner makes an abductive inference of the following type: If that novel word meant *X,* then it would be *relevant* to our ongoing intentional interactions (Nelson, 1996; Sperber & Wilson, 1986).

A variety of studies have shown that after children have begun progressing in the process of language acquisition, they learn new words best in joint attentional interactions, in which children and adults coordinate their attention to each other and an object of mutual interest. This coordination is evident when children engage in referential looking, or gaze alternation between the object and the adult's face (e.g., Bakeman & Adamson, 1984; Trevarthen & Hubley, 1978). These joint attentional interactions often take place during routine situations, such as bathing, feeding, diaper changing, book reading, and traveling in the car, that are recurrent activities in the child's daily experience

(Tomasello, 1992). These activities are in many ways analogous to the store scenario in that children are likely to understand their own and the adult's goals in the situation, and this understanding may enable children to infer the relevance of the adult's language to those goals. (As we discuss later, children with autism, in contrast, have difficulty engaging in joint attentional interactions and thus may experience language more often than not in situations analogous to the first scenario that we mentioned, in which the language comes from "out of nowhere.")

One such study was conducted by Tomasello and Todd (1983), who documented that mother–child dyads who spent more time in joint attentional activities during the 12- to 18-month period had children with larger vocabularies at 18 months of age (see also Smith, Adamson, & Bakeman, 1988, and Tomasello, Mannle, & Kruger, 1986). The timing of adults' language in these activities is important as well. In two correlational and experimental studies, Tomasello and Farrar (1986) found that mothers who used their language to follow into their child's attention (i.e., to talk about an object that was *already* the focus of the child's interest and attention) had children with larger vocabularies than mothers who used their language in an attempt to direct the child's attention to something new (see also Akhtar, Dunham, & Dunham, 1991; Dunham, Dunham, & Curwin, 1993).

These studies demonstrate the importance of joint attentional activities and adult language that is sensitive to the child's current focus of attention in the language acquisition of children 18 months of age or older—an age by which many children have already become quite adept at word learning. A remaining question thus is whether these relations hold at even younger ages, when language skills are beginning to emerge just after the child's first birthday. This is more than just a question of whether relations can be demonstrated earlier; it also involves the issue of whether children's earliest language skills emerge out of the prelinguistic joint attentional activities just described or whether they arise from some other source.

The study of most direct relevance to this question is that of Carpenter, Nagell, and Tomasello (1998), who followed 24 infants longitudinally, at monthly intervals, from 9 to 15 months of age. At each monthly session infants interacted naturalistically with their mothers for 10 minutes, and from these interactions the following measures were computed: 1) the amount of time each mother–infant dyad spent in joint attentional engagement and 2) the percentage of maternal utterances that followed into the infants' focus of attention. At these same monthly sessions the mothers also reported, via a structured checklist, each of the words that their infants had mastered in comprehension and production (they also reported the different gestures their infants produced). Two main findings emerged. First, mother–infant dyads who spent more time in joint attentional engagement at 12 months of age had infants who used more gestures and comprehended more language in the months immediately following. A similar relation emerged a few months later between joint attentional engagement and language production. Second, mothers who followed into their infant's attentional focus with referential words at 12 months of age had infants with larger comprehension vocabularies in the months immediately following (with a similar relation to language production again showing up a bit later). When both of these variables—time in joint attentional engagement and mother's follow-in language—were used together in multiple regression equations, more than half of the variance in infants' language comprehension and production was predicted at several points during the period from 12 to 15 months of age, with each variable accounting for significant amounts of unique variance.

Several other findings of this study are important. First, a number of other social-cognitive measures (e.g., gaze following, imitative learning, gestural communication) of these infants were taken as well. All 24 of the infants had engaged meaningfully in these other joint attentional activities before they actually began producing conventional language. This fact, coupled with the fact that the emergence of linguistic skills was correlated with mother–infant joint attentional interactions, suggests that language skills indeed may be seen as emerging out of nonlinguistic joint attentional activities. In the most radical view of this process, children's nonlinguistic joint attentional activities may be said to come to be supplemented by linguistically mediated joint attentional activities. Second, two measures of infants' non–social-cognitive development (involving their knowledge of objects and space) were also taken. These mostly emerged in an uncorrelated fashion with language and the other joint attentional activities. This finding provides evidence that the relation between the emergence of joint attentional engagement and language is not just the result of some generalized developmental advance (e.g., in attention span). The relations among these social behaviors are much more intimately linked than that.

Finally, it is also noteworthy that the relation between maternal follow-in language and infants' language became weaker as infants grew older. This is an intriguing finding because it suggests the possibility—explored and supported later in this chapter—that mothers' use of language that follows into the infants' attentional focus is a kind of scaffolding for early language, which helps infants who are just getting started to discern the mother's communicative intentions and so to enter into a state of joint attentional focus. This kind of scaffolding, however, may not be necessary as the child grows older and becomes more skillful at determining communicative intentions in less child-friendly linguistic interactions. Something similar, but different, may occur with joint attentional activities as older children learn to establish and maintain joint attentional interactions on the basis of language itself, for example, using language to jointly attend with an adult to some past event that is no longer perceptually present (Tomasello, 1988).

The clear finding of the Carpenter, Nagell, and Tomasello (1998) study—which confirms the findings of similar studies of slightly older children—is that children's emerging ability to engage in nonlinguistically mediated joint attentional activities with adults at approximately 1 year of age is integrally related to their emerging linguistic skills. This finding is important because it demonstrates that the well-known age correspondence between joint attentional skills and language (which emerge, respectively, in the months before and after the child's first birthday) is not a coincidence. This finding presents an immediate and serious problem for theories of early language acquisition that do not focus on the social dimension of the process. For theories that focus primarily on the cognitive dimensions of word learning (e.g., Markman, 1989) or on the learning processes involved (Smith, Jones, & Landau, 1996), the question is why does language acquisition begin when it does? Why does it begin directly on the heels of the emergence of joint attentional skills? Any answer that invokes non–social-cognitive or learning processes—for example, that children at this age for the first time become able to conceptualize or to learn new sorts of things in general—must then answer the question of why early language emerges in a correlated fashion with these nonlinguistic social-cognitive and social-interactive skills. To our knowledge, none of the existing theories of early language acquisition—other than the social-pragmatic theory as espoused by Bruner (1983), Nelson (1985), Tomasello (1992, in press), and others—can account for these findings.

LEARNING LANGUAGE IN THE FLOW OF SOCIAL INTERACTION

A number of studies have thus established that very young language learners benefit from adult language models that follow into their already-established focus of attention on an object. Children, however, soon come to be able to determine adults' communicative intentions in a much wider variety of communicative contexts in which they have to do much more social-cognitive work. It does happen with some frequency that in Western middle-class culture, an adult holds up or points to an object while telling the child its name. The social dimensions of this process are manifest: The child must somehow determine the focus of the adult's attention. In this case, though, the social-cognitive task would seem to be at least relatively straightforward because such things as following gaze direction are so basic for infants.

It turns out, however, that in many cultures of the world adults do not engage in this kind of naming game with young children (Brown, in press). Moreover, even in Western middle-class culture, adults do not frequently use this naming game with words other than object labels; for example, they use verbs most often to regulate or anticipate children's behavior, not to name actions for them (Tomasello & Kruger, 1992). It would seem bizarre indeed if an adult were to exclaim to a child: "Look, this is an instance of putting. Look at me putting this here." Instead children typically hear common verbs as an adult directs their behavior in such utterances as "Put your toys away" while pointing to the toy box. It is clear that in such cases, the social-pragmatic cues that might indicate the adult's intended referent for the child are much more subtle, complex, and variegated than in the ostensive context. Indeed, they even change in fundamental ways from situation to situation: The adult requests that the child eat peas by directing the spoon at the child's face, requests that the child give something by holding out a hand, and requests the putting away of toys by pointing to the destination desired. Thus, there is no standardized "original naming game" for verbs and many other types of early words (e.g., prepositions) as there is for object labels for some children (Tomasello, 1995b).

A number of studies have demonstrated experimentally that children can indeed learn new words in a variety of fairly complex social-interactive situations. Children learn new words not just when adults stop and name objects for them but also in the ongoing flow of social interaction in which both they and the adult are trying to do things. In none of these cases can the child count on the adult following into the child's already-established focus of attention, but rather the child must adapt to the adult's focus of attention. For example, Baldwin (1993a, 1993b) taught 19-month-old children new words in two new situations. In one situation the adult followed into the child's focus of attention, and, as in other studies, children learned the new word quite well. Children, however, also learned new words in a situation in which the adult labeled an object the child was not already looking at, thus requiring the child to look up and then determine the adult's attentional focus.

In addition, Tomasello and colleagues (see Tomasello, in press, for a review) have conducted a series of studies that demonstrate the same point even more dramatically. The basic idea in all cases is to set up situations in which adults talk to children as they engage in various games, with novel words being introduced as naturally as possible into the ongoing flow of the game. In all cases multiple potential referents are available, that is, there are multiple novel referents for which the child has no existing name. Various social-pragmatic cues to the adult's intended referent are provided in different studies to see whether children are sensitive to them. The studies are designed so that neither the adult's gaze direction nor any of the well-known word-learning constraints that various investigators have proposed (e.g., whole object, mutual exclusivity, syntactic bootstrapping; Markman, 1989) will be helpful to the child in distinguishing among possible referents. In all these studies the children ranged from 18 to 24 months of age, and in all cases the majority of children learned the novel words in comprehension, production, or both. To give a feel for the kinds of situations in which children successfully read the adult's (E's) communicative intentions and so learn the new word, we summarize some different situations here. In each case, the original study gives all of the details of control conditions and so forth (there is also an overall summary with many details of these and other similar studies in Tomasello, in press).

- E announced her intention to "find the toma" and then searched in a row of buckets containing novel objects, rejecting some objects by scowling and replacing them until she found the one she wanted (indicated by a smile and the termination of search). Children learned the new word for the object that E's smile indicated was the one intended, no matter how many rejected objects intervened in the search (Tomasello & Barton, 1994).
- E had the child find four different objects in four different hiding places, one of which was a distinctive toy barn. Once the child had learned which objects went with which places, E announced her intention to "find the gazzer." She then went to the toy barn, but it turned out to be "locked." She frowned and proceeded to another hiding place to find another toy. Later, when children were asked to pick out the gazzer, they did so even though they had never seen the object after they had heard the new word (Study 1 of Akhtar & Tomasello, 1996; see also Study 2 of Akhtar & Tomasello, 1996, in which a similar procedure was used for verb learning).
- E announced her intention to "dax Mickey Mouse" and then proceeded to perform one action accidentally and another intentionally (or sometimes in the reverse order). Children learned the word for the intentional, not the accidental, action regardless of which came first in the sequence (Tomasello & Barton, 1994).
- A child, her mother, and E played with three novel objects; then the mother left the room, and the child and E played with a fourth object. When the mother returned, she looked at the four objects together and exclaimed "Oh look! A modi! A modi!" Understanding that the mother was likely to be excited about the object she was seeing for the first time, children learned the new word for that object (Akhtar, Carpenter, & Tomasello, 1996).

The point of these studies was to investigate something of the range of situations in which children might be able to discern the adult's communicative intentions and to learn the new word. Although any one of these studies might be explained in other ways (e.g., Samuelson & Smith, 1998), in our view when they are considered as a group, the most plausible explanation is that by the time children are 18–24 months of age, they have a deep and flexible understanding of other individuals as intentional beings. Thus, they are quite skillful at determining the adult's communicative intentions in a wide variety of novel communicative situations. Children's assumption that the adult's language is relevant to their ongoing social and instrumental activities is simply the natural expression of this intentional understanding.

In all cases, no matter what the situation, children must be able to do two things to acquire a communicative symbol. First, they must be able to determine adults' communicative intentions. This involves understanding the adult's intentions toward my attention, that is, understanding what the adult wants me to focus on. This is arguably a more difficult task than determining the adult's intentions toward, say, a ball, which are much more straightforward. Understanding communicative intentions involves a kind of intentional embedding: understanding his or her intentions toward my attention (Sperber & Wilson, 1986). This understanding allows children to begin to comprehend novel language. Second, to produce conventional linguistic symbols, children must engage in a process of role-reversal imitation in which they use the newly acquired symbol toward the adult in the same way and for the same communicative purpose that the adult used it toward them. Again this process of role-reversal imitation is more complex than imitating, say, the adult's action on a ball. Imitatively learning a communicative convention means imagining myself in the adult's role and enacting that action. Thus, learning a new word requires both a special form of the understanding of intentions—understanding communicative intentions—and a special form of cultural learning—role-reversal imitation.

Children get much better at this cultural learning process during the second and third years of life. Initially, at 1 year of age, they are able to learn new language mostly in highly repetitive and predictable social interactions in which the adult follows into their attentional focus. As children become more skillful at determining adult communicative intentions in a wider variety of interactive situations, however, highly structured formats with highly sensitive adults become less crucial to the process. The child must establish joint attention in more active ways by determining the adult's attentional focus in a variety of sociocommunicative contexts. Of possible relevance to this account is the finding that some children acquire their native language in cultures in which there is very little of the heavy scaffolding and attentional sensitivity that characterize many Western middle-class families. Although quantitative studies have yet to be done, by some accounts these children seldom acquire large numbers of words before their second birthdays (de Leon, personal communication, 1998). If this is true, the implication is that these children acquire the vast majority of their language only after they are able to be more active in determining adult communicative intentions within the flow of ongoing social interaction—as in the verb learning of Western middle-class children and in the experimental studies cited previously.

SOCIAL-COGNITIVE FOUNDATIONS

The social-cognitive foundation for language learning is thus the same, with a few twists, as the social-cognitive foundation for children's other joint attentional activities that first emerge around 1 year of age (e.g., gaze following, social referencing, imitative learning of instrumental actions, perception of intentional action). All of these skills and activities emerge in rough developmental synchrony because all of them reflect the infant's emerging ability to understand other individuals as intentional agents whose attention, emotion, and behavior to outside objects may be actively followed into and shared (Carpenter, Nagell, & Tomasello, 1998; Tomasello, 1995a). This social-cognitive revolution at the infant's first birthday sets the stage for the second year of life in which children culturally learn—imitatively—the use of all kinds of tools and artifacts, with linguistic symbols being one example. This imitative learning is not just a mimicking of adult movements and is not just a reproducing of interesting environmental effects by whatever means imaginable; instead it is a reproduction of the adult's intentional relations to the world. In imitative learning, the child perceives the adult's overt actions as composed of both a goal and a means for attaining that goal and then the child actively chooses the adult's means of goal attainment in contrast to others the child might have chosen. The clearest indications of this type of intentional understanding were shown by Meltzoff (1995), who found that 18-month-old infants imitatively learned actions that adults intended to perform on objects, even when the adult was unsuccessful in performing them, and by Carpenter, Akhtar, and Tomasello (1998), who found that 14- to 18-month-old infants imitated adults' intentional actions on objects and ignored their accidental actions.

Our view is thus that the acquisition of linguistic symbols begins during this same developmental period quite simply because comprehending and producing language relies on the same basic understanding of individuals as intentional agents as do all of the other social-cognitive and cultural learning skills that emerge at this same age. Language tends to follow the emergence of the more straightforward expressions of joint attention skills such as gaze following and imitation because it requires a special application of these skills both to understand the special form of intentions known as communicative intentions and to engage in the special form of imitative learning known as role-reversal imitation. Thus, we believe that disruptions to the foundational joint attentional skills that normally emerge at 1 year of age will have dire consequences for many aspects of children's language acquisition and use.

CHILDREN WITH AUTISM

Children with autism grow up in the same structured social world as do typically developing children. Despite early proposals to the contrary, there is no evidence that children with autism receive less (or more) social stimulation or worse (or different) parenting than other children (see Cantwell, Baker, & Rutter, 1978b, for a review, and Sigman & Capps, 1997, for discussion). Yet many children with autism never acquire any productive language, and the language of those who do acquire some language is different in many specific ways from that of typical children (this is discussed later in this chapter; see also Frith, 1989, for a review). Consequently, according to the social-pragmatic approach to language acquisition, if these children's structured social worlds are the same, then there must be something atypical about the ability of children with autism to tune into the social world in which they live (via joint attention), to understand the communicative intentions of those who speak to them, and/or to engage in role-reversal imitation of linguistic symbols. In the remainder of this chapter we review briefly the abilities of children with autism in each of these areas. We then examine studies that have investigated the relations between these abilities and children's language, and we discuss the implications of deficits in each of these areas for other aspects of language development.

Tuning into the Social World

From very early in life, typical infants are especially attuned to social stimuli (e.g., Morton & Johnson, 1991). Although few studies have been done on very young children with autism because diagnosis is rarely made before age 3 years or so, there is some evidence that these children show differences in orientation to social stimuli compared with both typical children and children with developmental delays as early as 1 year of age. For example, children with autism do not orient to certain speech sounds—their mother's voice (Klin, 1991) or their own names (Dawson, Meltzoff, & Osterling, 1995; Osterling & Dawson, 1994)—as readily as do other children. (See Chapter 2 for further discussion of early characteristics.) They thus may miss many opportunities to learn new language because they may not attend to much of the speech directed to them.

Similarly, children with autism do not tune into other people in the more active ways that typical children do. Whereas children with autism are social to some degree—for example, they participate in social interactions and games (Dawson, Hill, Spencer, Galpert, & Watson, 1990; Mundy, Sigman, & Kasari, 1990; Sigman, Mundy, Sherman, & Ungerer, 1986) and may form secure attachments to caregivers (Capps, Sigman, & Mundy, 1994; Rogers, Ozonoff, & Maslin-Cole, 1991)—these children nevertheless interact with others in fundamentally different ways from other children. Most importantly, children with autism generally do not actively share interest and attention with others, nor do they respond to others' bids to share interest and attention with them. Many studies (see Charman, in press, for a review) have found deficits in a variety of joint attentional skills: *referential looking* (i.e., gaze alternation between object and adult; this is the basis of the joint attentional interactions discussed previously; Charman et al., 1997; Lewy & Dawson, 1992; Mundy, Sigman, Ungerer, & Sherman, 1986; Wetherby, Prizant, & Hutchinson, 1998), *declarative pointing and showing* (Baron-Cohen, 1989; Loveland & Landry, 1986; Sigman et al., 1986; Wetherby et al., 1998; Wetherby & Prutting, 1984), *looking where others look and point* (Baron-Cohen, 1989; Leekam, Baron-Cohen, Perrett, Milders, & Brown, 1997), and *social referencing* (Sigman, Kasari, Kwon, & Yirmiya, 1992).

These deficits are not a result of an inability to perform the specific behaviors involved. That is, although children with autism show no differences in amount of overall gaze toward the faces of other people compared with other children (Dawson et al., 1990), they make eye contact in different situations and in different ways. For example, children with autism look to adults' faces as often as other children during face-to-face social games (Sigman et al., 1986). When play includes objects, however, children with autism do not usually alternate gaze between objects and the adult's face (i.e., engage in joint attention). In addition, when they do happen to look to the adult's face, they neither follow the adult's gaze nor use the adult's facial expressions to influence their own behavior to new objects (social referencing); they also do not combine positive affective expressions with their gaze in the way typical children do (Dawson et al., 1990). Similarly, although children with autism often gesture to others imperatively to request objects or actions from them (often with accompanying gaze alternation between the object they are gesturing about and the other's face), they only very rarely gesture declaratively, simply to indicate an object in order to share something about it with the other person (Baron-Cohen, 1989; Curcio, 1978; Wetherby et al., 1998; Wetherby & Prutting, 1984).

This deficit in joint attentional skills is evident very early in development—even before diagnosis is made (Baron-Cohen, et al., 1996; Osterling & Dawson, 1994)—and persists throughout childhood (Baron-Cohen, 1989; Landry & Loveland, 1988), although the specific joint attentional deficits present may change with development (Mundy, Sigman, & Kasari, 1994). It reliably differentiates children with autism from children with various other developmental delays (Mundy et al., 1986; Mundy et al., 1990; Wetherby et al., 1998). It is an open question at this point whether lack of joint attention is itself a primary deficit in autism or whether it is instead a consequence of earlier-emerging, more basic deficits such as difficulties with interpersonal relatedness or affective sharing (Hobson, 1993; Mundy & Sigman, 1989) or shifting attention between two stimuli (Courchesne et al., 1994; see also Chapter 8). Either way, the result is that children are prevented from following into and directing others' attention and interest to objects in their shared world. As we discuss later, this difficulty has dire consequences for these children's acquisition of language.

Communicative Intentions and Role-Reversal Imitation

Because joint attention is a precursor of understanding others' communicative intentions and engaging in role-reversal imitation, these latter skills also are likely to be impaired in children with autism. There is very little direct experimental evidence, however, concerning either of these skills in these children. We are aware of no studies of these children's understanding of others' communicative intentions in word-learning situations, similar to Tomasello and colleagues' (e.g., Tomasello & Barton, 1994) studies of typically developing children, for example. There is some evidence that suggests that children with autism may have difficulty understanding others' *behavioral* intentions (Phillips, Baron-Cohen, & Rutter, 1992, 1998); if this is true, then it is likely that this difficulty extends to understanding others' communicative intentions as well.

Similarly, very few studies of children with autism have included tasks designed to measure children's ability to reverse roles when imitating. These children generally show impaired performance on traditional imitation tasks (see Smith & Bryson, 1994, for a review), so the more difficult role-reversal imitation may be even more problematic for them. There is suggestive evidence that this may be the case. Ohta (1987), for example, tested relatively high-functioning children with autism (with a mean chronological age of 10 years) on several gesture imitation tasks. On some of these tests, children with autism sometimes made a distinctive type of error that other children rarely made. For instance, when the modeled action was "waving with the open palm facing the subject," some children with autism waved with their own palm facing themselves (as opposed to palm facing the experimenter); that is, they reproduced the action exactly as they saw it. Smith and Bryson (1998) and Whiten and Brown (1998) reported similar results for some of their gesture imitation tasks.

Relation Between Social-Cognitive Skills and Language

Joint attention and the other social-cognitive skills just discussed all have several things in common. First, to varying degrees, they all rely on children's ability to take the perspective of their social partners toward some object or event, or toward themselves. Second, they require children to attribute to others such mental states as attention, interest, affect, intentions, and prior experience in relation to the object or event at hand. Third, they reflect children's ability, and motivation, to share in those mental states with others. Finally, in typically developing children, at least, the skills are theoretically (and empirically, in the case of joint attention) demonstrated to be essential to typical language development. Deficits in these skills thus would be expected to result in a wide range of problems for language acquisition (see Chapter 5 for further discussion).

That children with autism have difficulties with both language and joint attentional skills is already suggestive of a link between social-cognitive skills and language, but there is more specific and direct evidence as well. Individual differences in the joint attentional skills of children with autism correlate with individual differences in language skills. This would not have to be the case because it easily could be that a certain level of joint attentional skill is needed for basic language abilities, but then further levels of joint attentional skill result in no further increases in language abilities. It is also the case that skills of other types are necessary for typical language abilities (e.g., skills of concept formation and categorization), and these could easily mitigate quantitative correlations between joint attention skills and language development. Still, a number of studies have shown that these two key skills do indeed correlate strongly.

Robust, positive correlations (ranging from $r = .43$ to $r = .94$) consistently are found between various measures of joint attention and various measures of children's language. Several researchers (e.g., Landry & Loveland, 1988; Mundy et al., 1990; Mundy, Sigman, Ungerer, & Sherman, 1987; Wetherby et al., 1998; see also Chapter 4) have found correlations between children's overall joint attention scores (and individual components of those scores) and measures of concurrent and later receptive and expressive vocabulary sizes. It is interesting to note that Mundy and colleagues (1994) also found that children's joint attention scores were negatively correlated with parents' reports of disturbances (including odd prosody and echolalia) in their children's language. Furthermore, the relation between joint attention and language extends beyond vocabulary size, as strong, positive relations also are found between 1) joint attention and acquisition of grammar (Rollins & Snow, in press, found that 89% of the variance in children's syntactic development was explained by joint attention scores) and 2) joint attention and correct use of *I/you* pronouns (Landry & Loveland, 1988; Loveland & Landry, 1986). These joint attention–language correlations are specific to joint attention and are not a reflection of general social ability: Few relations are found in any of these studies between general social interaction or communicative behavior regulation (i.e., requesting) measures and language.

In addition to correlations between joint attention and language, several studies have found correlations between imitation, another important social-cognitive skill, and language development for children with autism. These children's vocal and gestural imitative skills are positively related to their verbal and nonverbal communication skills (Abrahamsen & Mitchell, 1990; Curcio, 1978; Dawson & Adams, 1984).

There are thus correlational relations between various social-cognitive skills and language development in children with autism. Most of the relations are with children's vocabulary size, a somewhat blunt measure of children's communicative competence, but there is evidence that these social-cognitive skills also are important in other, very specific areas of language acquisition and use by children with autism. For example, another parallel between joint attention and language concerns the function of joint attention and language. Children with autism tend to talk less often for the purpose of sharing or seeking information than for the purpose of expressing needs and wants (Stone &

Caro-Martinez, 1990; Tager-Flusberg, 1992, 1993; Wetherby et al., 1998; Wetherby & Prutting, 1984). This is not surprising given that 1) the function of joint attention is to share something—affect, interest, and attention—about objects with others and 2) children with autism gesture more for imperative purposes than declarative ones.

Another interesting characteristic of the language of children with autism that reflects joint attention deficits is these children's tendency occasionally to learn words for incorrect referents. Baron-Cohen, Baldwin, and Crowson (1997), in a replication of Baldwin's (1993a, 1993b) discrepant labeling studies, found that children with autism did not use the adult's gaze direction to learn new words, instead learning the new word for the object they themselves were looking at when the word was uttered. Because of the tendency of these children not to use joint attention behaviors to establish reference and because adults occasionally label objects that are not already in the child's focus of attention, it is not surprising that there are abundant examples of "metaphorical speech" in children with autism (Baron-Cohen et al., 1997; Kanner, 1973). These types of errors can be avoided if caregivers follow into children's focus of attention when using new words: Watson (1998) found that language comprehension of children with autism was positively correlated with frequency of maternal follow-in language and negatively correlated with maternal directing language (as is the case with typically developing children). Thus, whereas these children may learn words in scaffolded interactions in which adults follow into their focus of attention, they are less able to do this in less ostensive contexts, when they must determine and use the speaker's perspective.

Therefore, children's ability or tendency to engage in joint attention is related to their language skills in many ways. A similar pattern is found for deficits in understanding others' communicative intentions. For children who do not understand communicative intentions, in the extreme case, language would simply be semirandom sounds that came out of others' mouths (the sounds would not be completely random because sometimes they might be associated with certain objects or situations). If such children were to speak at all, their speech would be limited to a small number of familiar nouns or phrases, learned associatively or through training and reinforcement, which more often than not would involve highly motivating, imperative situations (e.g., "I want juice"); this type of speech is characteristic of a subset of children with autism. If children understood a little more about others' intentions with regard to language—that is, others' *informative intention* but not their *communicative intention* (see, e.g., Happé, 1993)—then language would have more meaning but nevertheless would be incomprehensible in some very specific circumstances. For example, such children would not understand that there can be another level to language—the level of communicative intention—and this would be manifest by their tendency to mistakenly interpret all language literally. Thus, these children should show specific difficulties with comprehension of such figurative aspects of language as metaphors, irony, sarcasm, jokes, and lies—but should not have difficulties with similes or other literal language, because in the latter cases, understanding the added layer of communicative intention is not necessary. There is abundant evidence of these specific strengths and weaknesses in the comprehension of children with autism (e.g., Happé, 1993; see also Frith, 1989, for further discussion). Similar results are found with production of language as well: Eales (1993) has demonstrated that although the inappropriateness of execution of informative intentions of adults with autism was no different from that of adults with receptive language disorder, adults with autism produced significantly more utterances reflecting failures of communicative intentions and relevance than did the other adults.

A similar pattern also is found for role-reversal imitation. The tendency of children with autism to engage in echolalia, or direct imitation of others' speech, is well known, and we would argue that this tendency is a reflection of these children's ability to imitate but not to engage in role-reversal imitation—these children learn words and phrases exactly as they hear them. Echolalia may be used communicatively by children with autism (Prizant & Duchan, 1981), but it clearly does not involve flexible, reciprocal understanding of language. Echolalia decreases as children's language level increases (McEvoy, Loveland, & Landry, 1988).

In many cases, early speech (i.e., in the one- and two-word stages) learned via simple imitation might be indistinguishable from speech learned via role-reversal imitation. Once children begin including personal pronouns and other deictic words (i.e., words whose meaning changes depending on context; e.g., *I/you, this/that*) in their speech, however, the type of imitation used to learn the words becomes more obvious.[1] If children then use the same form the speaker did in these cases, saying, for example, "You want candy," to ask for candy, this provides a clear indication of imitation without speaker–listener role reversal. Children with autism often make these types of errors. Furthermore, there is experimental evidence that children with autism can comprehend *me/you* pronouns in others' speech but have difficulty then using those pronouns in their own speech (i.e., reversing the listener's and speaker's roles). Jordan (1989) demonstrated that children with autism responded correctly to instructions such as "Put the hat on you/me" but did not usually respond with the correct pronoun when completing the speaker's statement, e.g., "Look! The dog has jumped on . . . ?" Most of children's "errors" in this case were caused by substituting the experimenter's or their own name (appropriately; e.g., if the dog jumped on the child, the child used his or her name instead of

[1]Even during the early stages of language development, intonation may be a distinguishing factor: When children use questioning intonation when they are making a statement (e.g., "Want cookie?" to indicate that they want a cookie), this is undoubtedly an example of echolalia. These question–statement reversals are common in children with autism (Tager-Flusberg, 1993).

the experimenter's name) for the pronoun, a strategy that does not require role reversal of adults' language.

We have emphasized so far the importance of several early social-cognitive skills for language acquisition. Related to each of the social-cognitive deficits we have discussed is the well-known deficit in theory of mind (ToM) exhibited by children with autism (Baron-Cohen, Tager-Flusberg, & Cohen, 1993). Several researchers (e.g., Baron-Cohen, 1988; Frith, 1989; Tager-Flusberg, 1993, 1997) have described theoretical and empirical relations between ToM abilities and various aspects of (more advanced) language use. For example, an understanding of others' thoughts, beliefs, knowledge, interests, emotions, and other mental states is particularly important in the area of pragmatics. Children with autism have been shown to have deficits in a wide range of pragmatic skills: For example, they do not take into account what is new, interesting, or important to the listener; they ask socially inappropriate and embarrassing questions; and they use pedantic speech. Both the narratives of children with autism (see Loveland & Tunali, 1993, for a review) and the instructions they give to others (Loveland, Tunali, McEvoy, & Kelley, 1989) also are inadequate, in general, for the same sort of reason: These children do not take into account what listeners know or do not know. Indeed, direct relations have been found between ToM and such aspects of language as understanding of figurative language (Happé, 1993), narrative skills (Tager-Flusberg & Sullivan, 1995), and various pragmatic skills (Eisenmajer & Prior, 1991).

There are several other characteristics of the language of children with autism that may result from difficulties with ToM, perspective taking, and keeping track of what the listener knows. For example, children with autism use fewer words for mental states than do other children (e.g., Tager-Flusberg, 1992). Furthermore, although the form of the syntax of children with autism is in general unimpaired (Cantwell, Baker, & Rutter, 1978a; Tager-Flusberg et al., 1990), their use of various syntactic forms differs markedly from that of other children in specific ways that reflect difficulties understanding that others may have different knowledge and points of view from their own (see Tager-Flusberg, 1997, for a review). Children with autism also often do not choose pragmatically loaded words (e.g., *a/the, this/that*) and forms (e.g., past/present tense) correctly (Bartolucci, Pierce, & Streiner, 1980), and they also do not stress important parts of sentences communicatively (e.g., Fine, Bartolucci, Ginsberg, & Szatmari, 1991).

CLINICAL AND EDUCATIONAL IMPLICATIONS

The joint attention deficits in autism are well known and are already often a target of intervention programs. In addition to promoting joint attentional skills per se, therapists should work with caregivers on establishing routine interactions (see Wetherby, 1986, and Chapter 9 for further discussion) and on following into their child's focus of attention when using new language (or at least work on not directing children's attention to something new as often; Watson, 1998) because children with autism undoubtedly need both kinds of scaffolding even more than typical beginning language learners do. Following into the focus of attention of these children is especially important because they do not respond to others' initiations well—when adults attempt to direct their attention to new objects, they usually do not follow (McArthur & Adamson, 1996; Leekam et al., 1997). Although it is possible to draw these children's attention to a new object by using literal instead of conventional methods (McArthur & Adamson, 1996), once this is accomplished, it is important to encourage the sharing of attention with other people, perhaps through the use of the kinds of tricks that parents of typical infants use when joint attention is first developing (e.g., bringing the object into the joint line of regard of the child and the adult; Bruner, 1983).

In addition to joint attention, we believe that other factors are important in language acquisition: understanding communicative intentions and role-reversal imitation. These skills should also be targeted for intervention. For example, work on understanding others' communicative intentions could begin with work on understanding others' behavioral intentions (e.g., encouraging children to figure out why others behave the way they do, calling attention to others' accidents and mistakes). Work on imitation should be extended beyond having children mimic simple actions or vocalizations without perspective taking. An important accompaniment to traditional imitation tasks is the addition of tasks that require some form of role reversal, such as a hiding/finding game in which the child plays one role and then at a later time is asked to play the game in the other role.

Finally, it is important for clinicians and parents to think about language and communication in a more cultural, social-pragmatic way, as opposed to teaching and rewarding associations between words and objects (see Seibert & Oller, 1981; Wetherby, 1986; and Chapter 9). Only with such an approach will children be able to learn language flexibly and pragmatically.

DIRECTIONS FOR FUTURE RESEARCH

There is a lot that is not yet known about the important abilities discussed in this chapter. More information is needed about all of these abilities in children with autism and in other children. For joint attention, it is necessary to know *why* children with autism do not tend to engage in joint attentional behaviors. Various theories have been proposed (see, e.g., Courchesne et al., 1994; see also Chapter 7) but little testing of the underlying mechanisms of joint attention has been conducted. For communicative intentions, tests of the prediction that even highly verbal children with autism would have difficulties in the different kinds of word-learning studies conducted by Baldwin (1993a, 1993b) and Tomasello and colleagues (e.g., Akhtar & Tomasello, 1996; Tomasello & Barton, 1994; see also Tomasello, Call, & Gluckman, 1997) would be valuable. For role-reversal imitation, direct tests of this ability are needed, both for gestural/object imitation and for imitation of language. It also would be interesting to see whether the same relations between deficits in these skills and specific weaknesses in language are apparent in other populations, such as blind children.

CONCLUSIONS

Several reviews of language in autism (e.g., Baron-Cohen, 1988; Frith, 1989; Tager-Flusberg, 1993) have proposed that the specific pattern of strengths and weaknesses shown by people with autism in their language development fits well with a ToM explanation. We agree that having a ToM is necessary to produce appropriate narratives, to understand figurative language, and to engage in relevant, interesting conversation with others. We also point out, however, that earlier in the process of language acquisition, when children are just beginning to learn words and other linguistic symbols, deficits in other, more foundational social-cognitive skills—specifically, joint attention, understanding of others' communicative intentions, and role-reversal imitation—can explain many other selective impairments in the language of children with autism and that these skills, especially understanding others' communicative intentions, still are important in later language as well.

REFERENCES

Abrahamsen, E.P., & Mitchell, J.R. (1990). Communication and sensorimotor functioning in children with autism. *Journal of Autism and Developmental Disorders, 20,* 75–85.

Akhtar, N., Carpenter, M., & Tomasello, M. (1996). The role of discourse novelty in early word learning. *Child Development, 67,* 635–645.

Akhtar, N., Dunham, F., & Dunham, P.J. (1991). Directive interactions and early vocabulary development: The role of joint attentional focus. *Journal of Child Language, 18,* 41–49.

Akhtar, N., & Tomasello, M. (1996). Twenty-four-month-old children learn words for absent objects and actions. *British Journal of Developmental Psychology, 14,* 79–93.

Bakeman, R., & Adamson, L. (1984). Coordinating attention to people and objects in mother–infant and peer–infant interactions. *Child Development, 55,* 1278–1289.

Baldwin, D. (1993a). Early referential understanding: Young children's ability to recognize referential acts for what they are. *Developmental Psychology, 29,* 1–12.

Baldwin, D. (1993b). Infants' ability to consult the speaker for clues to word reference. *Journal of Child Language, 2,* 395–418.

Baron-Cohen, S. (1988). Social and pragmatic deficits in autism: Cognitive or affective. *Journal of Autism and Developmental Disorders, 18,* 379–402.

Baron-Cohen, S. (1989). Perceptual role taking and protodeclarative pointing in autism. *British Journal of Developmental Psychology, 7,* 113–127.

Baron-Cohen, S., Baldwin, D., & Crowson, M. (1997). Do children with autism use the speaker's direction of gaze strategy to crack the code of language? *Child Development, 68,* 48–57.

Baron-Cohen, S., Cox, A., Baird, G., Swettenham, J., Nightingale, N., Morgan, K., Drew, A., & Charman, T. (1996). Psychological markers in the detection of autism in infancy in a large population. *British Journal of Psychiatry, 168,* 158–163.

Baron-Cohen, S., Tager-Flusberg, H., & Cohen, D.J. (1993). *Understanding other minds: Perspectives from autism.* New York: Oxford University Press.

Bartolucci, G., Pierce, S., & Streiner, D. (1980). Cross-sectional studies of grammatical morphemes in autistic and mentally retarded children. *Journal of Autism and Developmental Disorders, 10,* 39–50.

Bloom, L. (1993). *The transition from infancy to language: Acquiring the power of expression.* New York: Cambridge University Press.

Brown, P. (in press). The conversational context for language acquisition: A Tzeltal (Mayan) case study. In M. Bowerman & S. Levinson (Eds.), *Language acquisition and conceptual development.* Cambridge, England: Cambridge University Press.

Bruner, J.S. (1975). The ontogenesis of speech acts. *Journal of Child Language, 2,* 1–20.

Bruner, J.S. (1983). *Child's talk: Learning to use language.* New York: W.W. Norton.

Cantwell, D., Baker, L., & Rutter, M. (1978a). A comparative study of infantile autism and specific developmental receptive language disorder: IV. Analysis of syntax and language function. *Journal of Child Psychology and Psychiatry and Allied Disciplines, 19,* 351–362.

Cantwell, D.P., Baker, L., & Rutter, M. (1978b). Family factors. In M. Rutter & E. Schopler (Eds.), *Autism: A reappraisal of concepts and treatment* (pp. 269–296). New York: Plenum.

Capps, L., Sigman, M., & Mundy, P. (1994). Attachment security in children with autism. *Development and Psychopathology, 6,* 249–261.

Carpenter, M., Akhtar, N., & Tomasello, M. (1998). Fourteen- to 18-month-old infants differentially imitate intentional and accidental actions. *Infant Behavior and Development, 21,* 315–330.

Carpenter, M., Nagell, K., & Tomasello, M. (1998). Social cognition, joint attention, and communicative competence from 9 to 15 months of age. *Monographs of the Society for Research in Child Development, 63*(4, Serial No. 255).

Charman, T. (in press). Specifying the nature and course of the joint attention impairment in autism in the preschool years: Implications for diagnosis and intervention. *Autism: The International Journal of Research and Practice.*

Charman, T., Swettenham, J., Baron-Cohen, S., Cox, A., Baird, G., & Drew, A. (1997). Infants with autism: An investigation of empathy, pretend play, joint attention, and imitation. *Developmental Psychology, 33,* 781–789.

Chomsky, N. (1986). *Knowledge of language.* Berlin: Praeger.

Courchesne, E., Townsend, J., Akshoomoff, N.A., Saitoh, O., Yeung-Courchesne, R., Lincoln, A.J., James, H.E., Haas, R.H., Schreibman, L., & Lau, L. (1994). Impairment in shifting attention in autistic and cerebellar patients. *Behavioral Neuroscience, 108,* 848–865.

Curcio, F. (1978). Sensorimotor functioning and communication in mute autistic children. *Journal of Autism and Childhood Schizophrenia, 8,* 281–292.

Dawson, G., & Adams, A. (1984). Imitation and social responsiveness in autistic children. *Journal of Abnormal Child Psychology, 12,* 209–225.

Dawson, G., Hill, D., Spencer, A., Galpert, L., & Watson, L. (1990). Affective exchanges between young autistic children and their mothers. *Journal of Abnormal Child Psychology, 18,* 335–345.

Dawson, G., Meltzoff, A., & Osterling, J. (1995, March). *Children with autism fail to orient to naturally occurring social stimuli.* Paper presented at the meeting of the Society for Research in Child Development, Indianapolis.

Dunham, P.J., Dunham, F.S., & Curwin, A. (1993). Joint attentional states and lexical acquisition at 18 months. *Developmental Psychology, 29,* 827–831.

Eales, M.J. (1993). Pragmatic impairments in adults with childhood diagnoses of autism or developmental receptive language disorder. *Journal of Autism and Developmental Disorders, 23,* 593–617.

Eisenmajer, R., & Prior, M. (1991). Cognitive linguistic correlates of 'theory of mind' ability in autistic children. *British Journal of Developmental Psychology, 9,* 351–364.

Fine, J., Bartolucci, G., Ginsberg, G., & Szatmari, P. (1991). The use of intonation to communicate in pervasive developmental disorders. *Journal of Child Psychology and Psychiatry and Allied Disciplines, 32,* 771–782.

Frith, U. (1989). A new look at language and communication in autism. *British Journal of Disorders of Communication, 24,* 123–150.

Happé, F.G.E. (1993). Communicative competence and theory of mind in autism: A test of relevance theory. *Cognition, 48,* 101–119.

Hobson, R.P. (1993). *Autism and the development of mind.* Mahwah, NJ: Lawrence Erlbaum Associates.

Jordan, R.R. (1989). An experimental comparison of the understanding and use of speaker–addressee personal pronouns in autistic children. *British Journal of Disorders of Communication, 24,* 169–179.

Kanner, L. (1973). *Childhood psychosis: Initial studies and new insights.* New York: John Wiley & Sons.

Klin, A. (1991). Young autistic children's listening preferences in regard to speech: A possible characterization of the symptom of social withdrawal. *Journal of Autism and Developmental Disorders, 21,* 29–42.

Landry, S.H., & Loveland, K.A. (1988). Communication behaviors in autism and developmental language delay. *Journal of Child Psychology and Psychiatry and Allied Disciplines, 29,* 621–634.

Leekam, S., Baron-Cohen, S., Perrett, D., Milders, M., & Brown, S. (1997). Eye-direction–detection: A dissociation between geometric and joint attention skills in autism. *British Journal of Developmental Psychology, 15,* 77–95.

Lewy, A.L., & Dawson, G. (1992). Social stimulation and joint attention in young autistic children. *Journal of Abnormal Child Psychology, 20,* 555–566.

Loveland, K.A., & Landry, S.H. (1986). Joint attention and language in autism and developmental language delay. *Journal of Autism and Developmental Disorders, 16,* 335–349.

Loveland, K., & Tunali, B. (1993). Narrative language in autism and the theory of mind hypothesis: A wider perspective. In S. Baron-Cohen, H. Tager-Flusberg, & D. Cohen (Eds.), *Understanding other minds: Perspectives from autism* (pp. 247–266). New York: Oxford University Press.

Loveland, K., Tunali, B., McEvoy, R.E., & Kelley, M.L. (1989). Referential communication and response adequacy in autism and Down's syndrome. *Applied Psycholinguistics, 10,* 301–313.

Markman, E. (1989). *Categorization and naming in children.* Cambridge: MIT Press.

McArthur, D., & Adamson, L.B. (1996). Joint attention in preverbal children: Autism and developmental language disorder. *Journal of Autism and Developmental Disorders, 26,* 481–496.

McEvoy, R.E., Loveland, K.A., & Landry, S.H. (1988). The functions of immediate echolalia in autistic children: A developmental perspective. *Journal of Autism and Developmental Disorders, 18,* 657–668.

Meltzoff, A.N. (1995). Understanding the intentions of others: Re-enactment of intended acts by 18-month-old children. *Developmental Psychology, 31*(5), 1–16.
Morton, J., & Johnson, M. (1991). CONSPEC and CONLEARN: A two-process theory of infant face recognition. *Psychological Review, 98,* 164–181.
Mundy, P., & Sigman, M. (1989). Specifying the nature of the social impairment in autism. In G. Dawson (Ed.), *Autism: Nature, diagnosis, and treatment* (pp. 3–21). New York: Guilford Press.
Mundy, P., Sigman, M., & Kasari, C. (1990). A longitudinal study of joint attention and language development in autistic children. *Journal of Autism and Developmental Disorders, 20,* 115–128.
Mundy, P., Sigman, M., & Kasari, C. (1994). Joint attention, developmental level, and symptom presentation in autism. *Development and Psychopathology, 6,* 389–401.
Mundy, P., Sigman, M., Ungerer, J., & Sherman, T. (1986). Defining the social deficits of autism: The contribution of nonverbal communication measures. *Journal of Child Psychology and Psychiatry and Allied Disciplines, 27,* 657–669.
Mundy, P., Sigman, M., Ungerer, J., & Sherman, T. (1987). Nonverbal communication and play correlates of language development in autistic children. *Journal of Autism and Developmental Disorders, 17,* 349–364.
Nelson, K. (1985). *Making sense: The acquisition of shared meaning.* San Diego: Academic Press.
Nelson, K. (1996). *Language and cognitive development.* Cambridge, England: Cambridge University Press.
Ohta, M. (1987). Cognitive disorders of infantile autism: A study employing the WISC, spatial relationship conceptualization, and gesture imitation. *Journal of Autism and Developmental Disorders, 17,* 45–62.
Osterling, J., & Dawson, G. (1994). Early recognition of children with autism: A study of first birthday home videotapes. *Journal of Autism and Developmental Disorders, 24,* 247–257.
Phillips, W., Baron-Cohen, S., & Rutter, M. (1992). The role of eye contact in goal detection: Evidence from normal infants and children with autism or mental handicap. *Development and Psychopathology, 4,* 375–383.
Phillips, W., Baron-Cohen, S., & Rutter, M. (1998). Understanding intention in normal development and in autism. *British Journal of Developmental Psychology, 16,* 337–348.
Pinker, S. (1995). *The language instinct.* New York: William Morrow & Co.
Prizant, B.M., & Duchan, J.F. (1981). The functions of immediate echolalia in autistic children. *Journal of Speech and Hearing Disorders, 46,* 241–249.
Quine, W. (1960). *Word and object.* Cambridge, MA: Harvard University Press.
Rogers, S.J., Ozonoff, S., & Maslin-Cole, C. (1991). A comparative study of attachment behavior in young children with autism or other psychiatric disorders. *Journal of the American Academy of Child and Adolescent Psychiatry, 30,* 483–488.
Rollins, P.R., & Snow, C.E. (in press). Shared attention and grammatical development in typical children and children with autism. *Journal of Child Language.*
Samuelson, L.K., & Smith, L.B. (1998). Memory and attention make smart word learning: An alternative account of Akhtar, Carpenter, and Tomasello. *Child Development, 69,* 94–104.
Seibert, J.M., & Oller, D.K. (1981). Linguistic pragmatics and language intervention strategies. *Journal of Autism and Developmental Disorders, 11,* 75–88.
Sigman, M., & Capps, L. (1997). *Children with autism: A developmental perspective.* Cambridge, MA: Harvard University Press.
Sigman, M.D., Kasari, C., Kwon, J., & Yirmiya, N. (1992). Responses to the negative emotions of others by autistic, mentally retarded, and normal children. *Child Development, 63,* 796–807.

Sigman, M., Mundy, P., Sherman, T., & Ungerer, J. (1986). Social interactions of autistic, mentally retarded, and normal children and their caregivers. *Journal of Child Psychology and Psychiatry and Allied Disciplines, 27,* 647–656.

Smith, C.B., Adamson, L. B., & Bakeman, R. (1988). Interactional predictors of early language. *First Language, 8,* 143–156.

Smith, I.M., & Bryson, S.E. (1994). Imitation and action in autism: A critical review. *Psychological Bulletin, 116,* 259–273.

Smith, I.M., & Bryson, S.E. (1998). Gesture imitation in autism: Nonsymbolic postures and sequences. *Cognitive Neuropsychology, 15*(6), 747–770.

Smith, L., Jones, S., & Landau, B. (1996). Naming in young children: A dumb attentional mechanism? *Cognition, 60,* 143–171.

Sperber, D., & Wilson, D. (1986). *Relevance: Communication and cognition.* Cambridge, MA: Harvard University Press.

Stone, W.L., & Caro-Martinez, L.M. (1990). Naturalistic observations of spontaneous communication in autistic children. *Journal of Autism and Developmental Disorders, 20,* 437–454.

Tager-Flusberg, H. (1992). Autistic children's talk about psychological states: Deficits in the early acquisition of a theory of mind. *Child Development, 63,* 161–172.

Tager-Flusberg, H. (1993). What language reveals about the understanding of minds in children with autism. In S. Baron-Cohen, H. Tager-Flusberg, & D.J. Cohen (Eds.), *Understanding other minds: Perspectives from autism* (pp. 138–157). New York: Oxford University Press.

Tager-Flusberg, H. (1997). Language acquisition and theory of mind: Contributions from the study of autism. In L.B. Adamson & M.A. Romski (Eds.), *Communication and language acquisition: Discoveries from atypical development* (pp. 135–160). Baltimore: Paul H. Brookes Publishing Co.

Tager-Flusberg, H., Calkins, S., Nolin, T., Baumberger, T., Anderson, M., & Chadwick-Dias, A. (1990). A longitudinal study of language acquisition in autistic and Down syndrome children. *Journal of Autism and Developmental Disorders, 20,* 1–21.

Tager-Flusberg, H., & Sullivan, K. (1995). Attributing mental states to story characters: A comparison of narratives produced by autistic and mentally retarded individuals. *Applied Psycholinguistics, 16,* 241–256.

Tomasello, M. (1988). The role of joint attentional processes in early language development. *Language Sciences, 10,* 69–88.

Tomasello, M. (1992). The social bases of language acquisition. *Social Development, 1,* 67–87.

Tomasello, M. (1995a). Joint attention as social cognition. In C. Moore & P. Dunham (Eds.), *Joint attention: Its origins and role in development* (pp. 103–130). Mahwah, NJ: Lawrence Erlbaum Associates.

Tomasello, M. (1995b). Pragmatic contexts for early verb learning. In M. Tomasello & W. Merriman (Eds.), *Beyond names for things: Young children's acquisition of verbs* (pp. 115–146). Mahwah, NJ: Lawrence Erlbaum Associates.

Tomasello, M. (1996). The cultural roots of language. In B.M. Velichkovsky & D.M. Rumbaugh (Eds.), *Communicating meaning: The evolution and development of language* (pp. 275–308). Mahwah, NJ: Lawrence Erlbaum Associates.

Tomasello, M. (in press). Perceiving intentions and learning words in the second year of life. In M. Bowerman & S. Levinson (Eds.), *Language acquisition and conceptual development.* Cambridge, England: Cambridge University Press.

Tomasello, M., & Barton, M. (1994). Learning words in non-ostensive contexts. *Developmental Psychology, 30,* 639–650.

Tomasello, M., Call, J., & Gluckman, A. (1997). Comprehension of novel communicative signs by apes and human children. *Child Development, 68,* 1067–1080.

Tomasello, M., & Farrar, M.J. (1986). Joint attention and early language. *Child Development, 57,* 1454–1463.

Tomasello, M., & Kruger, A.C. (1992). Joint attention on actions: Acquiring verbs in ostensive and non-ostensive contexts. *Journal of Child Language, 19,* 311–334.

Tomasello, M., Kruger, A.C., & Ratner, H.H. (1993). Cultural learning. *Behavioral and Brain Sciences, 16,* 495–552.

Tomasello, M., Mannle, S., & Kruger, A. (1986). The linguistic environment of one to two year old twins. *Developmental Psychology, 22,* 169–176.

Tomasello, M., & Todd, J. (1983). Joint attention and lexical acquisition style. *First Language, 4,* 197–212.

Trevarthen, C., & Hubley, P. (1978). Secondary intersubjectivity: Confidence, confiding and acts of meaning in the first year. In A. Lock (Ed.), *Action, gesture, and symbol: The emergence of language* (pp. 183–229). San Diego: Academic Press.

Watson, L.R. (1998). Following the child's lead: Mothers' interactions with children with autism. *Journal of Autism and Developmental Disorders, 28,* 51–59.

Wetherby, A.M. (1986). Ontogeny of communicative functions in autism. *Journal of Autism and Developmental Disorders, 16,* 295–316.

Wetherby, A.M., Prizant, B.M., & Hutchinson, T.A. (1998). Communicative, social/affective, and symbolic profiles of young children with autism and pervasive developmental disorders. *American Journal of Speech-Language Pathology, 7,* 79–91.

Wetherby, A.M., & Prutting, C.A. (1984). Profiles of communicative and cognitive-social abilities in autistic children. *Journal of Speech and Hearing Research, 27,* 364–377.

Whiten, A., & Brown, J.D. (1998). Imitation and the reading of other minds: Perspectives from the study of autism, normal children and non-human primates. In S. Braten (Ed.), *Intersubjective communication and emotion in ontogeny: A sourcebook* (pp. 198–227). Cambridge, England: Cambridge University Press.

Wittgenstein, L. (1953). *Philosophical investigations.* New York: Macmillan.

4

Joint Attention, Social Orienting, and Nonverbal Communication in Autism

Peter Mundy and Jennifer Stella

Autism is a biologically based disorder that may be more prevalent than once thought, occurring at a rate of 1 in 1,000 (Bryson, 1996). It is characterized by impaired social development (Bailey, Philips, & Rutter, 1996; Kanner, 1943). Rather than display a "pervasive lack of responsiveness to others" (American Psychiatric Association, 1980), however, people with autism are now understood to display a *pattern of strengths and weaknesses* in the acquisition of social and communication skills, which changes with development (Mundy & Sigman, 1989a). Understanding the nature of this pattern of strengths and weaknesses may be fundamental to research and intervention with these children.

In preverbal children, the communication disturbance of autism is exemplified by a failure to adequately develop joint attention skills. These skills involve the tendency to use eye contact, affect, and gestures for the singularly social purpose of sharing experiences with others. Prototypical of joint attention behavior is the act of pointing or showing to share one's pleasure in a toy. Alternatively, less impaired is the use of eye contact and gestures to regulate the behavior of others for more instrumental purposes. These behaviors include requesting aid in obtaining objects or even displaying attachment/reunion behaviors after a caregiver separation (Curcio, 1978; Loveland & Landry, 1986; Mundy, Sigman, Ungerer, & Sherman, 1986; Sigman & Mundy, 1989; Wetherby, Prizant, & Hutchinson, 1998).

Portions of this chapter have been reprinted from "On the nature of communication and language impairment in autism," Mundy, P., & Markus, J., *Mental Retardation and Developmental Disabilities Research Reviews, 343–349,* Copyright © 1997, Wiley-Liss, Inc. a subsidiary of John Wiley & Sons, Inc.; adapted by permission.

Preparation of this manuscript was supported in part by National Institute on Deafness and Other Communication Disorders Grant No. 00484 and by a grant from the Florida State Department of Education to the University of Miami Center for Autism and Related Disabilities.

Numerous observations suggest that joint attention disturbance may reflect a fundamental component of the etiology of autism (Mundy, 1995; Mundy & Markus, 1997). Research also suggests that an understanding of the nature of joint attention disturbance may be critical to sound clinical practice with young children with autism (Mundy & Crowson, 1997). Measures of joint attention appear to be among the more powerful early diagnostic indicators of autism (see Mundy & Crowson, 1997, for a review). Moreover, individual differences in joint attention skill development are important prognostic indicators for cognitive, language, and social development among children with autism (Mundy, Sigman, & Kasari, 1990, 1994; Sigman & Ruskin, 1997). Finally, research on joint attention development has begun to contribute to the understanding of the complex network of neurological processes that may be involved in autism (Caplan et al., 1993; Mundy, Card, & Fox, 1999).

In children with autism who display functional speech, strengths and weaknesses in communication skills are also apparent. The processes that enable adequate phonological, syntactic, and semantic usage of language may only be mildly impaired (Volden & Lord, 1991). Alternatively, a disturbance of the pragmatics of language usage is a prominent feature of autism (Eales, 1993; Happé, 1993; Surian, Baron-Cohen, & Van der Lely, 1996; Tager-Flusberg, 1993). The pragmatics of language refers to a broad array of skills involved in prosody, appropriate turn taking, politeness, and topic maintenance in conversation. Pragmatics also involves the critical ability to signal and interpret unspoken premises, as with figures of speech (e.g., metaphor), with nonverbal behaviors, or by relying on the context of a communicative interaction. Just as with research on joint attention disturbance, it has been well documented that verbal pragmatic disturbance in children with autism not only plays a critical role in the process of social-interaction disturbance that children with autism experience but also reflects potentially a key to understanding the very nature of the disorder (Eales, 1993; Happé, 1993; Surian et al., 1996; Tager-Flusberg, 1993).

This brief synopsis indicates that a comprehensive model of autism ultimately will need to address both linguistic pragmatic difficulties and the very early onset of preverbal sociocommunicative deficits that are characteristic of the syndrome. In the course of debate that is necessary to develop this model, fundamental issues must be raised and examined. These issues concern not only autism but also the nature of the ontogeny of the human capacity for complex social-communication. Two of these issues are highlighted in this review.

One issue concerns the nature of the neurological disturbance that leads to the sociocommunicative disturbance of autism. The status of the neuroscience of social behavior is not sufficiently articulated to allow anything but an oversimplified modeling of the neurology of autism. Nevertheless, the neurological functions associated primarily with frontal cortical and medial temporal systems are likely foci for the types of sociocommunicative disturbance displayed by individuals with autism (e.g., Bachevalier, 1994; Damasio & Maurer, 1978; Dawson, 1996; Minshew, 1996; Mundy, 1995; Pennington & Ozonoff, 1996). Of course, there is considerable debate as to whether functional disturbances of these systems are primary in the etiology of autism or secondary upstream effects of impaired functions in more caudal brain systems (Courchesne, Chisum, & Townsend, 1994; Damasio & Maurer, 1978; see also Chapter 8).

Another issue concerns the functional, or psychological, nature of the neurological disturbance in autism. Three prominent models propose to account for the social communication disturbance of autism while sharing a common focus on frontal processes. These include the theory of mind (ToM) model, the executive function model (see Chapter 5), and the social orienting model.[1] The ToM model suggests that one aspect of frontal process may be dedicated to a facility for social cognition necessary for estimating the psychological status of others, such as their beliefs. According to this model the sociocommunicative disturbance of autism may be understood in terms of an impairment in the functions of this social-cognitive facility (Baron-Cohen et al., 1994).

The executive function model suggests that social-cognitive and sociocommunicative impairment in autism does not derive from a system dedicated to social cognition. Rather, the sociocommunicative disturbance of autism is viewed as one manifestation of an impairment in frontally mediated executive cognitive processes. The fundamental function of these is to select appropriate goal-directed actions from an array of competing action potentials (Pennington & Ozonoff, 1996).

A critical assumption of the third model, the social orienting model, is that the earliest forms of sociocommunicative impairment of autism may not be completely understood in terms of either of the cognitive mechanisms espoused in the ToM or executive function models. The social orienting model suggests that prior to the emergence of cognition as the primary regulator of behavior, frontally mediated neuroaffective motivation systems prioritize social information processing in human development. A deficit in these systems is thought to contribute to initial as well as subsequent social and cognitive disturbances in autism (e.g., Dawson & Lewy, 1989; Fotheringham, 1991; Hobson, 1993; Mundy, 1995).

Each model provides a different and valuable perspective on the nature of autism and on sociocommunicative skill acquisition more generally. This chapter provides an overview of the similarities and differences among these models. We also note that a collective view of these models gives rise to a consideration of how related neurological processes may serve different functions at different stages in the development of autism.

---

[1]The first use of the term *social orienting* to describe deficits in autism may be attributed to Dawson, Meltzoff, and Osterling (1995).

THEORY OF MIND AND SOCIOCOMMUNICATIVE DISTURBANCE IN AUTISM

Consider a possible newspaper headline, "Iraqi Head Seeks Arms" (Pinker, 1994). Adequate lexical development and an understanding of grammar alone do not allow for the correct interpretation of this statement. Rather, some additional cognitive, pragmatic facility that goes beyond the neural systems that may be specific to the grammar of language development is assumed to play a role in correctly conveying and recognizing the ambiguous communicative intentions that are frequently embedded in language (Pinker, 1994).

Children with autism display a poor facility for the pragmatics of language (Frith, 1989). To understand this feature of autism, some have turned to theory and research on the nature of social-cognition. The capacity for social-cognition may be an important, if not defining, feature of primate and especially human neurobehavioral evolution (Cosmides, 1989; Whiten & Byrne, 1988). In keeping with this evolutionary psychological view, a modular perspective on cognition has been adapted to suggest that the capacity to understand the intentions of others follows its own proprietary developmental course, with brain mechanisms responsible for apprehending mental states separate from brain mechanisms related to nonsocial cognition (e.g., Baron-Cohen, 1995; Leslie & Thaiss, 1992). This dedicated socio-neuro-cognitive mechanism has various descriptions (Baron-Cohen, 1995) but will be referred to here as the *ToM module* (Leslie, 1987).

Hypothetically, the ToM module employs a special type of cognition called *metarepresentation.* Metarepresentational ability allows one to mentally depict the psychological status of others, such as their thoughts and beliefs. It is called *metarepresentation* because it involves the capacity of one individual to mentally represent the mental representations of another individual. The development of metarepresentation involves the onset of a critical "decoupling" mechanism that enables the child to keep cognitive representations organized so that his or her own thoughts and feelings can be easily distinguished from representations of others' thoughts and feelings (Leslie, 1987, 1993). According to the ToM model, a disturbance in this metarepresentational thought process gives rise to the social and pragmatic deficits of people with autism (Baron-Cohen, 1995; Frith, 1989; Leslie, 1987; Tager-Flusberg, 1993). The logic here is that if children with autism have difficulty thinking about others' psychological status, then it would be unlikely that they would correctly identify the communicative intent of the author of the headline "Iraqi Head Seeks Arms." A host of other types of pragmatic errors would also be evident, such as difficulties with understanding figures of speech (e.g., idioms), difficulty in gauging the timing constraints of discourse, or difficulty in perceiving the informational needs of others as well as conventions of topic maintenance. According to the ToM, most, if not all, of the social deficits of autism may be understood in terms of this type of social-cognitive disturbance (Baron-Cohen, 1995).

Numerous experimental studies support the hypothesis that children with autism have difficulty on ToM measures (Baron-Cohen, 1995). In the prototypical "false belief paradigm," a child is asked to watch an agent ("Sally") hide an object in one of two hiding places (Place 1 versus Place 2). Sally then leaves the room, and another agent ("Anne") moves the object from Place 1 to Place 2. When Sally returns, the child must answer the question, "Where will Sally look for the object?" To answer this question correctly the child must disregard his or her own knowledge of where the object really is (Place 2) and *think about where Sally thinks* the object is. The metarepresentational component of this task has been italicized. Children typically develop the ability to solve this type of problem between 3 and 5 years of age. People with autism, however, manifest robust difficulty with false belief and related ToM tasks relative to language and IQ-score matched controls (see Baron-Cohen, 1995, for a review). Theoretically, this is because these individuals lack the requisite metarepresentational cognitive functions required to think about others' thoughts (Leslie, 1987). The argument for the modularity or the dedicated nature of this type of social-cognitive process has been made on numerous grounds (Leslie, 1993). The most important observation may be that representational deficits are more likely to be manifested by children with autism on social-cognitive tasks rather than analogous non–social-cognitive tasks (e.g., Leekam & Perner, 1991; Leslie & Thaiss, 1992; Scott & Baron-Cohen, 1996).

ToM-related ability has been directly linked to the degree to which pragmatic skill deficits are displayed among people with autism (Happé, 1993; Surian et al., 1996). Research has also begun to suggest that specific neural subsystems may be involved in thinking about the thoughts, beliefs, and feelings of others (Baron-Cohen et al., 1994; Fletcher et al., 1995). Using single photon emission computerized tomography data, Baron-Cohen and colleagues (1994) have reported that the right orbital frontal region may be involved in the processing of mental state terms. Fletcher and colleagues (1995) presented six male volunteers with ToM tasks while examining their brain activity with functional neuroimaging. These men were presented with ToM stories in which they were asked to think of the answers to questions about the internal motivations, beliefs, or thoughts of the protagonists. They were also presented with stories that required them to think of the answers to questions about causality of physical events or to answer question about sequences of unrelated sentences. The results indicated that thinking about the answers to the ToM vignettes involved cortical activity in the left medial frontal gyrus (Brodmann area 8) to a significantly greater extent than did thinking about the answers to the physical stories or unrelated sentence questions (Fletcher et al., 1995). It is interesting to note that the authors observed that this area had been linked, in comparative and human studies, to facility with conditional learning

(Petrides, 1990). The potential importance of the latter observation is made clear in the discussion of the executive function model.

The ToM model is seminal to the current understanding of language and communication disturbance in autism. It has been directly linked to the significant phenomenon of pragmatic communication disturbance in this syndrome. Moreover, preliminary data on the brain mechanisms that may be specific to ToM functions have also been presented. Several problems, however, arise with this model. Research suggests that ToM task deficits may not be as specific to autism as once thought (Peterson & Siegal, 1995; Yirmiya, Erel, Shaked, & Solomonica-Levi, 1998). It is also debatable whether the ToM model can explain the early forms of sociocommunicative disturbance displayed by children with autism (Leslie & Happé, 1989; Mundy & Sigman, 1989b; see also Chapter 5). Furthermore, it is not clear whether the ToM model can explain a class of phenomena referred to as *executive function deficits* in autism (Bishop, 1993; Pennington & Ozonoff, 1996). Alternatively, executive function deficits may contribute to an explanation of difficulties in ToM functions, as well as pragmatic communication disturbance, in people with autism (Hughes & Russell, 1993; Ozonoff, 1995; Pennington & Ozonoff, 1996; see also Chapter 5).

EXECUTIVE FUNCTIONS AND SOCIOCOMMUNICATIVE DISTURBANCE

A critical difference between the executive function model and the ToM model is that in the former the fundamental disturbance of autism is not considered to be specific to a neurologically dedicated system for social cognition. Rather, a more general cognitive disturbance in so-called executive functions is viewed as central to autism. Hypothetically, executive functions involve a system of frontal neurological processes that are behaviorally manifested in the related capacities to 1) initiate behaviors while inhibiting competing responses that may interfere with effective problem solving; 2) regulate attention to filter distractions during problem solving and shift attention across relevant stimulus components; and 3) upload and manipulate mental representations to bring them to bear in a task-effective fashion (Ozonoff, 1995; Pennington & Ozonoff, 1996). Central to executive function is the notion of appropriate action selection in the face of competing but context-inappropriate responses. Action selection is thought to be dependent on the integration of behavioral constraint and activation parameters that flow from memory, perception, and affective or motivation systems (Pennington & Ozonoff, 1996).

Studies indicate that people with autism display difficulties with appropriate action selection in the face of competing response potentials (Hughes & Russell, 1993; see Pennington & Ozonoff, 1996, for a review). Moreover, several researchers have argued that instead of a disturbance in a ToM module, autistic difficulties on false belief and related social-cognitive tasks may be explained in terms of this type of more general executive function difficulty (Frye, Zelazo, & Palfai, 1995; Hughes & Russell, 1993; Pennington & Ozonoff, 1996).

For example, recall that to solve the Sally-Anne false belief task, the child must *disregard his or her own knowledge* of where the object really is (Place 2), and *think about where Sally thinks* the object is. Notice that we have now italicized two operations in this task sequence, 1) the executive function of inhibiting a competing response and 2) metarepresentation. The executive function model suggests that children with autism have difficulty with the former and fail false belief and related social-cognitive tasks because of this difficulty. Similarly, they may be unable to correctly interpret the statement, "Iraqi Head Seeks Arms," because they cannot disregard the false, literal meaning in favor of the correct, nonliteral inference. A key diagnostic feature of autism that involves the singular pursuit of a limited, idiosyncratic set of interests may also be explained in terms of executive function disturbance (Hughes & Russell, 1993; Ozonoff, 1995).

One study has, in fact, suggested that the normal course of ToM development is associated with executive function development. Frye and colleagues (1995) demonstrated that in typical 3- to 5-year-olds, performance on a nonsocial sorting task that measured ability to select appropriate actions in the face of competing responses was significantly correlated with the development of ToM in the form of false belief task performance. In addition to being consistent with the executive function model, this observation is intriguing for another reason. A link exists between the type of executive function isolated in the work of Frye and colleagues (1995) and the neurological concomitants of ToM performance. Recall that ToM performance was linked to activity in left medial frontal circuits (Brodmann area 8; Fletcher et al., 1995). Fletcher and colleagues (1995) also noted that Petrides (1990) had connected activity in this subsystem to conditional associate learning. The primary task demand of this type of learning is the inhibition of competing responses to efficiently solve a problem. Indeed, the task used by Petrides (1990) was very similar to the task employed by Frye and colleagues (1995). Thus, the neurological linkage between frontal process and ToM performance observed by Fletcher and colleagues (1995) may overlap with frontal correlates of the types of processes that are central to the executive function model.

The executive function model poses a reasonable alternative to the ToM model of social-cognitive and sociocommunicative pathology in autism. This model, however, may have difficulty explaining the observation that children with autism manage nonsocial representational tasks better than analogous false belief tasks (Leslie, 1993). It may also have difficulty explaining why children with autism display even more basic social-cognitive difficulties, such as more difficulty using mental as opposed to physical state words (Baron-

Cohen et al., 1994; Tager-Flusberg, 1993). Furthermore, although executive function tasks may be correlated with ToM tasks, they do not explain all of the variability in the latter (Frye et al., 1995). Also, some people with autism spectrum disorder (ASD) may display executive function disturbance but not ToM disturbance (Ozonoff, 1995). These observations suggest that an executive function disturbance and a ToM impairment may have partially independent paths of effects on the poor sociocommunicative skills of autism. Thus, a combination of the executive function and ToM models provides a clearer picture of the sociocommunicative disturbance of autism. It is unlikely, though, that even a combination of these compelling models may provide a complete explanation of the earliest forms of sociocommunicative disturbance observed in autism.

SOCIAL ORIENTING AND SOCIOCOMMUNICATIVE DISTURBANCE IN AUTISM

Recall that preverbal children with autism display a deficit in joint attention skills but not in more instrumental sociocommunicative behaviors, such as those involved in nonverbal requesting. For example, children with autism will rarely use eye contact and gestures such as showing or pointing to share attention regarding an active wind-up toy. When the toy is moved out of reach, though, they are as likely to use eye contact and pointing to elicit aid obtaining the object as will comparison children (e.g., Mundy et al., 1994).

This seemingly simple observation may be fundamental to an understanding of autism. Joint attention behaviors reflect the tendency of children to socially orient while engaged in observing an object or event to share their experience of the object or event with others (Mundy, 1995). This capacity usually emerges between 6 and 12 months. Thus, observations of joint attention impairment in autism suggest that the pathological processes fundamental to this disorder may be manifestly active in the first year of life (Mundy & Sigman, 1989b). Consistent with this notion, first birthday videotape data suggest that 12-month-old children with autism display evidence of a disturbance in joint attention and social orienting (Osterling & Dawson, 1994). Measures of joint attention skills have also contributed to the very early identification of autism at 18 months in a sample of 16,000 children (Baron-Cohen et al., 1996).

Several other observations attest to the importance of joint attention deficits. These deficits are observed in young children regardless of IQ score and are related to parents' reports of symptom intensity (Mundy et al., 1994). Individual differences in joint attention skill development also appear to be singularly powerful in predicting language development among these children (Mundy et al., 1990; Sigman & Ruskin, 1997). Indeed, joint attention skill development is considered to be integral to language, social, and cognitive development among all children (Tomasello, 1995; see also Chapter 3), not just children with autism. For example, joint attention skills have been observed to predict language development from 6 months through the second year in typical samples (Morales, Mundy, & Rojas, 1998; Mundy & Gomes, 1998) and to predict individual differences in childhood IQ scores from 13 months in a high-risk sample (Ulvund & Smith, 1996).

Attempts have been made to explain joint attention disturbance in terms of dysfunction in ToM (Baron-Cohen, 1995; Leslie & Happé, 1989) or in cognitive executive functions (McEvoy, Rogers, & Pennington, 1993). With evidence of the emergence of this domain in the first year of life, however, it may be less than parsimonious to explain impairments in such an early-emerging facet of behavior solely in terms of later-developing, complex cognitive functions. Alternatively, several researchers have suggested that joint attention deficits may be understood as part of a fundamental social-approach, or social-orienting, impairment (Dawson & Lewy, 1989; Fotheringham, 1991; Hobson, 1993; Mundy, 1995). These models vary in the hypothesized mechanisms of impairment. Yet, they agree that a primary social-orienting impairment may have enormous ramifications for the subsequent development of social, cognitive, and even neurological disturbance in autism. To illustrate this point, consider the basic assumptions of one of these social-orienting models (Mundy, 1995; Mundy & Crowson, 1997; Mundy, Sigman, & Kasari, 1993).

Like the ToM and executive function models, it is assumed that the social communication pathology of autism, including joint attention disturbance, derives in part from neurological impairment that involves frontal cortical processes. Three studies, using electroencephalogram (EEG) (Mundy et al., 1999), positron emission tomography (Caplan et al., 1993), and behavioral measures (McEvoy et al., 1993), have directly linked joint attention development to frontal processes. In this model, though, it is also assumed that frontal systems may play different functional roles at different points in development. In particular, the types of functions proposed by the ToM model and executive function model are thought to require a degree of cognitive maturation and information acquisition that is not likely to be fully available in the first 12 months of life when joint attention skills are beginning to develop.

Alternatively, the terminology of the executive function model (Pennington & Ozonoff, 1996) may be used to suggest that early in life frontal action selection functions may be more dependent on behavioral constraint and activation parameters that flow from affective and motivational parameters than on cognitive memory parameters. That is, prior to the effects of more cognitive constraint parameters, frontally mediated action selection is constrained by a motivational executive system that serves to prioritize perceptual inputs that are most significant to the development of the infant (Derryberry & Reed, 1996; Mundy, 1995; Tucker, 1992). In particular, this system prioritizes social perceptual input and social information processing, via social orienting, from early on in the development of the child. One mechanism of this prioritization may involve the attribution of positive valence to the perception of social information, possibly by way of temporal/midbrain systems involving the amygdala (LeDoux, 1989), as well as brain stem nuclei (e.g., nucleus ambiguous) (Derryberry & Reed, 1996).

Several studies provide evidence for a basic social-orienting disturbance in autism. Klin (1991) reported that the typical preference for speech and speech-like sounds, which is usually displayed by infants in the first months of life, was not present in any of the children with autism that he observed. It was, however, present in all of the matched controls with developmental delays observed in the study.

In an intriguing study, Dawson, Meltzoff, and Osterling (1995) examined the degree to which children with autism, Down syndrome, or typical development oriented (displayed a head turn) toward social stimuli (hands clapping or a voice calling the child's name) and nonsocial stimuli (a musical jack-in-the-box being played or a rattle being shaken). The results indicated that the children with autism more often failed to orient to both types of stimuli. Their failure to orient to social stimuli, however, was significantly more extreme than their impaired orienting to nonsocial stimuli. Furthermore, individual differences in difficulty with social orienting but not object orienting were significantly related to a measure of joint attention among the children with autism. A disturbance in social orienting among children with autism has also been observed in first birthday videotape data (Osterling & Dawson, 1994). Finally, individual differences in social orienting have long-term stability and predict the degree to which children with autism process the nonverbal affective information presented by others (Dissanayake, Sigman, & Kasari, 1996). In addition to providing some support for a social-orienting impairment model, these observations may not easily be explained in terms of current ToM or executive function models (see Baron-Cohen, 1995, for an alternative view).

What might be the ramifications of an early social-orienting disturbance? Another assumption of the model is that experience drives a substantial portion of postnatal brain development. This occurs through the competitive enhancement of active neural connections and the culling of less-active connections (Huttenlocher, 1994). We also assume that, to some degree, the human neurobehavioral system is self-organizing. One component of this self-organizing system is the aforementioned prioritization of social information processing. In an experience-expectant fashion (Greenough, Black, & Wallace, 1987), this drives the early developing neuroarchitecture along paths that typically emphasize social-cognitive development (Cosmides, 1989). In the child with autism, however, the lack of this self-organizing feature leads to increasingly deviant development of neurobehavioral systems over time. Thus, autism may be characterized by primary neurobiological deficits, which lead to less than optimal behavioral proclivities in the first months of life (e.g., a lack of early social orienting), which, in turn, lead to secondary neurological disturbance via a negative feedback system. In this system the lack of social orienting and social information processing contributes to a dynamic alteration of the typical, experience-driven mechanisms of neural activation and culling. Hence, the lack of early social orienting and processing contributes to subsequent disruptions of neurobehavioral development (Mundy & Crowson, 1997). This notion has implications for early intervention that are considered later in this chapter.

In this model, joint attention skill measures are viewed as a sensitive index of social-orienting disturbance. Hence, one aspect of sociocommunicative pathology in autism (i.e., joint attention deficits) may be traced directly to this hypothesized social-orienting disturbance (Mundy, 1995). It is not clear, though, whether all subsequent executive function, social-cognitive, and sociocommunicative deficits flow directly from this early source. Nevertheless, some interesting hypotheses follow from this model.

Frontally mediated social-orienting processes may contribute to the observation that children with autism vary from aloof to active but odd in their social communication style. Dawson, Klinger, Panagiotides, Lewy, and Castelloe (1995) have reported that variability in frontal activity (EEG power) was related to these social style differences among people with autism. Another observation that the social-orienting disturbance in autism is most severe in the preschool years may be linked to the observation of a transient component of frontal metabolic activity disturbance, which improves between the ages of 6 and 7 in children with autism (Zilbovicius et al., 1995). Hence, there may be an early critical period for the process involved in social orienting impairment in autism. This possibility may be important in considering reports of positive early intervention effects with autism (Mundy & Crowson, 1997).

It is also likely that an early disturbance of social orienting could influence executive function and ToM development. With regard to the former, perhaps the frontal executive motivation system that prioritizes orienting to social stimuli *primes* the development of the more general executive capacity to engage action selection in the face of competing response potentials. Presumably, early in life, infants are frequently confronted with a choice between attending to competing social exteroceptive stimuli, nonsocial exteroceptive stimuli, and/or proprioceptive stimuli. It may be that the activation of an intrinsically motivated social-orienting system yields, as an important byproduct, early practice (hence neuro-organization) associated with selecting an action (social orienting) in the face of exteroceptive and proprioceptive stimuli that compete for attention. Without such practice contributing to adequate neural self-organization, the later-emerging, cognitive executive functions of the frontal system may not develop normally in children with autism (see Hughes & Russell, 1993, for an alternative hypothesis).

Similarly, it may be that a relative failure to process social information early on gives rise to a cognitive system that has insufficient information and experience to develop facility with ToM functions and social-cognition (Mundy et al., 1993; Mundy, 1995). Indeed, research with children with sensory impairments strongly suggests that sufficient social input is required for typical ToM development as measured on false belief tasks (Peterson & Siegal, 1995). Moreover, a disturbance of joint attention development, secondary to a social-orienting impairment, may deprive children with autism of early, critical social interactive experiences. Theoretically, the negative feedback of such a loss during a critical period of cognitive development may distort typical symbolic and social-cognitive development (Mundy et al., 1993; Werner & Kaplan, 1963) as well as contribute to the language delays that are symptomatic of this syndrome (Mundy et al., 1990; Sigman & Ruskin, 1997).

Finally, we have hypothesized that attenuated social orienting may be associated with a reciprocal augmentation of nonsocial information processing in autism. Such a reciprocal function may assist in explaining the relative success of people with autism in nonsocial problem-solving situations (Mundy, 1995). In this model, the development of social-information processing is separable from the development of object-oriented information processing. In many people these systems are balanced. In some people, however, these systems are *adaptively* imbalanced. For example, a bias toward visuospatial analysis and object-oriented information processing may often yield a cognitive style useful in engineering or the physical sciences. An extreme version of this type of imbalance, with insufficient social information processing proclivities, however, may lead to the style of maladaptive development seen in ASDs. This model may assist understanding why children with autism display strengths in some forms of cognition but not in social cognition (see Baron-Cohen & Hammer, 1997; Baron-Cohen, Wheelwright, Stott, Bolton, & Goodyear, 1997; Mundy, 1995).

IMPLICATIONS FOR CLINICAL PRACTICE, THEORY, AND RESEARCH

The foregoing discussion provides what may be a useful theoretical integration of viewpoints on early and later sociocommunicative disturbance in autism. What, though, of more practical matters? Are there implications of all of this theory for clinical practice with children with autism? To address this important issue we focus on the domain we know best, joint attention disturbance in autism.

Consider the research on early intervention with children with autism. Studies have begun to indicate that highly structured, intensive early intervention may lead to significant developmental gains for many children with autism (Birnbrauer & Leach, 1993; Bondy & Frost, 1995; Harris, Handleman, Gordon, Kristoff, & Fuentes, 1991; Koegel & Koegel, 1995; Laski, Charlop, &

Schreibman, 1988; Lovaas, 1987; Rogers, 1996; Sheinkopf & Siegel, 1998). Several researchers, though, have recognized that the assessments that have been used in this type of research, especially the outcome measures, may be less than optimal (Lovaas, 1987; Schopler, Short, & Mesibov, 1989). This is because outcome has primarily been assessed in terms of global measures of IQ or general measures of social or adaptive skills (e.g., Koegel & Frea, 1993; Lovaas, 1987). These types of measures are important and reflect a logical starting point in intervention research with autism. These measures alone, however, may lack precision and sensitivity in evaluating intervention effects because they do not incorporate recent empirical and theoretical insights on the nature of autism. To improve the precision and sensitivity of outcome assessment, it may be useful to integrate research on the nature of the sociocommunicative disturbance of autism with research on early intervention.

In particular, it seems likely that measures of joint attention and other nonverbal sociocommunicative skills may be especially important in the development and evaluation of early intervention methods for young children with autism. As suggested in portions of the foregoing review, these measures appear to tap into a cardinal component of the early social disturbance of autism. In particular, these measures have been directly related to neurological, cognitive, and affective processes that may play a role in autism. Mundy and Crowson (1997) have presented an extended discussion of the implications of joint attention skills research and social-orienting theory for early intervention with children with autism. Here, three examples of these implications are provided, including discussions of the recovery intervention hypothesis and of the pivotal skill intervention hypothesis as well as of a model of early intervention effects with children with autism.

The Recovery Intervention Hypothesis

Some researchers have claimed that early intervention may lead not only to developmental and intellectual gains but also to recovery from autism (Lovaas, 1987; McEachin, Smith, & Lovaas, 1993). To unequivocally test the "recovery hypothesis," however, it is necessary to evaluate interventions with measures that address the cardinal social and social-cognitive symptoms of the syndrome. The inference of recovery with regard to specific social skill deficits cannot be made from either general measures of social development or IQ in studies of children with autism. This is because research indicates that specific and critical social and cognitive deficits may remain among children with autism who have high IQ scores (e.g., Mundy et al., 1994; Ozonoff, 1995; Sigman, Yirmiya, & Capps, 1995). Furthermore, research suggests that children with autism may display significant gains in some social domains while continuing to have difficulty with other critical social skills (Volkmar, Cohen, Bregman, Hooks, & Stevenson, 1989). These observations suggest that it may be possible for some children with autism to respond to early intervention with important gains on general measures of IQ and social development yet also to exhibit important difficulties on specific social and cognitive skills.

To address this possibility, it is necessary to employ intervention outcome measures that are most sensitive to the specific social and cognitive processes that are central to the nature of autism. Measures of joint attention and social orienting certainly appear to fit this criterion, especially for the preschool period (Mundy & Crowson, 1997). In terms of the recovery hypothesis, then, the critical issue is not whether children in early intervention show more progress in joint attention development than do children with autism who have received less early intervention. Rather, the essential issue is whether children in early intervention achieve a level of facility with critical nonverbal social-communication skills, such as initiating joint attention, that is comparable to children without autism matched for mental age. It may be that evaluations of early interventions in the future will provide an affirmative answer to this question for at least some children with autism. If this can be demonstrated, then early intervention research stands to have an enormous effect on the basic research enterprise, as such a finding would likely lead to a serious reconsideration of the nature of autism.

The Pivotal Skill Hypothesis

Another example of the potential utility of research on nonverbal communication skills for early intervention efforts comes from a consideration of the pivotal skill hypothesis. According to this hypothesis, interventions that lead to change in one or two pivotal behaviors may then lead to important collateral changes in a broader range of atypical behaviors within the syndrome of autism (Koegel & Frea, 1993). In this regard, the literature on nonverbal sociocommunicative development suggests that the tendency to initiate joint attention bids may constitute an important target for early intervention efforts (Mundy et al., 1994).

Theory and research suggest that if one can affect joint attention development in children, then this change may be expected to contribute to the development of symbolic abilities (Hobson, 1993; Mundy et al., 1993; Werner & Kaplan, 1963), the development of language abilities (Baldwin, 1995; Bates, Benigni, Bretherton, Camaioni, & Volterra, 1979; Bruner, 1975; Tomasello, 1988), and the development of general social-cognitive processes (Baron-Cohen, 1995; Bruner, 1975; Mundy, 1995; Tomasello, 1995). Finally, theory in autism has suggested that joint attention deficits may be a marker of a disturbance of systems that serve to motivate infants and young children to attend to and engage their social world (Mundy, 1995). This may be important because it also has been suggested that motivation to communicate may be considered to be an important target for early intervention programs with children with autism (Koegel & Koegel, 1995). Hence, a cogent argument can be made for joint attention as a pivotal skill arena, and this argument may be based as much on theory and research from typical development as on research specific to autism.

At this point it is worth noting a potential modification or extension of the pivotal skill hypothesis. To the extent that pivotal skills truly exist, in some cases the development of these skills may not lead directly to change in other domains. Instead, pivotal skill development may mark a readiness for change in other domains. That is, pivotal skill development may be an important indicator of individual differences among children in early intervention programs for children with autism. The identification of what may be called pivotal individual difference markers may be critical to a better understanding of why a specific form of early intervention appears to work for some but not all children (Birnbrauer & Leach, 1993; Lovaas, 1987). The identification of such markers may also be useful in individualized intervention planning decisions, such as when to move a child from a relatively intensive but restrictive style of intervention to a less intensive but perhaps more inclusive intervention context.

To suggest that joint attention is a pivotal skill domain without commenting on the potential for early interventions to effect change in this arena is less than useful. Fortunately, several groups are developing intervention technologies that may be specific to the development of joint attention and other prelinguistic communication skills (Bondy & Frost, 1995; Yoder, Warren, Kim, & Gazdag, 1994). Moreover, at least one study has been undertaken with children with autism in which joint attention skills were a clear focus of intervention (Lewy & Dawson, 1992).

Lewy and Dawson (1992) presented 21 young children with ASD and comparison children with either unpredictable or predictable social stimulation. In the unpredictable condition, an experimenter played with toys in a fashion that did not match the toy play activities of the child. In the predictable social stimulation condition, the experimenter imitated or approximated the toy play behavior of the child. The primary social behavior assessed in this study was joint attention acts defined in terms of alternating looking between toys and the experimenter, pointing to toys while looking at the experimenter, or showing toys. The results indicated that all of the groups, including the group of children with autism, displayed more joint attention behavior in the predictable (imitated) social condition than in the unpredictable condition. It is important to note that even in the predictable condition, the children with autism displayed significantly less joint attention behavior than did the comparison children. Nevertheless, this study and the literature associated with this study begin to articulate one approach that may be especially useful in targeting joint attention development as a pivotal skill arena in early intervention (Dawson & Lewy, 1989).

A Model of Autism and Intervention Effects

In all attempts to evaluate intervention effects, it is useful to consider primary and secondary aspects of behavior disturbance in autism. To understand this notion, recall the central thesis of social-orienting theory. In the pathological development of children with autism, a disturbance of a system of neurological processes that promote social orienting leads to an attenuation of the application of a child's developing cognitive capacities to social problem solving (Mundy, 1995). To the extent that this sequence of assumptions is valid, any early intervention program that sufficiently and regularly provides an external organizational scaffold that promotes the application of the child's cognitive and self-regulatory capacities to a wide variety of social interaction tasks may be of tremendous benefit to children with autism in the preschool period. Because of the way the brain develops, however, there may be something of an early critical period for the provision of such an organizational scaffold.

Brain development, as noted previously, is an interactive process with information from the environment directly affecting the postnatal shaping of neural connections, especially in the first few years of life (Huttenlocher, 1994). As noted in the foregoing discussion of the social orienting model, a fundamental component of autism may involve a disturbance of the neurological systems that typically promote or enable early social information processing in children. Several potential mechanisms for such a disturbance have been proposed (Courchesne et al., 1994; Dawson & Lewy, 1989; Hobson, 1993; Mundy, 1995). Such a disturbance may lead to an attenuation of the amount of social information that is provided as input to the developing nervous system of the child with autism. This, in turn, may have a negative effect on subsequent neurobehavioral development (Kraemer, 1985), especially as it applies to the social development of the child. That is, an attenuation of social information processing may deprive the developing child with autism of the amount of social information, or social stimulation, that is needed for the normal shaping of neurological connections that are involved in the early process of social neurobehavioral development.

This environmental neurological shaping process may be necessary to yield a neural architecture that will support subsequent elaboration of social-behavioral development. Without adequate early social input, the neurological and behavioral development of the child with autism may be deflected further and further from the normal path, and the child may display secondary forms of behavior disturbance that are directly related to development in the context of a severe attenuation of social input (Kraemer, 1985; Mundy & Sigman, 1989a). Thus, we are suggesting a cybernetic model of autism in which an initial neurological disturbance in children with autism feeds back on itself to give rise to additional, and perhaps pernicious, components of the neurodevelopmental disturbance (see Mundy & Crowson, 1997, for figurative illustration).

Accordingly, children with autism may be affected by initial pathological processes (IPPs; see Bachevalier, 1994; Baron-Cohen, 1995; Courchesne et al., 1994; Dawson & Lewy, 1989; Hobson, 1993; and Mundy, 1995, for possible contributors to IPPs). A primary manifestation of IPPs is an attenuation of the typical capacity of the child to attend to and process social information. During the first 2 years of life, this manifestation of IPPs begins to give rise to a secondary neurological disturbance (SND). This SND is the result of the interaction between the effects of IPPs and ongoing central nervous system developmental processes that may not be directly affected by IPPs. That is, SND is the increasingly abnormal neurobehavioral architecture that develops in children with autism because IPPs have an ongoing negative effect on the input of social information to the child necessary for normal central nervous system development. Without early intervention, SND has an increasingly negative effect on the development of the child, so that by age 5, the impact of the IPPs plus unchecked SND on the child with autism yields a maximally deviant path of development. Alternatively, with early intensive intervention that provides compelling social input to the child, the effects of SND are mitigated and the path of development of the child with autism deviates to a lesser extent from the typical path of development.

If this model is correct, then a major beneficial component of intensive early intervention may be to lessen the impact of attenuated social input on the developing nervous system of the child with autism, that is, to decrease the effects of processes associated with SND. Intensive early intervention may provide the child with experiential building blocks that have a direct and positive effect on neurological development. Moreover, if there is an early transient neurological component to autism, early intervention may provide children with autism with an experiential and neurological foundation that maximizes the likelihood that they will make developmental gains as they catch up and move toward a more typical neurodevelopmental path after the preschool period. According to this model, the types of early intervention may, to some degree, be less important than is the early application of any one of a number of different high-quality, structured, and intensive programs. This is because all intensive intervention is delivered in the context of social interaction. As long as these interactions are not aversive, the child in intensive early intervention can be provided with a requisite amount of social input that offsets the secondary neurodevelopmental disturbance that may be associated with attenuated social interaction in the early years of life.

CONCLUSIONS

Researchers in psychopathology typically agree that models that identify a single cause for atypical behavior are likely to be incomplete (Cicchetti, 1993). This is not to say that single-factor models are not valuable. The value of single-factor models, however, may only truly be realized when they are synthesized to yield a more divergent, rather than convergent, perspective on the processes involved in the ontogeny of pathology. This is clearly the case with respect to the state of research on autism. It is abundantly clear that higher-order cognitive dysfunctions play a critical role in autism (Minshew, 1996). In particular, at this time both an executive function disturbance and a form of higher-order representational impairment appear to be linked to the social-pragmatic disturbance of communication that is characteristic of the older child with autism (Leslie, 1993; Ozonoff, 1995). Furthermore, these impairments may be linked to functions of the frontal systems (Baron-Cohen et al., 1994; Fletcher et al., 1995). A complete understanding of the nature of this linkage, however, may not be clear unless the earliest manifest forms of sociocommunicative disturbance in autism are considered. These joint attention and social-orienting difficulties may also be related to an impairment involving frontal systems. It is unlikely, though, that these ontogenetically primary impairments may be explained simply by way of recourse to the constructs used to explain later-emerging cognitive deficits in autism. Instead, these early-emerging deficits challenge researchers to adopt a more developmental and dynamic systems approach to understanding the nature of autism. Such a perspective is a reminder that the behavioral function of a neurological subsystem may change during development. Moreover, a sufficiently powerful disturbance of early behavior may itself lead to subsequent disturbance in neurological and neurobehavioral development. Thus, a consideration of the dynamic interplay between initial biological insult and subsequent transactions with the environment may be crucial to an understanding of autism. It may also be that understanding of autism will play a critical role in acquiring a better understanding of the complex interaction that occurs between neural development and environmental constraint in the ontogeny of the quintessential human capacity for social communication and cognition.

REFERENCES

American Psychiatric Association. (1980). *Diagnostic and Statistical Manual on Mental Disorders* (3rd ed.). Washington, DC: Author.

Bachevalier, J. (1994). Medial temporal lobe structures and autism: A review of clinical and experimental findings. *Neuropsychologia, 32,* 627–648.

Bailey, A., Philips, W., & Rutter, M. (1996). Autism: Towards an integration of clinical, genetic, neuropsychological, and neurobiological perspectives. *Journal of Child Psychology and Psychiatry and Allied Disciplines, 37,* 89–126.

Baldwin, D. (1995). Understanding the link between joint attention and language. In C. Moore & C. Dunham (Eds.), *Joint attention: Its origins and role in development* (pp. 189–205). Mahwah, NJ: Lawrence Erlbaum Associates.

Baron-Cohen, S. (1995). *Mindblindness.* Cambridge, MA: MIT Press.

Baron-Cohen, S., Cox, A., Baird, G., Swettenham, J., Nightingale, N., Morgan, K.,

Drew, A., & Charman, T. (1996). Psychological markers in the detection of autism in infancy in a large population. *British Journal of Psychiatry, 168,* 158–163.
Baron-Cohen, S., & Hammer, J. (1997). Is autism an extreme form of the "male brain"? *Advances in Infancy Research, 11,* 193–217.
Baron-Cohen, S., Ring, H., Moriarty, J., Schmitz, B., Costa, D., & Ell, P. (1994). Recognition of mental state terms: Clinical findings in children with autism and a functional neuroimaging study of normal adults. *British Journal of Psychiatry, 165,* 640–649.
Baron-Cohen, S., Wheelwright, S., Stott, C., Bolton, P., & Goodyear, I. (1997). Is there a link between engineering and autism? *Autism, 1,* 101–109.
Bates, E., Benigni, L., Bretherton, I., Camaioni, L., & Volterra, V. (1979). *The emergence of symbols: Cognition and communication in infancy.* San Diego: Academic Press.
Birnbrauer, J., & Leach, D. (1993). The Murdoch Early Intervention Program after 2 years. *Behaviour Change, 10,* 63–74.
Bishop, D. (1993). Autism, executive functions and theory of mind: A neuropsychological perspective [Annotation]. *Journal of Child Psychology and Psychiatry and Allied Disciplines, 34,* 279–293.
Bondy, A., & Frost, L. (1995). Educational approaches in preschool. Behavior techniques in a public school setting. In E. Schopler & G. Mesibov (Eds.), *Learning and cognition in autism* (pp. 311–334). New York: Plenum Press.
Bruner, J. (1975). From communication to language: A psychological perspective. *Cognition, 3,* 255–287.
Bryson, S. (1996). Brief report: Epidemiology of autism. *Journal of Autism and Developmental Disorders, 26,* 165–168.
Caplan, R., Chugani, H., Messa, C., Guthrie, D., Sigman, M., Traversay, J., & Mundy, P. (1993). Hemispherectomy for early onset intractable seizures: Presurgical cerebral glucose metabolism and postsurgical nonverbal communication patterns. *Developmental Medicine and Child Neurology, 35,* 582–592.
Cicchetti, D. (1993). Developmental psychopathology: Reactions, reflections, projections. *Developmental Review, 13,* 471–502.
Cosmides, L. (1989). The logic of social exchange: Has natural selection shaped how humans reason?: Studies with the Wason selection task. *Cognition, 31,* 187–276.
Courchesne, E., Chisum, H., & Townsend, J. (1994). Neural activity-dependent brain changes in development: Implications for psychopathology. *Development and Psychopathology, 6,* 697–722.
Curcio, F. (1978). Sensorimotor functioning and communication in mute autistic children. *Journal of Autism and Childhood Schizophrenia, 8,* 281–292.
Damasio, A., & Maurer, R. (1978). A neurological model of childhood autism. *Archives of Neurology, 35,* 777–786.
Dawson, G. (1996). Brief report. Neuropsychology of autism: A report of the state of the science. *Journal of Autism and Developmental Disorders, 26,* 179–184.
Dawson, G., & Lewy, A. (1989). Arousal, attention, and the social-emotional impairments of individuals with autism. In G. Dawson (Ed.), *Autism: Nature, diagnosis, and treatment* (pp. 49–74). New York: Guilford Press.
Dawson, G., Klinger, L., Panagiotides, H., Lewy, A., & Castelloe, P. (1995). Subgroups of autistic children based on social behavior display distinct patterns of brain activity. *Journal of Abnormal Child Psychology, 23,* 569–583.
Dawson, G., Meltzoff, A., & Osterling, J. (1995, March). *Children with autism fail to orient to naturally occurring social stimuli.* Paper presented at the meeting of the Society for Research in Child Development, Indianapolis.

Derryberry, D., & Reed, M. (1996). Regulatory processes and the development of cognitive representations. *Development and Psychopathology, 8,* 215–234.

Dissanayake, C., Sigman, M., & Kasari, C. (1996). Long-term stability of individual differences in the emotional responsiveness of children with autism. *Journal of Child Psychology and Psychiatry and Allied Disciplines, 36,* 1–8.

Eales, M. (1993). Pragmatic impairments in adults with childhood diagnoses of autism or developmental receptive language disorder. *Journal of Autism and Developmental Disorders, 23,* 593–617.

Fletcher, P., Happé, F., Frith, U., Baker, S., Sloan, R., Frackowiak, R., & Frith, C. (1995). Other minds in the brain: A functional imaging study of "theory of mind" in story comprehension. *Cognition, 57,* 109–128.

Fotheringham, J. (1991). Autism: Its primary psychological and neurological deficit. *Canadian Journal of Psychiatry, 36,* 686–692.

Frith, U. (1989). A new look at language and communication in autism. *British Journal of Disorders of Communication, 24,* 123–150.

Frye, D., Zelazo, P., & Palfai, T. (1995). Theory of mind and rule based reasoning. *Cognitive Development, 10,* 483–527.

Greenough, W., Black, J., & Wallace, C. (1987). Experience and brain development. *Child Development, 58,* 539–559.

Happé, F.G.E. (1993). Communicative competence and theory of mind in autism: A test of relevance theory. *Cognition, 48,* 101–119.

Harris, S., Handleman, J., Gordon, R., Kristoff, B., & Fuentes, F. (1991). Changes in cognitive and language functioning of preschool children with autism. *Journal of Autism and Developmental Disorders, 21,* 281–290.

Hobson, R.P. (1993). *Autism and the development of mind.* Mahwah, NJ: Lawrence Erlbaum Associates.

Hughes, C., & Russell, J. (1993). Autistic children's difficulty with mental disengagement from an object: Its implications for theories of autism. *Developmental Psychology, 29,* 498–510.

Huttenlocher, P. (1994). Synaptogenesis in the human cerebral cortex. In G. Dawson & K. Fischer (Eds.), *Human behavior and brain development* (pp. 137–152). New York: Guilford Press.

Kanner, L. (1943). Autistic disturbances of affective contact. *Nervous Child, 2,* 217–250.

Klin, A. (1991). Young autistic children's listening preferences in regard to speech: A possible characterization of the symptom of social withdrawal. *Journal of Autism and Developmental Disorders, 21,* 29–42.

Koegel, L., & Koegel, R. (1995). Motivating communication in children with autism. In E. Schopler & G. Mesibov (Eds.), *Learning and cognition in autism* (pp. 73–87). New York: Plenum Press.

Koegel, R., & Frea, W. (1993). Treatment of social behavior in autism through the modification of pivotal social skills. *Journal of Applied Behavior Analysis, 26,* 369–377.

Kraemer, G. (1985). Effects of differences in early social experience on primate neurobiological-behavioral development. In M. Reite & T. Fields (Eds.), *The psychobiology of attachment and separation* (pp. 135–161). San Diego: Academic Press.

Laski, K., Charlop, M., & Schreibman, L. (1988). Training parents to use the natural language paradigm to increase their autistic children's speech. *Journal of Applied Behavior Analysis, 21,* 391–400.

LeDoux, J. (1989). Cognitive-emotional interactions in the brain. *Cognition and Emotion, 3,* 267–289.

Leekam, S., & Perner, J. (1991). Does the autistic child have a metarepresentational deficit? *Cognition, 40,* 203–218.

Leslie, A. (1987). Pretense and representation: The origins of "theory of mind." *Psychological Review, 94,* 412–426.

Leslie, A. (1993). What autism teaches us about metarepresentation. In S. Baron-Cohen, H. Tager-Flusberg, & D. Cohen (Eds.), *Understanding other minds: Perspectives from autism* (pp. 83–111). New York: Oxford University Press.

Leslie, A., & Happé, F.G.E. (1989). Autism and ostensive communication: The relevance of metarepresentation. *Development and Psychopathology, 1,* 205–212.

Leslie, A., & Thaiss, L. (1992). Domain specificity in conceptual development: Neuropsychological evidence from autism. *Cognition, 43,* 225–251.

Lewy, A., & Dawson, G. (1992). Social stimulation and joint attention in young autistic children. *Journal of Abnormal Child Psychology, 20,* 555–566.

Lovaas, O.I. (1987). Behavioral treatment and normal educational and intellectual functioning in young autistic children. *Journal of Consulting and Clinical Psychology, 55,* 3–9.

Loveland, K.A., & Landry, S.H. (1986). Joint attention and language in autism and developmental language delay. *Journal of Autism and Developmental Disorders, 16,* 335–349.

McEachin, J.J., Smith, T., & Lovaas, O.I. (1993). Long term outcome for children with autism who received early intensive behavioral treatment. *American Journal on Mental Retardation, 97,* 359–372.

McEvoy, R., Rogers, S., & Pennington, R. (1993). Executive function and social communication deficits in young autistic children. *Journal of Child Psychology and Psychiatry and Allied Disciplines, 34,* 563–578.

Minshew, N. (1996). Brief report: Brain mechanisms in autism: Functional and structural abnormalities. *Journal of Autism and Developmental Disorders, 26,* 205–209.

Morales, M., Mundy, P., & Rojas, J. (1998). Gaze following and language development in six- month-olds. *Infant Behavior and Development, 21,* 349–372.

Mundy, P. (1995). Joint attention, social-emotional approach in children with autism. *Development and Psychopathology, 7,* 63–82.

Mundy, P., Card, J., & Fox, N. (1999). *The development of joint attention and cortical activity in the second year.* Manuscript submitted for publication.

Mundy, P., & Crowson, M. (1997). Joint attention and early communication: Implications for intervention with autism. *Journal of Autism and Developmental Disorders.*

Mundy, P., & Gomes, A. (1998). Individual differences in joint attention skill development in the second year. *Infant Behavior and Development, 21,* 469–482.

Mundy, P., & Markus, J. (1997). On the nature of communication and language impairment in autism. *Mental Retardation and Developmental Disabilities Research Reviews, 3,* 343–349.

Mundy, P., & Sigman, M. (1989a). Specifying the nature of the social impairment in autism. In G. Dawson (Ed.), *Autism: Nature, diagnosis, and treatment* (pp. 3–21). New York: Guilford Press.

Mundy, P., & Sigman, M. (1989b). The theoretical implications of joint attention deficits in autism. *Development and Psychopathology, 1,* 173–183.

Mundy, P., Sigman, M., & Kasari, C. (1990). A longitudinal study of joint attention and language development in autistic children. *Journal of Autism and Developmental Disorders, 20,* 115–128.

Mundy, P., Sigman, M., & Kasari, C. (1993). The theory of mind and joint attention deficits in autism. In S. Baron-Cohen, H. Tager-Flusberg, & D. Cohen (Eds.), *Understanding other minds: Perspectives from autism* (pp. 181–203). Oxford, England: Oxford University Press.

Mundy, P., Sigman, M., & Kasari, C. (1994). Joint attention, developmental level, and symptom presentation in young children with autism. *Development and Psychopathology, 6,* 389–401.

Mundy, P., Sigman, M., Ungerer, J., & Sherman, T. (1986). Defining the social deficits of autism: The contribution of nonverbal communication measures. *Journal of Child Psychology and Psychiatry and Allied Disciplines, 27,* 657–669.

Osterling, J., & Dawson, G. (1994). Early recognition of children with autism: A study of first birthday home videotapes. *Journal of Autism and Developmental Disorders, 24,* 247–257.

Ozonoff, S. (1995). Executive functions in autism. In E. Schopler & G. Mesibov (Eds.), *Learning and cognition in autism* (pp. 199–220). New York: Plenum Press.

Pennington, B., & Ozonoff, S. (1996). Executive functions and developmental psychopathology. *Journal of Child Psychology and Psychiatry and Allied Disciplines, 37,* 51–87.

Peterson, C., & Siegal, M. (1995). Deafness, conversation and theory of mind. *Journal of Child Psychology and Psychiatry and Allied Disciplines, 36,* 459–474.

Petrides, M. (1990). Non-spatial conditional learning impaired in patients with unilateral frontal but not temporal lobe excisions. *Neuropsychologia, 28,* 137–149.

Pinker, S. (1994). *The language instinct: How the mind creates language.* New York: HarperCollins.

Rogers, S. (1996). Brief report: Early intervention in autism. *Journal of Autism and Developmental Disorders, 26,* 243–246.

Schopler, E., Short, A., & Mesibov, G. (1989). Relation of behavioral treatment to "normal functioning": Comment on Lovaas. *Journal of Consulting and Clinical Psychology, 57,* 162–164.

Scott, F., & Baron-Cohen, S. (1996). Logical, analogical, and psychological reasoning in autism: A test of the Cosmides theory. *Development and Psychopathology, 8,* 235–245.

Sheinkopf, S., & Siegel, B. (1998). Home-based behavioral treatment of young children with autism. *Journal of Autism and Developmental Disorders, 28,* 15–23.

Sigman, M., & Mundy, P. (1989). Social attachments in autistic children. *Journal of the American Academy of Child and Adolescent Psychiatry, 28,* 74–81.

Sigman, M., & Ruskin, E. (1997). *Joint attention in relation to language acquisition and social skills in children with autism.* Paper presented at the meeting of the Society for Research in Child Development, Washington, DC.

Sigman, M., Yirmiya, N., & Capps, L. (1995). Social and cognitive understanding in high-functioning children with autism. In E. Schopler & G. Mesibov (Eds.), *Learning and cognition in autism* (pp. 159–176). New York: Plenum Press.

Surian, L., Baron-Cohen, S., & Van der Lely, H. (1996). Are children with autism deaf to Gricean maxims? *Cognitive Neuropsychiatry, 1,* 55–71.

Tager-Flusberg, H. (1993). What language reveals about the understanding of minds in children with autism. In S. Baron-Cohen, H. Tager-Flusberg, & D. Cohen (Eds.), *Understanding other minds: Perspectives from autism* (pp. 138–157). New York: Oxford University Press.

Tomasello, M. (1988). The role of joint attentional processes in early language development. *Language Sciences, 11,* 69–88.

Tomasello, M. (1995). Joint attention as social cognition. In C. Moore & P. Dunham (Eds.), *Joint attention: Its origins and role in development* (pp. 103–130). Mahwah, NJ: Lawrence Erlbaum Associates.

Tucker, D. (1992). Developing emotions and cortical networks. In M. Gunnar & C. Nelson (Eds.), *Minnesota Symposium on Child Psychology: Vol. 24. Developmental behavioral neuroscience* (pp. 75–128). Mahwah, NJ: Lawrence Erlbaum Associates.

Ulvund, S., & Smith, L. (1996). The predictive validity of nonverbal communication skills in infants with perinatal hazards. *Infant Behavior and Development, 19,* 441–449.

Volden, J., & Lord, C. (1991). Neologisms and idiosyncratic language in autistic speakers. *Journal of Autism and Developmental Disorders, 28,* 109–130.

Volkmar, F., Cohen, D., Bregman, J., Hooks, M., & Stevenson, J. (1989). An examination of social typologies in autism. *Journal of the American Academy of Child and Adolescent Psychiatry, 28,* 82–86.

Werner, H., & Kaplan, B. (1963). *Symbol formation: An organismic developmental approach to language and the expression of thought.* New York: John Wiley & Sons.

Wetherby, A., Prizant, B., & Hutchinson, T. (1998). Communicative, social-affective, and symbolic profiles of young children with autism and pervasive developmental disorder. *American Journal of Speech-Language Pathology, 7,* 79–91.

Whiten, A., & Byrne, R. (1988). The Machiavellian intelligence hypothesis. In A. Whiten & R. Byrne (Eds.), *Machiavellian intelligence: Social expertise and the evolution of intellect in monkeys, apes, and humans* (pp. 118–137). New York: Oxford University Press.

Yirmiya, N., Erel, O., Shaked, M., & Solomonica-Levi, D. (1998). Meta-analysis comparing theory of mind abilities of individual with autism, individuals with mental retardation, and normally developing individuals. *Psychological Bulletin, 124,* 283–307.

Yoder, P., Warren, S., Kim, K., & Gazdag, G. (1994). Facilitating prelinguistic communication in very young children with developmental disabilities II: Systematic replication and extension. *Journal of Speech and Hearing Research, 37,* 841–851.

Zilbovicius, M., Garreau, B., Samson, Y., Remy, P., Barthélémy, C., Syrota, A., & Lelord, G. (1995). Delayed maturation of the frontal cortex in childhood autism. *American Journal of Psychiatry, 152,* 248–252.

5

Intersubjectivity in Autism

The Roles of Imitation and Executive Function

Sally J. Rogers and Loisa Bennetto

The language and communication problems inherent in autism were among the first symptoms recognized as associated with the disorder (Kanner, 1943) and have figured preeminently in all theories of autism and conceptualizations about the nature of the disorder. For many years, autism was conceptualized by a variety of theorists primarily as a communication/language disorder (Churchill, 1978). An important paper in 1986 by Fein, Pennington, Markowitz, Braverman, and Waterhouse, however, challenged the field to reconsider the profound social deficits involved in autism and the possibility that social impairments could be primary. This paper was published at a time when the pragmatics orientation to language development also was emphasizing the origins of communication in social exchanges and relationships (Bruner, 1975). This emphasis on the functionalism of language and its embeddedness in social interaction contributed to a new wave of theorizing in autism.

The first strong theory to emerge from this reorientation focused on children's growing understanding of other minds. The experimental and theoretical work on theory of mind (ToM) in autism, as represented by the work of Baron-Cohen, Leslie, and Frith (1985), grew from the normative developmental research on social cognition occurring in the laboratories of Flavell, Botkin, Fry, Wright, and Jarvis (1968) and Perner, Leekam, and Wimmer (1987), among others. The rapid development of ideas and experimental paradigms resulting from this work provided the field with a rich example of the depth and breadth of knowledge that a developmental psychopathology approach could

This chapter was supported in part by the following: National Institute of Child Health and Human Development Grant No. PO1 HD35468-01, Bureau of Maternal and Child Health Grant No. MCJ08941301, and National Institute of Mental Health Grant No. RO3MH55366. Our thanks to the Developmental Psychobiology Research Group at the University of Colorado Health Sciences Center for their ongoing support of our work.

stimulate, with studies of typical and atypical development building from each other (Cicchetti, 1990). A burst of well-designed studies resulting in consistent and well-replicated findings concerning ToM deficits in autism put the spotlight on social cognition as a potential primary deficit in autism (Baron-Cohen, 1991; Perner, Frith, Leslie, & Leekam, 1989). In addition to the ToM work, language studies of autism were narrowing in on pragmatics as the area of major deficit in the communication/language domain (Tager-Flusberg, 1993). A strength of the ToM model was its ability to account for the pragmatics deficit in autism. The communication/language deficit in autism came to be seen as secondary, resulting from a more primary impairment in social cognition (Baron-Cohen, 1988). Although the ToM approach fits well with the symptoms seen in older children and adults with autism, it has trouble accounting for the very early symptoms of this disorder. A cognitive skill that typically develops in the fourth or fifth year of life lacks explanatory power for symptoms present in the first 12 months of life in children with autism (Osterling & Dawson, 1994).

In 1991 Rogers and Pennington proposed a developmental model for autism that could account for the earliest symptoms of this disorder. The paper highlighted several developmental domains that appeared to differentiate people with autism reliably from other clinical groups: imitation, emotional perception and responses, joint attention and communication, ToM, and executive function (EF). The authors then constructed a developmental model, heavily influenced by Stern's (1985) work, *The Interpersonal World of the Human Infant,* that could account for the full symptom picture in autism at various points in development. The authors suggested a developmental cascade in which impairments in imitation, emotional functioning, and EF could prevent the development of intersubjectivity as seen early on in joint attention and later in ToM, resulting in the social-cognitive, communicative, and repetitive characteristics that mark autism.

Several aspects of the model were original at the time compared with other theories about autism. The first original feature was a model for the mechanism by which an imitation deficit might significantly affect interpersonal development. The paper's second unique contribution involved a crucial role for EFs mediated by the prefrontal cortex in development of secondary intersubjectivity, particularly involving joint attention, symbolic play, and early language. The third main component of Rogers and Pennington's (1991) theory, although not unique to their work (Hobson, 1993), involved a possible primary impairment in the affective system as it relates to social life. Rogers and Pennington suggested a developmental cascade that could result in the deficits in joint attention, social referencing, communication, symbolic play, and repetitive restricted behaviors that define autism. A very important aspect of the Rogers and Pennington model, and one that set it apart from all others at that time, was its ability to account for the deficits in all three main symptom areas: social relatedness; communication; and restricted, repetitive behaviors. Another unique feature of the model was the suggestion that autism involved multiple primary deficits. Although this idea had been suggested prior to the 1991 paper (Goodman, 1989), no other theory had suggested what the multiple deficits might be and how they might interact in such a way that autism would be the outcome.

In this chapter, two aspects of the Rogers and Pennington model—imitation and EF—are revisited in light of the empirical work that has occurred since the early 1990s. We first discuss findings in those areas, then consider what implications those findings have for the original Rogers and Pennington model regarding the development of sociocommunicative aspects of autism. We end by considering the implications for both clinical intervention and future research.

IMITATION

In Rogers and Pennington's (1991) paper, the possibility of a core deficit in the capacity to imitate motor movements was suggested from the review of imitation studies that had been completed in autism at that time. Eight studies were identified that involved comparison of people who had autism with matched clinical control groups. Of these studies, seven of the eight reported autism-specific deficits in imitation skills. The one paper that reported no differences was found to have significant methodological flaws involving ceiling effects for the comparison groups. Because ceiling effects artificially restrict the variability of scores, the null conclusion of this study is open to question. Given the uniformity of the findings of the seven methodologically sound studies, Rogers and Pennington hypothesized that an impairment in the ability to imitate another person's movements was a core part of the neuropsychological profile of autism.

FINDINGS INVOLVING IMITATION IN AUTISM

Since 1991, two other groups have provided very similar conceptual accounts of the potential role of an imitation deficit in the intersubjective impairments involved in autism (Hobson, 1993; Meltzoff & Gopnik, 1993). Empirical support is also growing in the developmental literature regarding the effects of differences in early imitation skills on later parent–child relationships. Heimann (1989) reported that individual differences in the capacity of neonates to imitate several movements were correlated with mother–child interaction variables a few months later.

The 1991 paper stimulated new interest in the question of imitation in autism, and a handful of carefully done studies has been published since that time. Charman and colleagues have published two papers on imitation. Their first paper (Charman & Baron-Cohen, 1994), which reported no group differences, used infant level tasks of motor and vocal behavior with 7- to 15-year-old individuals who were verbal. Ceiling effects were present and may have masked group differences. Their second paper (Charman et al., 1997) involved a study of the youngest children with autism yet to appear in the literature. Ten 20-month-old high-functioning children with autism and matched groups of typical children and children with developmental delays participated. The tasks and method involved a rigorous paradigm first developed by Meltzoff (1988) consisting of a simple action on each of four novel objects. These toddlers with autism demonstrated significantly less imitation than did the comparison groups, even with age, nonverbal mental age (MA), and language skills co-varied. These authors proposed that imitation of very simple movements is most impaired early in the disorder and improves across childhood, as suggested by Rogers and Pennington in 1991.

Dawson, Meltzoff, Osterling, and Rinaldi (1999) examined both immediate and deferred imitation as part of a larger study of neuropsychological functioning in early autism. They examined 20 children with autism compared with matched groups of typical youngsters and those with developmental delays. The tasks included familiar and novel movements—actions on objects, hand imitations, and face imitations—developed by Meltzoff (1988) for studies of immediate and deferred toddler imitation. Children with autism demonstrated significantly less imitation on both immediate and deferred (10 minutes) tasks than did children in comparison groups, who did not differ from one another. Furthermore, immediate imitation scores were significantly related to performance on two neuropsychological measures: delayed nonmatch-to-sample (a task involving temporal and prefrontal areas) and delayed response (a prefrontal task).

Smith and Bryson (1998) reported a very carefully controlled study of 20 high-functioning older children with autism and matched clinical and typical groups. Tasks involved nonsymbolic hand postures, presented both singly and sequentially. Length of sequences was systematically varied, and control tests for recognition memory and manual dexterity were used. Findings demonstrated a significant impairment in the imitation of single hand postures in the group with autism, relative to both comparison groups, which did not differ. Even with manual dexterity differences co-varied out of the analyses, the group with autism continued to demonstrate imitation impairments. Unexpectedly, the group with autism did not demonstrate deficits on the sequential tasks. The authors discussed the possibility of a praxic deficit underlying the imitation problems in autism.

Loveland and colleagues (1994) reported a study of imitation of facial expressions in a group of 18 people with autism across a wide age range and a matched group with Down syndrome. All people were verbal with language levels of at least 36 months. They were presented with a model demonstrating five different emotional expressions (happy, angry, sad, surprised, and neutral) and instructed to imitate the model. Although subjects with autism did produce *recognizable* imitations with as much success as the comparison group, they produced a greater number of atypical imitations than the comparison group, with significantly more unusual and more mechanical expressions. The group with autism, however, had even more difficulty with producing correct facial expressions to verbal command than they did with imitation (another test of praxis). The authors suggested that motor planning and execution problems may be involved in the imitation problems of people with autism and that with development, the imitation deficit in autism may involve poor-quality rather than absent imitation.

Stone has continued her line of research regarding imitation deficits in autism with three studies, two involving parent report and one involving laboratory measures. In both parent report studies, parents of children with autism reported observing less imitative behavior from their children at home than did parents of children with mental retardation (Stone & Hogan, 1993; Stone & Lemanek, 1991), a finding also reported by Knott, Lewis, and Williams (1995) in their observational study of home interactions of children who had autism compared with children who had Down syndrome. Stone, Ousley, and Littleford (1997) reported two studies of imitation of body movements and actions on objects in young children with autism compared with matched groups of typical youngsters and those with delays. In the first study, children with autism demonstrated weaker imitation skills than controls. Results from the second study suggested that for all groups, imitation of body movements and actions on objects may represent independent dimensions that relate respectively to expressive language or play skills. Stone and her colleagues also found evidence of age-related improvements in the motor imitation skills of young children with autism.

The final study to be reviewed in this chapter involved high-functioning adolescents with autism on a set of tasks that examined single and sequential manual and face imitation as well as pantomime (Rogers, Bennetto, McEvoy, & Pennington, 1996). The study was designed to test two alternative hypotheses about the nature of the imitation deficit in autism: a symbolic hypothesis suggested by Baron-Cohen (1988) and an EF hypothesis suggested by Rogers and Pennington (1991). Autism-specific imitation impairments were demonstrated for single and sequential hand tasks and sequential face tasks. The subjects with autism performed *better* on meaningful, or symbolic, tasks than on nonmeaningful tasks, in contrast to Baron-Cohen's hypothesis. Performance on hand and face tasks was significantly correlated for the group with autism. Pantomime, with its close relationship to symbolic play and deferred imitation, was also examined, and subjects with autism performed significantly more poorly than controls on both single and sequential pantomime. Significant correlations between hand imitations and pantomime were found for the group with autism. Rogers and colleagues (1996) suggested that autism-related impairments in both imitation and pantomime (and, by implication, symbolic play deficits) may be due to an underlying dyspraxia in autism.

Praxis refers to the planning, execution, and sequencing of movements (Ayres, 1985); motor imitation and pantomime are considered classic tests of praxis. Praxis also appears to have direct brain–behavior relationships. Patients with left hemisphere lesions and lesions of the prefrontal cortex typically demonstrate significant impairments (apraxia) on tasks (Kimura & Archibald, 1974) like the ones administered in the Rogers and colleagues (1996) study. In fact, both the imitation and the pantomime tasks were taken from apraxia studies of adults with acquired brain injury. In apraxia, the deficits in planning, executing, and sequencing movements cannot be accounted for by other motor impairments.

To conclude, a number of studies of imitation in autism have been published since 1991, with marked improvements in conceptualization and methodology. The vast majority of these studies report autism-specific impairments in imitation skills. In the toddler studies, the frequency of production of imitations is decreased. In studies involving older children and adults with autism, the accuracy of the movements is impaired. In addition, several of the authors specifically targeted problems with motor execution, or dyspraxia, as a potential mechanism underlying the imitation deficit in autism. The possibility of specific motor involvement is of particular concern to sociocommunicative development. Social and communicative behaviors are largely motor behaviors, and thus generalized motor impairments have the potential of disrupting communication. At first glance, reports of motor coordination problems seem contrary to general beliefs about autism, which often include motor strengths in children. For many years, however, researchers have published papers describing difficulties with postural control, motor dyscoordination, and dyspraxia (Colbert, Koegler, & Markham, 1958; Damasio & Maurer, 1978; Ornitz, 1973; Wing, 1981). Papers examining other aspects of movement in people with autism have added further support to this idea.

FINDINGS INVOLVING MOTOR IMPAIRMENTS IN AUTISM

Kohen-Raz, Volkmar, and Cohen (1992) reported a pilot study involving 91 children with autism examined on a computerized measure of postural control. The group with autism was compared with three other groups: typically developing younger children, children with cognitive impairments, and adults with vestibular impairments. Although the groups were not matched and there were other methodological constraints, the group with autism showed striking differences on tasks involving standing balance on unstable surfaces. Children with autism showed poorer performance on simpler postures than on more difficult postures. The authors suggested that the children with autism were using primitive, somatosensory postural control systems (particularly implicating the cerebellum) rather than higher-level visually mediated vestibular control systems. Furthermore, the children demonstrated little improvement with age, and the severity of their postural deficits was associated with the severity of their autism.

Minshew, Goldstein, and Siegel (1997) examined motor performance in a neuropsychological study of 33 very high-functioning adolescents and adults with autism compared with typical controls in a matched pair design that included four different motor tests. Results demonstrated that a significant feature of the neuropsychological profile in autism involved an impairment in skilled motor abilities as demonstrated by difficulties with the grooved pegboard and the Trails A test, a replication of earlier findings by Rumsey and Hamburger (1988). Although Cornish and McManus (1996) used a similar measure and reported no autism-specific deficit, subject groups were not matched and the study was not as well controlled as in Minshew and colleagues (1997) and Rumsey and Hamburger (1988).

Smith and Bryson (1998) also administered a task of manual dexterity, grooved pegboard, to language-matched groups of children with autism and children with language impairments. Although their groups did not differ in handedness, the group with autism performed significantly more slowly than did the controls on this task. Furthermore, performance on the dexterity task accounted for a significant amount of the variability on the manual imitation performances of the subjects. These findings represent the first clear demonstration of the praxis hypothesis (DeMyer, Hingtgen, & Jackson, 1981; Rogers et al., 1996) of a particular motor difficulty in autism and its relation to imitation performance. The relationship between motor imitation skills and apraxia in autism was also examined by Seal and Bonvillian (1997), who reported a correlation between two measures of apraxia with the accuracy of manual language signs and the size of sign vocabulary in 14 students with autism.

Finally, three home videotape studies of infants later diagnosed with autism suggested that motor difficulties may be present very early in autism. Baranek (1999) reported a study of 32 infants 9–12 months of age, 11 of whom were later diagnosed with autism, 10 of whom had other kinds of developmental delays, and 11 of whom had typical development.

Retrospective analysis of home videotapes revealed unusual posturing in both clinical groups compared with the typical infants. Similarly, a French study by Adrien and colleagues (1992) using a similar method comparing videotapes of children with autism with normal infants revealed increased use of unusual postures in the infants with autism between 12 and 24 months when compared with controls. Finally, in their home videotape study, Osterling and Dawson (1999) described increases in repetitive motor behaviors in two clinical groups of 12-month-olds, those with autism and those with other developmental disorders, as compared with typical infants.

DYSPRAXIA

Another area of motor research in autism has involved clumsiness, an aspect of dyspraxia that is thought to reflect problems with motor planning and that is often reported in association with Asperger syndrome. This raises the question of discriminant validity of praxis problems in children with autism, because clumsiness is reported to be common in many childhood psychiatric disorders, including attention-deficit/hyperactivity disorder and developmental language disorders (Ghaziuddin, Butler, Tsai, & Ghaziuddin, 1994).

Ghaziuddin and colleagues (1994) compared 9 children who had autism with 11 children who had Asperger syndrome on standardized tests of motor function. Using the Bruininks-Oseretsky Test of Motor Proficiency (Bruininks, 1978) and looking at gross and fine motor skills separately, they found no group differences between the groups of children with autism and Asperger syndrome. Their performance was universally poor, however, with all 18 children scoring far below the norms for their age. Furthermore, scores on the motor tests were independent of IQ score. Thus, clumsiness was found to characterize virtually all of the individuals with high-functioning ASD. Ghaziuddin and colleagues were careful to point out that clumsiness is a very vague term and that the origins of clumsiness could lie in a variety of deeper dysfunctions in areas such as motor coordination, information processing, visuospatial perception, and sensory sensitivity. Demonstrating the presence of motor dysfunction in both groups tells little further about the source or the nature of those deficits. Manjiviona and Prior (1995) reported similar results using a different measurement of clumsiness. Both the majority of high-functioning children with autism and a similar group of children with Asperger syndrome showed significant levels of motor impairment in a variety of motor areas.

Hughes (1996) carried out a study of motor planning with a large group of children with autism and matched groups of typical youngsters and those with delays. In this paradigm, subjects were given a task that involved reaching for a rod, grasping it, and placing it on one of two color disk targets. Each end of the rod was a different color, and the examiner simply asked the subject to grasp the rod and place one color end on one of the color targets, specifying the colors involved. The outcome variable involved the hand position used to grasp the target, a measure of motor planning. Subjects with autism demonstrated significant abnormalities in the hand grasp they used to execute this task. This study demonstrated that even very simple tasks have significant components involving executive control, which improves in typical development from 2 to 4 years of age. Although both clinical groups were impaired compared with typical MA controls, subjects with autism performed more poorly than the comparison group with cognitive impairments.

Thus, there is an accumulating body of evidence that attests to motor difficulties in autism on nonimitative tasks that could play a role in the production of intentional, sequenced, coordinated movements needed to perform an imitation (Gonzalez-Rothi, Ochipa, & Heilman, 1991). As stated previously, however, motor performance is only one aspect of a chain of subcomponent behaviors involved in carrying out a motor imitation. As Rogers and colleagues (1996) and Smith and Bryson (1994) have indicated, there is a need for a new generation of imitation studies in autism that are focused less on molar questions and more on molecular questions involving the production of intentional actions, including imitated actions.

Bennetto, Pennington, and Rogers (1999) completed a study that examined components of imitation in a sample of 19 children and adolescents with high-functioning autism compared with 19 matched controls with dyslexia. This study assessed subjects' basic fine and gross motor functioning and body schema (i.e., cross-modal match between their own and another's body), as well as dynamic spatiotemporal representation, memory, and imitation of nonmeaningful hand and arm gestures. The individuals with autism demonstrated overall worse performance on the imitation tasks. Further analyses revealed a specific pattern of impairment, which was characterized by difficulty with the kinesthetic aspects of postures and movements, particularly during complex sequences. Subjects with autism also demonstrated impairments in basic motor skills, which appeared to account for some but not all of their imitation deficits. Subjects with autism did not, however, differ from control subjects on body schema, spatiotemporal representation, or memory, suggesting that their imitation deficits were not secondary to problems in these areas. This study is consistent with models of praxis deficits and further suggests that not all components of the imitation process are deficient in autism.

The literature has also suggested that praxic problems occur in children with a variety of disorders, raising the discriminant validity issue of whether an imitation deficit is specific to autism. The studies cited here have demonstrated that children with autism are more impaired in imitation and other motor skills than are children with other developmental delays. A developmental dyspraxia control group, however, will be important to add to future studies. Studies designed to examine the subcomponents of imitation or praxis, using dyspraxic matched controls, will go a long way to providing the data needed to construct neuropsychological models of the imitation deficit in autism. Existing neuropsychological models of praxis such as that of Gonzalez-Rothi and colleagues (1991) should help in the investigation of the phenomenon with greater sophistication.

EXECUTIVE FUNCTIONS

Given the previously discussed focus on motor difficulties in autism, there has been relatively little discussion about the brain–behavior relations involved. Although the cerebellum has been implicated in studies of postural control, other brain structures have been emphasized in existing work on apraxia and imitation (Damasio & Maurer, 1978; DeRenzi & Luchelli, 1988; Gonzalez-Rothi et al., 1991; Kimura & Archibald, 1974; Kolb & Milner, 1981). Rogers and Pennington (1991) also suggested that executive dysfunctions seen in other kinds of performance in autism may be involved in the imitation deficit as well. The three main aspects of the Rogers and Pennington model of autism—imitation, emotion sharing, and joint attention—all require the complex ability to form and coordinate representations of self with representations of another to guide behavior. In an effort to tie together the biological, neuropsychological, and behavioral levels of autism, Rogers and Pennington proposed that EFs of the prefrontal cortex may have a central role in the pathogenesis of autism. Since 1991, significant research on executive dysfunction in autism has been published. In the following sections we review this new evidence in light of the earlier hypothesis that the imitation/dyspraxia difficulties in autism may be due at least in part to executive dysfunction.

Findings Involving Executive Functions in Autism

At the time of the 1991 Rogers and Pennington paper, relatively little was known about the neuropsychological performance of individuals with autism, although a number of early descriptive and empirical papers had documented evidence consistent with EF impairment. This evidence included observations that individuals with autism had difficulties with abstract thinking (Scheerer, Rothman, & Goldstein, 1945), tendencies toward perseverative response patterns (e.g., Hermelin & O'Connor, 1970), and stimulus overselectivity (e.g., Lovaas & Schreibman, 1971). It was not until the mid-1980s, however, that empirical work directly addressing EF impairment was conducted (Rumsey, 1985; Steel, Gorman, & Flexman, 1984). In their 1991 paper, Rogers and Pennington reviewed seven studies that directly examined EFs in autism. These studies documented consistent evidence of EF deficits in high-functioning individuals with autism when compared with appropriately-matched control groups (Ozonoff, Pennington, & Rogers, 1991; Ozonoff, Rogers, & Pennington, 1991; Prior & Hoffman, 1990; Rumsey, 1985; Rumsey & Hamburger, 1988, 1990; Szatmari, Bartolucci, Bremmer, Bond, & Rich, 1989).

Although the evidence at the time was suggestive of an EF impairment in autism, Rogers and Pennington raised a number of theoretical and methodological challenges to an EF theory of autism:

1. *Timing:* For a deficit to have a causal role in the development of autism, it has to be present before the onset of the disorder and therefore present in the youngest children with the disorder. If an EF deficit is primary in autism, then it should be evident in the youngest children.
2. *Ecological validity:* It was not clear whether laboratory measures of EF accurately reflected subjects' actual adaptive functioning in life situations.

Similarly, relationships between EF and the main sociocommunicative symptoms in autism had not yet been demonstrated.

3. *Etiologic heterogeneity:* At the time Rogers and Pennington's paper appeared, autism was thought to arise from a variety of conditions. Suggesting a specific impairment in EF, however, implied a common final pathway. A related issue not discussed in the original paper is that of discriminant validity. An increasing number of studies have demonstrated EF impairments in other developmental disorders with very different behavioral phenotypes from autism.

In the following sections, we review the work that has been done in this area since the early 1990s to determine which questions have been answered, which remain, and which new questions have arisen. We also direct the reader to several excellent papers that outline and critique the role of EF in autism (Pennington & Ozonoff, 1996; Russell, 1997).

Performance on Global Tests of Executive Functions

Since 1991, several studies have further examined EFs in autism using traditional tasks like the Wisconsin Card Sorting Task (WCST; Grant & Berg, 1993) and the Tower of Hanoi (Shallice, 1982), which are complex tasks that assess planning, abstract thinking, inhibition of well-practiced responses, and cognitive flexibility. Because of the conceptual and verbal demands of many of the tests utilized, these studies have limited their focus to high-functioning individuals with autism.

A number of researchers have replicated earlier findings of EF deficits in studies of older children, adolescents, and adults with autism or Asperger syndrome relative to carefully matched controls, using a wide range of traditional EF tasks (Berthier, 1995; Ciesielski & Harris, 1997; Ozonoff & McEvoy, 1994; Ozonoff, Rogers, & Pennington, 1991; Szatmari, Tuff, Finlayson, & Bartolucci, 1990). Two groups of researchers found that matched groups with autism and Asperger syndrome were equally impaired relative to controls on the WCST and Tower of Hanoi, without significant differences between the performance of the two clinical groups (Ozonoff, Rogers, & Pennington, 1991; Szatmari et al., 1990). The one longitudinal study of high-functioning children demonstrated stable impairments in EF performance with little improvement over time on any of the tasks, pointing to a possible developmental ceiling on this type of ability (Ozonoff & McEvoy, 1994).

Ciesielski and Harris (1997) further explored the nature of these EF deficits by analyzing the tasks according to the degree of rule constraint, or internal structure, provided within the task. The group with autism showed a pattern of deficiencies that suggested that poorly defined rules were differentially harder for them, independent of their IQ scores. In such situations, they had notable difficulty disengaging from previous response patterns. In contrast, their best performances were on tasks with highly specific rules governing performance.

Two studies published by Minshew and colleagues (Minshew, Goldstein, Muenz, & Payton, 1992; Minshew et al., 1997) found that compared with typical controls, people with autism had a relatively impaired performance on a range of tests measuring complex memory and linguistic problem-solving skills but not on the WCST. Their results suggest a deficit in complex information processing but point to a lack of impairment and/or variability in EF.

Thus, there is relatively consistent evidence that on global tasks of EF, most but not all high-functioning people with autism and Asperger syndrome demonstrate deficits. Variability on EF tasks in autism may be due to IQ score differences and the amount of structure in the tasks, with more impairment on tasks with less clearly-defined rules.

Deconstructing Executive Function Deficits

In addition to variability in structure, EF tasks may encompass a variety of cognitive processes, including working memory, inhibition, attention to and appropriate response to feedback, and cognitive flexibility. Individuals with autism may therefore have impairments in all or only a subset of these components. If there is a distinct subset, then determining whether this subset is the same as that impaired in other groups with EF deficits may help address concerns about the discriminant validity of EF in autism. Studies have examined the subcomponent processes of working memory, inhibition, cognitive flexibility, generativity, and attention in autism. In the following sections we briefly review these studies as well as their implications for an EF model of autism.

Working Memory in Autism

Working memory refers to the simultaneous processing and storage of information during complex cognitive tasks (Baddeley & Hitch, 1974). More recently, it has been described as critical for integrating transient, context-specific information from diverse sources (Pennington & Ozonoff, 1996) and thus provides a theoretical tie between the demands of traditional EF tasks and social interactions. Studies of working memory have reported conflicting findings.

Two groups have reported an autism-specific deficit. Bennetto, Pennington, and Rogers (1996), examining verbal working memory in a group of high-functioning adolescents with autism and matched controls, reported intact rote memory, short- and long-term recognition, cued recall, and new learning ability but significant impairments on a variety of working memory tasks including temporal order memory, source memory, and supraspan free recall. Turner (1997) reported similar findings for both high- and low-functioning individuals using nonverbal working memory tasks. In contrast, two other groups have not found differences between children with autism and children with general intellectual impairments (Russell, Jarrold, & Henry, 1996; Sykes & Russell, 1997). This raises the question of whether working memory capacity is affected by neurological or cognitive impairment in general rather than by autism in particular.

An important implication of these studies is that individuals with autism have difficulty with standard EF tasks as well as with everyday problem solving because of difficulties with working memory. Thus, the construct of working memory may be quite helpful in devising treatment approaches that support EF (Ozonoff, 1998), as exemplified by the TEACCH (Treatment and Education of Autistic and related Communications Handicapped Children) program, which uses a variety of visual strategies to support sequencing, transitions, and task completion for people with autism (Mesibov, Schopler, & Hearsey, 1994). It is not clear, however, whether people with autism have more difficulties with working memory than do other people with cognitive impairments.

Inhibition in Autism

Inhibition refers to the ability to stop oneself from carrying out a well-practiced and "ready" response when that response is not adaptive. The nature of inhibitory functions in autism is somewhat inconclusive. The majority of studies report no autism-specific deficit on a variety of simple inhibition tasks (Bryson, 1983; Eskes, Bryson, & McCormick, 1990; Ozonoff, Strayer, McMahon, & Filloux, 1994), although Hughes (1996) reported autism-specific deficits on two tasks. In general, individuals with autism appear to demonstrate intact inhibition on relatively simple cognitive and motor tasks but may have more difficulty when required not only to inhibit but also to shift their attention or cognitive set to a new stimulus. Because impaired inhibitory mechanisms have been documented in individuals with other developmental disorders (e.g., attention-deficit/hyperactivity disorder, obsessive-compulsive disorder, schizophrenia), these studies may help to define a subtype of EF deficits specific to individuals with autism.

Cognitive Flexibility in Autism

Difficulty shifting attentional focus from one stimulus to another or from one idea to another has long been recognized as a symptom of executive dysfunction, which results in perseveration of thoughts and actions in people with frontal brain injury. Set shifting is an important component of many EF tasks, and this capacity has been specifically examined in people with autism. Both Hughes, Russell, and Robbins (1994) and Ozonoff and colleagues (1994) examined set shifting in children with autism compared with clinical controls known to have EF difficulties by experimentally isolating the set-shifting component of two simplified traditional neuropsychological tests. The results of both studies suggested that subjects with autism were differentially impaired relative to control groups. Courchesne and colleagues' (1994) work in attention shifting may be related to this impairment as well (see Chapter 8 for a discussion). Questions remain, however, about whether children with autism have difficulty shifting attention away from a salient cue, toward a new cue, or both.

Executive Function Studies of Preschool Children

Although the studies just discussed have demonstrated consistent EF impairment in older children, adolescents, and adults with autism, EF deficits in preschoolers have not been as consistently documented. The first paper on the subject (McEvoy, Rogers, & Pennington, 1993) reported EF deficits on a spatial reversal task in a group of young children with autism (mean age of 64 months), compared both with matched clinical and with typical comparison groups. The authors also found a significant relationship between performance on the spatial reversal task and measures of joint attention and social interaction. A near-replication of this study in a younger group of children (mean age 51 months), however, did not find autism-specific deficits on any of a number of EF tasks, although EF continued to be related to joint attention (Griffith, Pennington, Wehner, & Rogers, 1999). Lack of group differences in preschoolers with autism on EF tasks was also reported by Barth, Fein, and Waterhouse (1995). Dawson and colleagues (1998), however, reported that compared with a matched clinical and typical controls, preschoolers with autism performed worse on a task thought to tap dorsolateral prefrontal functioning (delayed response) as well as one thought to measure medial temporal lobe functioning (delayed nonmatching-to-sample). The authors found that the prefrontal task was significantly correlated with imitation performance but not with social behavior, whereas the medial temporal task was more consistently related to social deficits.

Implications of Executive Function Research

That executive dysfunction could be a significant deficit at least in older children and adults with autism, as suggested in the Rogers and Pennington (1991) paper, seems to be supported by the continuing studies and increasing refinement of the questions being asked. In terms of clinical relevance, the construct of executive dysfunction has been a very helpful one. Clinical interventions that attend to executive difficulties target variables such as increased structure, visual supports for working memory, visual systems for organization, and environmental supports for set shifting to help with transitions and change. These kinds of programs are currently considered recommended practices in preschool intervention for children with autism (Dawson & Osterling, 1997) and characterize some of the best known approaches to preschool intervention (Rogers, 1998).

At the level of theory, in question is the extent to which executive dysfunction can be characterized as one of the primary deficits in autism. The most damaging finding to the EF theory of autism comes from the preschool studies. If executive dysfunction is not present early in autism, then it can hardly have explanatory power for the development of the disorder. Furthermore, it is not yet known whether executive dysfunction distinguishes autism from other developmental disorders. And in most studies, there is no evidence that executive dysfunction as seen in laboratory paradigms is related to everyday functioning and everyday difficulties of people with autism. If executive dysfunction does not differentiate autism from other disorders, does not present clearly early in the disorder, and cannot be linked to specific symptoms that characterize autism, then it should not be considered a primary cause of symptoms of autism.

Is it time to discard the EF theory? Not yet, because in two areas of autistic symptomatology, executive dysfunction *has* been empirically linked: pragmatics of communication and imitation.

Relationships Between Executive Function and Pragmatics of Communication

Joint attention behavior is an extremely important aspect of early pragmatics of communication, and joint attention deficits are among the earliest symptoms of autism to appear. Relationships between performance on joint attention tasks and performance on EF measures were first hypothesized by Butterworth and Grover (1988) as they considered the cognitive demands of joint attention in an infant. Joint attention has powerful working memory demands, for the infant must hold on line the partner's attentional focus while seeking to coordinate it with the infant's own visual experience. There are also powerful inhibition and goal-seeking demands as the infant maintains the goal of shared attention until it is reached while inhibiting responses to other visual distractions. Finally, there are clear set-shifting demands on the infant.

Two studies have found autism-specific relationships between EF performance and joint attention in preschoolers with autism. McEvoy and colleagues (1993) found a significant relationship between performance on an EF task, spatial reversal, and social interaction and joint attention variables in young children with autism. This finding was replicated by Griffith and colleagues (1999), both cross-sectionally and longitudinally. Furthermore, matched control children with other kinds of developmental disorders did not demonstrate this relationship. Caplan and colleagues (1993) found a developmental association between joint attention and behavior flexibility in a sample of normally developing infants as well. Using different measures, however, Dawson and colleagues (1998) did not find this relationship.

The joint attention deficit in autism is considered by many to be a precursor of later ToM deficits. In fact, the ToM problems in autism often are believed to be responsible for many of the pragmatic problems that high-functioning adults with autism continue to demonstrate in communication (Tager-Flusberg, 1993). A variety of researchers have reported strong relationships between executive dysfunction and ToM performance in autism.

Ozonoff, Pennington, and Rogers (1991) and Russell, Mauthner, Sharpe, and Tidswell (1991) have demonstrated that for high-functioning subjects with autism and Asperger syndrome, performance on EF tasks was closely related to performance on both first- and second-order ToM tasks. Russell and colleagues have suggested that problems with ToM performance could be explained by difficulties with an EF capacity—difficulty disengaging from salient cues. Evidence from neuroimaging studies also links performance on ToM tasks with activity in the frontal cortex. Baron-Cohen and colleagues (1994) conducted a single photon emission computerized tomography study with typical subjects, which focused on several regions of interest in the frontal lobes. Their findings suggested possible involvement of the right orbitofrontal cortex in thinking about mental content. In another study of typical adults, Fletcher and colleagues (1995) noted changes in regional cerebral blood flow in the left medial prefrontal cortex during the processing of stories involving mental state attribution. Happé and colleagues (1996), however, examined activation in five adults with Asperger syndrome who demonstrated no task-related change in this region, despite normal activation in adjacent areas.

Thus, there are indications that EF performance is indeed tied to everyday difficulties in two main symptom areas for people with autism, which are considered key for sociocommunicative development: joint attention behavior, a main deficit in young children with autism, and ToM abilities, a strong discriminator of autism in older children and adults. The field needs creative new research approaches to explore these relationships further and significant theory building to flesh out the promises and questions that this line of work has initiated (e.g., Mundy & Markus, 1997).

Relationships Between Executive Function and Imitation

Relationships between frontal lobe functioning and imitation/pantomime skills have been demonstrated in studies of adults with brain injury (Kolb & Milner, 1981), which influenced Rogers and Pennington's (1991) hypothesis concerning ties between imitation and EF in autism. Thus far, two studies have examined the hypothesized relationship in autism. Rogers and colleagues (1996) conducted a study of imitation and pantomime skills in high-functioning adolescents with autism, using a clinical comparison group with learning disabilities. Their findings suggested a possible relationship between EF and certain imitation tasks, particularly those that required holding a sequence of movements on line. Dawson and colleagues (1998) reported significantly positive correlations between immediate imitation tasks and both frontal and temporal lobe measures. There is currently a press, however, to learn more about motor problems in autism, and the extent to which imitation difficulties are part of a dyspraxia versus part of a more global motor impairment remains to be seen. Dyspraxia in autism is a common clinical finding. The extent to which executive dysfunction can explain the imitation/pantomime difficulties is an open question.

Implications of Imitation/Praxis Research on Sociocommunicative Development in Autism

As of 2000, there was virtually no empirical data on possible relationships among imitation, joint attention, emotion sharing, and ToM. Such studies are underway. Without such data, clinical evidence and developmental theories must serve to suggest how an imitation/praxis deficit very early in life could disrupt sociocommunicative development.

The first and more obvious potential impact involves the ability to speak. Speech involves production of a complex series of sequenced oral-motor movements, first learned through motor imitation of another person. Verbal dyspraxia has long been recognized as a cause of expressive speech impairments in children and, in its most severe form, can prevent the acquisition of speech in children with normal intelligence who comprehend speech. We hypothesize that one reason for the lack of speech development in some children with autism is an underlying oral-motor dyspraxia.

Bringing the concept of verbal apraxia into the Denver Model (Rogers et al., in press) treatment approach for young children with autism led us to add imitation training as well as other standard oral-motor therapy approaches aimed at treating oral dyspraxia to our ongoing reactive communication interventions. These interventions consisted of a variety of reactive developmentally based approaches focused on developing both nonverbal and verbal intentional communication strategies in the children. The addition of imitation training significantly increased our success at developing speech as a primary communication system in previously nonverbal young children with autism (Rogers, Hall, Osaki, Reaven, & Herbison, in press).

Although the concepts related to verbal dyspraxia are useful in understanding lack of speech development in some children with autism, they do not address the deeper level of communicative impairment that young children with autism demonstrate. Dyspraxia does not explain the lack of awareness of communication, the lack of dyadic exchange, or the lack of early nonverbal signaling in autism that typical infants develop in the first year of life. Research suggests that these deficits are already present by 12 months of age in most infants who will later be diagnosed with autism (Baranek, 1999; Osterling & Dawson, 1999). Can an impairment in the ability to imitate other people's movements provide explanatory power at this level? Several different theorists have answered in the affirmative. Infant imitation allows for infant and parent behavior to become coupled, synchronous, and reciprocal, even in the neonatal period.

In Stern's (1985) model, sharing emotions during the 3- to 6-month-old period is a main vehicle for interpersonal development. Emotion studies have demonstrated that assuming physical emotion postures and expressions actually induces an emotional experience and emotion sharing (Adelmann & Zajonc, 1989; Hatfield, Cacioppo, & Rapson, 1994; McIntosh, 1996). Meltzoff and Gopnik (1993) have provided a detailed theoretical account of the role of imitation in developing self–other awareness during infancy. They suggested that infants' imitation of emotional expressions creates an internal affective state that matches the partner's, giving the infant an internal sense of matching between self and other (and that corresponds to physical matchings of self and other)—the experience of emotional mirroring. Thus, through imitation the infant is experiencing the synchrony between self and other's internal and external states. An important implication of this model is that the correspondence of self and other is coming from an internal sense, the way it "feels" to be in relationship with another. These correspondences between body movements and internal experiences allow the slightly older infant to read the intentions behind others' movements, which allows for sharing of intentions as well as emotions and foci of attention, thus laying down the bedrock of communication. Meltzoff and Gopnik suggested that having a sense of internal correspondence between self and others' intentions is a midpoint on the way to a sense of correspondence of mental states of self and other. These authors suggested that in autism, a primary deficit in imitation blocks the child from developing the "like-me" sense at the level of body correspondences, emotional correspondences, and attentional correspondences. The child with autism is unable to use imitation as a tool for constructing internal self–other correspondences at the level of affect or mind.

A major problem with this model is that autism is not that simple. It is not a complete absence of self–other correspondences. Many children with autism eventually develop joint attention behaviors, speech, some level of sharing of experiences, and affect. Many people with autism eventually pass ToM tasks. People with autism are not devoid of social knowledge, interest, and reciprocal social relations. There is tremendous individual variability in the social area in autism. What is needed is a model that allows for the existence of imitative behavior and joint attention behavior in older, higher-functioning people with autism while still accounting for continuing difficulties in social relatedness, pragmatics, and intersubjectivity. Such a model, suggested by Rogers (1999) and reviewed in the following paragraphs, leans heavily on the fascinating area referred to as *emotional contagion* (Hatfield et al., 1994). Emotional contagion is the "the tendency to automatically mimic and synchronize facial expressions, vocalizations, postures, and movements with those of another person and consequently to converge emotionally" (p. 5). The behaviors involved in emotional contagion are seen as relatively automatic, unintentional, and largely inaccessible to awareness. This automatic synchrony of movements allows for the transmission of emotions between the partners. People's ongoing emotional experience is thus constantly influenced by the activity or feedback from the partner's movements, as well as from afferent feedback from their own emotional expressions, body postures, and vocal tones. The coordinated body movements literally create synchronous emotional experiences that are experienced as shared between the partners.

It is interesting to consider the concept of *social relatedness* in light of emotional contagion. Abnormalities in relatedness are the sine qua non of autism, but the term *relatedness* is rarely defined. We suggest that *relatedness* is a kind of interpersonal synchrony—of bodies, voices, movements, expressions, and synchronized or complimentary feeling states. It is the interpersonal coordination that people feel, see, and hear through the matching of their movements (face, body, voice) with those of their social partners. Typical relatedness may be a background experience that people do not notice until it is disrupted. Even mild disruptions of physical coordination with social partners, as seen in problems with the timing, grading, or inaccuracies of matching movements, could impede emotional synchrony and give one the sense that something is "off."

We are hypothesizing that a severe praxic and imitative deficit in an infant could markedly impair the physical coordinations involved in social exchanges. In so doing, the deficit would interfere with the establishment and maintenance of emotional connectedness between two people engaged in a typical social exchange. Furthermore, it would interfere with the social cascade from primary to secondary intersubjectivity and later with shared attention, shared intention, and intentional communication. Could severe dyspraxia be *the* primary deficit in autism? We would argue no. Infants with other disabilities, particularly blindness and severe cerebral palsy, do not receive cross-modal visual–physical matching experiences between infant and parent. Early on, blind infants do have some shared characteristics with infants who have autism, and difficulties with relatedness may mark the early months (Fraiberg, 1977). Blind infants and their parents, however, develop compensatory mechanisms, such as using voice, language, and touch, through which emotions can be shared, connectedness can be experienced, and intersubjective knowledge can be developed. Similarly, the movements of infants with severe cerebral palsy are not synchronous with those of their social partners. Yet interpersonal relatedness can be established and emotional contagion can be experienced through eye contact, facial expressions, sounds, conversations—the matching of the vitality affects (Stern, 1985) through whatever routes are available. As one communicates with a person who has severe motor impairments that might affect relatedness, one gradually begins to ignore asynchronies and attend to whatever interpersonal coordinations are present. Both in blindness and in cerebral palsy, infants find other routes than imitative body movements for establishing and maintaining affective connections with their social partners. Thus, a praxis deficit is not sufficient for explaining the intersubjective deficit in autism (though it may play an important role in lack of speech development in some children with autism). The affective system in autism must be looked at as well, an area that has more questions than answers at present.

CLINICAL AND EDUCATIONAL IMPLICATIONS

Emphasis on imitation as a core part of autism treatment has been described for many years by a variety of theoretically differing models. Imitation training is a fundamental part of Lovaas's (1981) behavior therapy, which provides a detailed approach for teaching imitation to young children with autism. Kaufman (1976) placed considerable emphasis on imitation in his work with his young son, the approach used by the Options Institute. Dawson and Galpert (1990) provided an empirical study of the increase in social behavior, including imitation, of children with autism under conditions in which an adult is imitating the child. Finally, Greenspan and Wieder (1997) emphasized the importance of imitation during floortime activities with children with autism.

Adding direct instruction in imitating motor movements to our ongoing work with natural language and augmentative language approaches in the Denver Model of intervention (Rogers et al., in press) has had tremendous impact on the progress of very young children with very severe autism. Our approach now combines direct imitation instruction approaches with more child-centered language approaches: interactive child-centered social routines built on repeated joint action games, focused on imitating the child (*sensory social routines,* in our terminology) and developing affectively rich, dyadic interactions (see Chapters 9 and 12). Since we added direct instruction programs to our treatment model in the late 1980s, most of the young children with a primary diagnosis of autism instructed in this way (between 50 and 100) have learned to imitate a variety of motor movements. These imitations are not simply "parlor tricks" but are useful skills that children exhibit in imitation of movements associated with preschool songs in group instruction; in imitation of toy play with adults and peers; in imitation of peers in open-ended play using sand, water, paint, and other typical preschool materials; and in following routines with objects, such as cleaning up after activities. Parents have also reported unprompted increases in sibling imitations at home.

Furthermore, given our hypothesis that the reason for lack of speech is due *in part* to severe oral-motor dyspraxia, our curriculum focuses heavily on teaching nonverbal children who can imitate hand and body movements to imitate a variety of oral-facial movements to develop intentional control of the musculature. (This is used *in addition* to child-centered language development approaches and augmentative communication approaches.) With this approach, we are much more successful at helping completely nonverbal young children to develop useful speech by the age of 5. This is not unique to our approach; other programs that emphasize imitation (motor or vocal) as the bedrock of their beginning treatment report similar outcomes (Lovaas, 1987;

McGee, 1997). Thus, direct instruction in imitation skills, as Dawson and Osterling suggested in their 1997 chapter, is considered by many to be part of the recommended practices in early intervention for young children with autism.

DIRECTIONS FOR FUTURE RESEARCH

One challenge to the field is to understand the mechanisms underlying the difficulty in imitating movements that people with autism have. Three areas need to be examined. The first has to do with understanding the mechanisms for the imitation deficit. The component parts of carrying out a motor imitation are many. One must visually perceive the movement and encode it in working memory. One must transfer the visual stimulus to a proprioceptive stimulus and map it onto one's body. One must then formulate a movement plan, execute it, monitor it as it is being executed by matching the felt movement to the remembered visual stimulus, and correct any errors that are perceived. Finally, one must match not only the movement pattern but also the *vitality affects* (Stern, 1985). This wonderful term describes the affective contours of a movement, which include the rhythm, speed, flow, and other aspects of the movement that convey the emotional tone accompanying the movement. To do this, one must have received the affective message in the movement as one saw it and encode the visual stimuli onto an affective map as well. Future research needs to explore which aspects of motor imitation are impaired in autism.

Second, the imitation deficit in autism needs to be understood in relation to other movement disorders. Other groups of children come into the world with motor systems that may be much more impaired than those of children with autism. The motor skills of people with autism, including imitation, need to be examined in relation to matched groups with developmental dyspraxia, cerebral palsy, and other kinds of motor impairments to reveal whether there is any unique aspect of the deficit in autism.

The dyspraxia hypothesis might lead one to theorize that the underlying problem is a movement problem. Rogers and Pennington (1991) suggested a union of movement and emotion in typical interpersonal relations and an impairment in this unity of motor-affective body coordination in people with autism. Movement is the messenger of emotion; coordinated movements between social partners maintain the emotional connectedness that occurs in an interaction, in infancy, and throughout life. Thus, in addition to focusing very closely on the motoric capacity of people with autism to respond to other people's movements, research also will have to step back to examine the relationship between motor skills and affect in people interacting in an affective relationship. This will have to be examined in people with various motor difficulties as well as in people with autism to understand how individuals with various motor disabilities compensate to participate in coordinated affective interpersonal exchanges.

Finally, relationships between imitation/praxis skills and other aspects of sociocommunicative functioning need to be examined. In the same way that EF studies have examined ties with joint attention, ToM, symbolic play, and pragmatics of communication, the hypothesized relations involving imitation and sociocommunicative development will have to be examined empirically. Given the nature of the model, longitudinal studies will be critical for understanding the role of imitation in early development.

CONCLUSIONS

In this chapter, two aspects of the Rogers and Pennington (1991) model, involving the roles of EF and imitation deficits in the pathogenesis of autism, were revisited in light of the empirical work that has occurred in the 1990s. Empirical evidence supporting significant deficits in these two areas in autism continues to be published, with the vast majority of studies in both areas demonstrating autism-specific deficits, both across the age span and across functioning levels. Studies are underway in various laboratories to understand the nature of these impairments at a deeper level and the implications of these impairments on the day-to-day life of people with autism.

Two particular aspects of Rogers and Pennington's (1991) theory are challenged by the research findings. One involves the role of EF in the development of autism. Studies of EFs in preschoolers with autism are mixed. If EFs are not differentially impaired in autism early in life, then they cannot be primary to the disorder. Further studies of young children with autism will determine whether the EF deficit is to have a primary or secondary role in neuropsychological models of autism.

A second aspect challenged by research findings is the idea that the imitation deficit represents a delay rather than a deviation in development. Rogers and Pennington (1991) originally hypothesized that children with autism would eventually learn to imitate motor movements. Studies involving imitation skills of higher-functioning older children, adolescents, and adults with autism report continuing problems with accuracy and quality of imitation. This indicates what may be a lifelong impairment, present in the youngest children with autism examined (20 months), virtually universal in the groups studied, and persistent across development. The imitation deficit thus continues to meet most of the criteria of a primary neuropsychological deficit. Questions of specificity still need to be answered.

These findings require an elaboration of Rogers and Pennington's (1991) developmental model. The infant or young child with autism is unable to match the partner imitatively and reciprocally; consequently, he or she does not have ongoing experiences of emotional contagion and the sense of self–other correspondences that develop from physical and affective sharing. As development occurs, the degree of imitative ability that develops in autism varies from one person to the next because of individual differences in development and treatment. The child with autism may learn to imitate many movements, but the ongoing praxis problems prevent the automatic, smooth, synchronous, continuous motor matching of a partner. The continuing problems in imitation involving timing, speed, grading, and movement impede the establishment of emotional synchrony, and these two components lie behind the "relatedness" deficit in autism. Moments of such relatedness can be created through carefully constructed interpersonal experiences (Dawson & Galpert, 1990; Rogers, 1998). Furthermore, the potential for increased synchrony improves as coordination of movements improves, as long as the environment provides continuing experiences of interpersonal matchings and as long as the person with autism has not "given up" on ever connecting with the social world.

We are suggesting that the social cascade can occur, in partial, fragmented ways, for people with autism. Partial improvements in imitation would lead to partial experiences of emotional contagion and moments of affective coordination of self and other. This, in turn, would allow for partial development of intersubjective and intentional awareness, including some aspects of joint attention, empathy, symbolic play, and intentional communication. We are suggesting, however, that the synchrony of movements, voices, and expressions will continue to be impaired in autism, even among high-functioning individuals. This will result in continuing difficulties in interpersonal relatedness, limiting the person with autism's access to internal states of other people through emotion contagion and synchrony and preventing comprehensive development of intersubjective knowledge and emotional attunements. This model thus allows for individual differences within autism while accounting for the chronicity of the interpersonal symptoms.

REFERENCES

Adelmann, P.K., & Zajonc, R.B. (1989). Facial efference and the experience of emotion. *Annual Review of Psychology, 40,* 249–280.

Adrien, J.L., Perrot, A., Sauvage, D., Leddet, I., Larmande, C., Hameury, L., & Barthélémy, C. (1992). Early symptoms in autism from family home movies: Evaluation and comparison between 1st and 2nd year of life using I.B.S.E. scale. *Acta Paedopsychiatrica, 55,* 71–75.

Ayres, A.J. (1985). *Developmental dyspraxia and adult onset apraxia.* Torrance, CA: Sensory Integration International.

Baddeley, A.D., & Hitch, G.J. (1974). Working memory. In G.H. Bower (Ed.), *The psychology of learning and motivation* (Vol. 8, pp. 47–89). San Diego: Academic Press.

Baranek, G. (1999). Autism during infancy: A retrospective video analysis of sensory-motor and social behaviors at 9–12 months of age. *Journal of Autism and Developmental Disorders, 29*(3), 213–224.

Baron-Cohen, S. (1988). Social and pragmatic deficits in autism: Cognitive or affective? *Journal of Autism and Developmental Disorders, 18,* 379–402.

Baron-Cohen, S. (1991). Do people with autism understand what causes emotion? *Child Development, 62,* 385–395.

Baron-Cohen, S., Leslie, A.M., & Frith, U. (1985). Does the autistic child have a "theory of mind"? *Cognition, 21,* 37–46.

Baron-Cohen, S., Ring, H., Moriarty, J., Schmitz, B., Costa, D., & Ell, P. (1994). The brain basis of the theory of mind: The role of the orbitofrontal region. *British Journal of Psychiatry, 165,* 640–649.

Barth, C., Fein, D., & Waterhouse, L. (1995). Delayed match-to-sample performance in autistic children. *Developmental Neuropsychology, 11,* 53–69.

Bennetto, L., Pennington, B.F., & Rogers, S.J. (1996). Intact and impaired memory functions in autism. *Child Development, 67,* 1816–1835.

Bennetto, L., Pennington, B.F., & Rogers, S.J. (1999). *A componential approach to imitation movement deficits in autism.* Manuscript submitted for publication.

Berthier, M.L. (1995). Hypomania following bereavement in Asperger's syndrome: A case study. *Neuropsychiatry, Neuropsychology, and Behavioral Neurology, 8,* 222–228.

Bruininks, R.H. (1978). *Bruininks-Oseretsky Test of Motor Proficiency: Examiner's manual.* Circle Pines, MN: American Guidance Service.

Bruner, J. (1975). The ontogenesis of speech acts. *Journal of Child Language, 2,* 1–19.

Bryson, S.E. (1983). Interference effects in autistic children: Evidence for the comprehension of single stimuli. *Journal of Abnormal Psychology, 92,* 250–254.

Butterworth, G., & Grover, L. (1988). The origins of referential communication in human infancy. In L. Weiskrantz (Ed.), *Thought without language.* Oxford, England: Clarendon.

Caplan, R., Chugani, H.T., Messa, C., Guthrie, D., Sigman, M., de Traversy, J., & Mundy, P. (1993). Hemispherectomy for intractable seizures: Presurgical cerebral glucose metabolism and postsurgical nonverbal communication. *Developmental Medicine and Child Neurology, 35,* 582–592.

Charman, T., & Baron-Cohen, S. (1994). Another look at imitation in autism. *Development and Psychopathology, 6,* 403–414.

Charman, T., Swettenham, J., Baron-Cohen, S., Cox, A., Baird, G., & Drew, A. (1997). Infants with autism: An investigation of empathy, pretend play, joint attention, and imitation. *Developmental Psychology, 33*(5), 781–789.

Churchill, D.W. (1978). Language: The problem beyond conditioning. In M. Rutter & E. Schopler (Eds.), *Autism: A reappraisal of concepts and treatment* (pp. 71–84). New York: Plenum.

Cicchetti, D. (1990). Perspectives on the interface between normal and atypical development. *Development and Psychopathology, 2*(4), 329–334.

Ciesielski, K.T., & Harris, R.J. (1997). Factors related to performance failure on executive tasks in autism. *Child Neuropsychology, 3,* 1–12.

Colbert, E.G., Koegler, R.R., & Markham, C.H. (1958). Toe walking in childhood schizophrenia. *Journal of Pediatrics, 53,* 219–220.

Cornish, K.M., & McManus, I.C. (1996). Hand preference and hand skill in children with autism. *Journal of Autism and Developmental Disorders, 26*(6), 597–610.

Courchesne, E., Townsend, J., Akshoomoff, N.A., Saitoh, O., Yeung-Courchesne, R., Lincoln, A.J., James, H.E., Haas, R.H., Schreibman, L., & Lau, L. (1994). Impairment in shifting attention in autistic and cerebellar patients. *Behavioral Neuroscience, 108,* 848–865.

Damasio, A.R., & Maurer, R.G. (1978). A neurological model for childhood autism. *Archives of Neurology, 35,* 777–786.

Dawson, G., & Galpert, L. (1990). Mothers' use of imitative play for facilitating social responsiveness and toy play in young autistic children. *Development and Psychopathology, 2,* 151–162.

Dawson, G., Meltzoff, A.N., Osterling, J., & Rinaldi, J. (1998). Neuropsychological correlates of early symptoms of autism. *Child Development, 69*(5), 1276–1285.

Dawson, G., & Osterling, J. (1997). Early intervention in autism. In M.J. Guralnick (Ed.), *The effectiveness of early intervention* (pp. 307–326). Baltimore: Paul H. Brookes Publishing Co.

DeMyer, M.K., Hingtgen, J.N., & Jackson, R.K. (1981). Infantile autism reviewed: A decade of research. *Schizophrenia Bulletin, 7,* 388–451.

DeRenzi, E., & Luchelli, F. (1988). Ideational apraxia. *Brain, 111,* 1173–1185.

Eskes, G.A., Bryson, S.E., & McCormick, T.A. (1990). Comprehension of concrete and abstract words in autistic children. *Journal of Autism and Developmental Disorders, 20,* 61–73.

Fein, D., Pennington, B.F., Markowitz, P., Braverman, M., & Waterhouse, L. (1986). Toward a neuropsychological model of infantile autism: Are the social deficits primary? *Journal of the American Academy of Child and Adolescent Psychiatry, 25*(2), 198–212.

Flavell, J., Botkin, P.T., Fry, C.L., Wright, J.W., & Jarvis, P.E. (1968). *The development of role-taking and communication skills in children.* New York: John Wiley & Sons.

Fletcher, P.C., Happé, F., Frith, U., Baker, S.C., Dolan, R.J., & Frackowiak, R.S.J. (1995). Other minds in the brain: A functional imaging study of "theory of mind" in story comprehension. *Cognition, 57,* 109–128.

Fraiberg, S. (1977). *Insights from the blind: Comparative studies of blind and sighted infants.* New York: New American Library.

Ghaziuddin, M., Butler, E., Tsai, L., & Ghaziuddin, N. (1994). Is clumsiness a marker for Asperger syndrome? *Journal of Intellectual Disability Research, 38,* 519–527.

Gonzalez-Rothi, L.J., Ochipa, C., & Heilman, K.M. (1991). A cognitive neuropsychological model of limb praxis. *Cognitive Neuropsychology, 8,* 443–458.

Goodman, R. (1989). Infantile autism: A syndrome of multiple primary deficits. *Journal of Autism and Developmental Disorders, 19,* 409–424.

Grant, D., & Berg, F. (1993). *Wisconsin Card Sorting Test.* Odessa, FL: Psychological Assessment Resources.

Greenspan, S.I., & Wieder, S. (1997). An integrated developmental approach to interventions for young children with severe difficulties in relating and communicating. In S.I. Greenspan, K. Kalmanson, R. Shahmoon-Shanok, S. Wieder, G.G. Williamson, & M. Anzalone (Eds.), *Assessing and treating infants and young children with severe difficulties in relating and communication* (pp. 5–17). Washington, DC: ZERO TO THREE: National Center for Infants, Toddlers, and Families.

Griffith, E.M., Pennington, B.F., Wehner, E.A., & Rogers, S.J. (1999). Executive functions in young children with autism. *Child Development, 70*(4), 817–832.

Happé, F., Ehlers, S., Fletcher, P., Frith, U., Johannson, M., Gillberg, C., Dolan, R., Frackowiak, R., & Frith, C. (1996). "Theory of mind" in the brain: Evidence from a PET scan study of Asperger syndrome. *Neuroreport, 8,* 197–201.

Hatfield, E., Cacioppo, J.T., & Rapson, R.L. (1994). *Emotional contagion.* New York: Cambridge University Press.

Heimann, M. (1989). Neonatal imitation, gaze aversion, and mother–infant interaction. *Infant Behavior and Development, 12,* 495–505.

Hermelin, B., & O'Connor, N. (1970). *Psychological experiments with autistic children.* New York: Pergamon.

Hobson, R.P. (1993). *Autism and the development of mind.* Mahwah, NJ: Lawrence Erlbaum Associates.
Hughes, C. (1996). Control of action and thought: Normal development and dysfunction in autism. A research note. *Journal of Child Psychology and Psychiatry and Allied Disciplines, 37,* 229–236.
Hughes, C., Russell, J., & Robbins, T.W. (1994). Evidence for a central executive dysfunction in autism. *Neuropsychologia, 32,* 477–492.
Kanner, L. (1943). Autistic disturbances of affective contact. *Nervous Child, 2,* 217–250.
Kaufman, B. (1976). *Son-rise.* New York: HarperCollins.
Kimura, D., & Archibald, Y. (1974). Motor functions of the left hemisphere. *Brain, 97,* 337–350.
Knott, F., Lewis, C., & Williams, T. (1995). Sibling interaction of children with learning disabilities: A comparison of autism and Down's syndrome. *Journal of Child Psychology and Psychiatry and Allied Disciplines, 36,* 965–976.
Kohen-Raz, R., Volkmar, F.R., & Cohen, D.J. (1992). Postural control in children with autism. *Journal of Autism and Developmental Disorders, 22,* 419–432.
Kolb, B., & Milner, B. (1981). Performance of complex arm and facial movements after focal brain lesions. *Neuropsychologia, 19,* 505–514.
Lovaas, O.I. (1981). *Teaching developmentally disabled children: The me book.* Baltimore: University Park Press.
Lovaas, O.I. (1987). Behavioral treatment and normal educational and intellectual functioning in young autistic children. *Journal of Consulting and Clinical Psychology, 55*(1), 3–9.
Lovaas, O.I., & Schreibman, L. (1971). Stimulus over-selectivity of autistic children in a two stimulus situation. *Behavior Research and Therapy, 9,* 305–310.
Loveland, K., Tunali-Kotoski, B., Pearson, D., Brelsford, K., Ortegon, J., & Chen, R. (1994). Imitation and expression of facial affect in autism. *Development and Psychopathology, 6,* 433–444.
Manjiviona, J., & Prior, M. (1995). Comparison of Asperger syndrome and high-functioning autistic children on a test of motor impairment. *Journal of Autism and Developmental Disorders, 25*(1), 23–40.
McEvoy, R.E., Rogers, S., & Pennington, B.F. (1993). Executive function and social communication deficits in young autistic children. *Journal of Child Psychology and Psychiatry and Allied Disciplines, 34,* 563–578.
McGee, G. (1997). *The Walden Toddler and Preschool Project.* Paper presented at the National Early Childhood Technical Assistance System conference on early intervention for young children with autism, Denver.
McIntosh, D.N. (1996). Facial feedback hypothesis: Evidence, implications, and directions. *Motivation and Emotion, 20*(2), 121–147.
Meltzoff, A. (1988). Infant imitation after a 1-week delay: Long-term memory for novel acts and multiple stimuli. *Developmental Psychology, 24,* 470–476.
Meltzoff, A., & Gopnik, A. (1993). The role of imitation in understanding persons and developing a theory of mind. In S. Baron-Cohen, H. Tager-Flusberg, & D.J. Cohen (Eds.), *Understanding other minds* (pp. 335–366). Oxford, England: Oxford University Press.
Mesibov, G., Schopler, E., & Hearsey, K.A. (1994). Structured teaching. In E. Schopler & G. Mesibov (Eds.), *Behavioral issues in autism* (pp. 195–207). New York: Plenum.
Minshew, N.J., Goldstein, G., Muenz, L.R., & Payton, J.B. (1992). Neuropsychological functioning in nonmentally retarded autistic individuals. *Journal of Clinical and Experimental Neuropsychology, 14,* 749–761.

Minshew, N.J., Goldstein, G., & Siegel, D.J. (1997). Neuropsychologic functioning in autism: Profile of a complex information processing disorder. *Journal of the International Neuropsychological Society, 3,* 303–316.

Mundy, P., & Markus, J. (1997). On the nature of communication and language impairment in autism. *Mental Retardation and Developmental Disabilities Research Reviews, 3,* 349.

Ornitz, E.M. (1973). Childhood autism: A review of the clinical and experimental literature. *California Medicine, 118,* 21–47.

Osterling, J., & Dawson, G. (1994). Early recognition of children with autism: A study of first birthday home videotapes. *Journal of Autism and Developmental Disorders, 24,* 247–257.

Osterling, J., & Dawson, G. (1999, April). *Early recognition of infants with autism versus mental retardation.* Paper presented at the biennial meeting of the Society for Research in Child Development, Albuquerque, New Mexico.

Ozonoff, S. (1998). Assessment and remediation of executive dysfunction in autism and Asperger syndrome. In E. Schopler, G.B. Mesibov, & L. Kunce (Eds.), *Asperger syndrome or high-functioning autism?* (pp. 263–292). New York: Plenum.

Ozonoff, S., & McEvoy, R.E. (1994). A longitudinal study of executive function and theory of mind development in autism. *Development and Psychopathology, 6,* 415–431.

Ozonoff, S., Pennington, B.F., & Rogers, S J. (1991). Executive function deficits in high-functioning autistic individuals: Relationship to theory of mind. *Journal of Child Psychology and Psychiatry and Allied Disciplines, 32,* 1081–1105.

Ozonoff, S., Rogers, S.J., & Pennington, B.F. (1991). Asperger's syndrome: Evidence of an empirical distinction from high-functioning autism. *Journal of Child Psychology and Psychiatry and Allied Disciplines, 32,* 1107–1122.

Ozonoff, S., Strayer, D.L., McMahon, W.M., & Filloux, F. (1994). Executive function abilities in autism and Tourette syndrome: An information processing approach. *Journal of Child Psychology and Psychiatry and Allied Disciplines, 35,* 1015–1032.

Pennington, B.F., & Ozonoff, S. (1996). Executive functions and developmental psychopathology. *Journal of Child Psychology and Psychiatry and Allied Disciplines, 37,* 51–87.

Perner, J., Leekam, S.R., & Wimmer, H. (1987). Three-year-olds' difficulty with false belief: The case for a conceptual deficit. *British Journal of Developmental Psychiatry, 5,* 125–137.

Perner, J., Frith, U., Leslie, A.M., & Leekam, S.R. (1989). Exploration of the autistic child's theory of mind: Knowledge, belief, and communication. *Child Development, 60,* 689–700.

Prior, M., & Hoffman, W. (1990). Brief report: Neuropsychological testing of autistic children through an exploration with frontal lobe tests. *Journal of Autism and Developmental Disorders, 20,* 581–590.

Rogers, S.J. (1998). Neuropsychology of autism in young children and its implications for early intervention. *Mental Retardation and Developmental Disabilities Research Reviews, 4,* 104–112.

Rogers, S.J. (1999). An examination of the imitation deficit in autism. In J. Nadel & G. Butterworth (Eds.), *Imitation in infancy* (pp. 254–283). Cambridge, England: Cambridge University Press.

Rogers, S.J., Bennetto, L., McEvoy, R., & Pennington, B.F. (1996). Imitation and pantomime in high-functioning adolescents with autism spectrum disorders. *Child Development, 67,* 2060–2073.

Rogers, S.J., Hall, T., Osaki, D., Reaven, J., & Herbison, J. (in press). The Denver Model: A comprehensive, integrated educational approach to young children with autism and their families. In S. Harris & J. Handleman (Eds.), *Preschool education programs for children with autism* (2nd ed.). Austin, TX: PRO-ED.

Rogers, S.J., & Pennington, B.F. (1991). A theoretical approach to the deficits in infantile autism. *Development and Psychopathology, 3,* 137–162.

Rumsey, J.M. (1985). Conceptual problem-solving in highly verbal, nonretarded autistic men. *Journal of Autism and Developmental Disorders, 15,* 23–36.

Rumsey, J.M., & Hamburger, S.D. (1988). Neuropsychological findings in high-functioning men with infantile autism, residual state. *Journal of Clinical and Experimental Neuropsychology, 10,* 201–221.

Rumsey, J.M., & Hamburger, S.D. (1990). Neuropsychological divergence of high-level autism and severe dyslexia. *Journal of Autism and Developmental Disorders, 20,* 155–168.

Russell, J. (1997). How executive disorders can bring about inadequate "theory of mind." In J. Russell (Ed.), *Autism as an executive disorder* (pp. 256–304). New York: Oxford University Press.

Russell, J., Jarrold, C., & Henry, L. (1996). Working memory in children with autism and with moderate learning disabilities. *Journal of Child Psychology and Psychiatry and Allied Disciplines, 37,* 673–686.

Russell, J., Mauthner, N., Sharpe, S., & Tidswell, T. (1991). The "windows task" as a measure of strategic deception in preschoolers and autistic subjects. *British Journal of Developmental Psychology, 9,* 331–349.

Scheerer, M., Rothman, E., & Goldstein, K. (1945). A case of "idiot savant": An experimental study of personality organization. *Psychological Monographs, 58,* 1–63.

Seal, B.C., & Bonvillian, J.D. (1997). Sign language and motor functioning in students with autistic disorder. *Journal of Autism and Developmental Disorders, 27*(4), 437–466.

Shallice, T. (1982). Specific impairments of planning. *Philosophical Transactions of the Royal Society of London, Series B: Biology Sciences, 298,* 199–209.

Smith, I.M., & Bryson, S.E. (1994). Imitation and action in autism: A critical review. *Psychological Bulletin, 116,*(2), 259–273.

Smith, I., & Bryson, S. (1998). Gestures imitation in autism: Nonsymbolic postures and sequences. *Cognitive Neuropsychology, 15*(6), 747–770.

Steel, J.G., Gorman, R., & Flexman, J.E. (1984). Neuropsychiatric testing in an autistic mathematical idiot-savant: Evidence for nonverbal abstract capacity. *Journal of the American Academy of Child Psychiatry, 23,* 704–707.

Stern, D.N. (1985). *The interpersonal world of the human infant.* New York: Basic Books.

Stone, W.L., & Hogan, K.L. (1993). A structured parent interview for identifying young children with autism. *Journal of Autism and Developmental Disorders, 23,* 639–652.

Stone, W.L., & Lemanek, K.L. (1991). Parental report of social behaviors in autistic preschoolers. *Journal of Autism and Developmental Disorders, 20,* 513–522.

Stone, W.L., Ousley, O.Y., & Littleford, C.D. (1997). Motor imitation in young children with autism: What's the object? *Journal of Abnormal Child Psychology, 25,* 475–485.

Sykes, E., & Russell, J. (1997, April). *Planning problems in autism: Can they be explained by an impairment in working memory?* Poster session presented at the biennial meeting of the Society for Research in Child Development, Washington, DC.

Szatmari, P., Bartolucci, G., Bremmer, R., Bond, S., & Rich, S. (1989). A follow-up study of high functioning autistic children. *Journal of Autism and Developmental Disorders, 19,* 213–225.

Szatmari, P., Tuff, L., Finlayson, M.A.J., & Bartolucci, G. (1990). Asperger's syndrome and autism: Neurocognitive aspects. *Journal of the American Academy of Child and Adolescent Psychiatry, 29,* 130–136.

Tager-Flusberg, H. (1993). What language reveals about the understanding of minds in children with autism. In S. Baron-Cohen, H. Tager-Flusberg, & D.J. Cohen, (Eds.), *Understanding other minds: Perspectives from autism* (pp. 138–157). Oxford, England: Oxford University Press.

Turner, M. (1997, April). *Working memory and strategy use in high-functioning and learning disabled individuals with autism.* Poster session presented at the biennial meeting of the Society for Research in Child Development, Washington, DC.

Wing, L. (1981). Asperger's syndrome: A clinical account. *Psychological Medicine, 11,* 115–129.

6

Understanding the Nature of Communication and Language Impairments

Amy M. Wetherby, Barry M. Prizant, and Adriana L. Schuler

The acquisition of communication and language is a major challenge faced by children with autism spectrum disorder (ASD). The significance of this challenge is reflected in conceptualizations of autism, which include impairments of verbal and nonverbal communication as a primary diagnostic feature (American Psychiatric Association, 1994). The level of communicative competence attained by individuals with autism has been found to be an important predictor of more positive outcomes (Garfin & Lord, 1986; McEachin, Smith, & Lovaas, 1993). The presence of fluent speech, defined as using multiword combinations spontaneously, communicatively, and regularly, before the age of 5 continues to be a good prognostic indicator of subsequent IQ scores, language measures, adaptive skills and academic achievement in adolescence (Lord & Paul, 1997). The severity of the communicative impairment may be one of the greatest sources of stress for families (Bristol, 1984). Therefore, enhancement of communication and language abilities needs to be a major focus in education and clinical intervention for children with autism and their families.

This chapter provides a review of the research on the nature of communication and language impairments in autism. Several different explanatory theories are examined to offer a better understanding of the profile of strengths and weaknesses in communication, language, and related abilities. Clinical implications for earlier identification, documentation of meaningful outcomes, and decision making about efficacy of intervention are discussed, and directions for future research are suggested.

NATURE OF THE COMMUNICATION AND LANGUAGE IMPAIRMENT IN AUTISM

Major advances have been made in delineating and understanding the communication and language difficulties of children with autism since the 1980s. This progress has resulted in a greater emphasis on early sociocommunicative patterns in the diagnostic criteria (American Psychiatric Association, 1994). The communication and language impairments of children with autism range from failure to develop any functional speech to the development of functional but idiosyncratic use of spontaneous speech and language (Lord & Paul, 1997). At least one third (Bryson, 1996) to one half (Lord & Paul, 1997) of children and adults with autism have no speech. For both verbal and nonverbal individuals, impairments in social aspects of language and related cognitive skills are the most salient (Lord & Paul, 1997; Wetherby, Schuler, & Prizant, 1997).

Research since the 1980s has identified communication deficits in children with autism that fall into two major areas: 1) the capacity for joint attention, which reflects difficulty coordinating attention between people and objects, and 2) the capacity for symbol use, which reflects difficulty learning conventional or shared meanings for symbols and is evident in acquiring language as well as symbolic play. The following section reviews research exploring the capacity for joint attention and symbol use in children with autism.

Capacity for Joint Attention

A deficit in joint attention is a core feature of autism in the diagnostic criteria of the *Diagnostic and Statistical Manual of Mental Disorders, Fourth Edition* (DSM-IV; APA, 1994), and includes a limited inclination to share enjoyment, interests, or achievements with other people. It is not that children with autism do not communicate but, rather, that they do not readily communicate for social goals or purposes. That is, they communicate predominantly or exclusively to regulate the behavior of others to get them to do something (request) or to stop doing something (protest). What is lacking is the use of communication for joint attention to draw another's attention to an object or event (comment or label) (Curcio, 1978; Loveland & Landry, 1986; McHale, Simeonsson, Marcus, & Olley, 1980; Sigman, Mundy, Sherman, & Ungerer, 1986; Wetherby, Prizant, & Hutchinson, 1998; Wetherby & Prutting, 1984; Wetherby, Yonclas, & Bryan, 1989). This deficit in communicating for joint attention appears to be a hallmark of autism and is not characteristic of children with developmental language disorders or mental retardation. Because the ability to communicate for joint attention emerges before words in typical development, this type of deficit may represent a fundamental or core impairment of autism (Mundy, Sigman, & Kasari, 1990; Sigman et al., 1999) and should be evident in very young children (Wetherby & Prizant, 1992; Wetherby et al., 1998). Furthermore, Mundy and colleagues (1990) found that measures of gestural joint attention (e.g., showing or pointing to direct attention) at initial testing were a significant predictor of language development 13 months later for preschool children with autism, whereas none of the other nonverbal measures, initial language scores, mental age, chronological age, or IQ scores were significant predictors. These findings were further substantiated in a larger follow-up study examining the communicative behaviors and language skills of more than 50 children with autism between the ages of 10 and 13 (Sigman et al., 1999). Limitations in joint attention were closely linked with deficits in play, emotional responsiveness, and peer interactions. Accumulated data suggest that the failure to acquire gestural joint attention may be a critical milestone that impairs language development and may be an important target for early communication intervention (see Chapter 4).

Research has examined contributions of social-affective and attentional mechanisms to the joint attention deficits in autism. Competence in sharing affective states is evident in a young child's ability to orient to social stimuli, to coordinate eye gaze between the object of focus and the caregiver, to display positive and negative affect directed to the caregiver, and to read and interpret the affective expressions of the caregiver (Prizant & Wetherby, 1990). Although there are clinical descriptions of children with autism who have pronounced deficits in the ability to share affective states, there is little empirical research in this area (APA, 1994; Dawson, Hill, Spencer, Galpert, & Watson, 1990). Children with autism have been found to display less eye gaze directed to people and less positive affect during interactions with unfamiliar adults (Snow, Hertzig, & Shapiro, 1987). Dawson and colleagues (1990) found that children with autism did not differ significantly in the frequency of gaze at their mothers' faces or displays of positive affect but showed significantly less positive affect coordinated with eye gaze and were much less likely to respond to their mothers' smile than were typical children. The frequency of gaze that children with autism directed to their mothers was significantly correlated with receptive and expressive language. These findings indicate that at the root of their language difficulties, children with autism have a substantial deficit in sharing positive affect, even when interacting with familiar adults.

Joint attention and shared positive affect may well be interrelated and both require that the proper attention is allocated to people as well as objects or events. Kasari, Sigman, Mundy, and Yirmiya (1990) compared affect displays of children communicating for joint attention with affect displays during behavior regulation. They found that typically developing children showed positive affect during episodes of sharing attention on objects or events, whereas children with autism showed lower levels of shared affect and did not show this integration of shared affect and joint attention. Children with autism show deficits in responding to as well as initiating bids for shared attention. McArthur and Adamson (1996) found that when a child with autism interacted with an adult who was calling the child's attention to an object or event to establish shared attention, episodes of joint attention were rare. During these adult-initiated episodes of joint attention, the children with autism displayed significantly less attention directed to the adult partner as well as to the objects of reference than did children with developmental language disorders matched on chronological and nonverbal mental age. The authors concluded that the difficulties of children with autism in acquiring shared meanings of cultural conventions may be traced to more basic limitations in the allocation of attention between people and objects.

The constellation of joint attention deficits may be rooted in an early failure to orient to social stimuli. Dawson, Meltzoff, Osterling, Rinaldi, and Brown (1998) found that children with autism more frequently failed to orient to social as well as nonsocial stimuli, compared with children with Down syndrome or typical development, but that this failure was much more pronounced for social stimuli. Moreover, responses to social stimuli were found to be delayed in timing. The failure to orient to social stimuli was significantly correlated with performance on a shared attention task in which the child was asked to follow the gaze and the point of the experimenter in reference to an object in front of or behind the child. Dawson and colleagues concluded that the shared attention impairments in children with autism are a result of a more basic failure to selectively attend to social stimuli (see Chapter 4 for a more detailed discussion of this theory).

Joint attention is an attentional state during which the child and partner share a site of interest (Adamson & Chance, 1998) and is thought to be an important milestone in the development of language. This coordination of attention provides a critical moment for language learning when the caregiver models language that interprets and relates the child's experience to the environment. The capacity for joint attention reflects the culmination of four developmental components: orienting and attending to a social partner, coordinating attention between people and objects, sharing affect or emotional states with people, and ultimately being able to draw others' attention to objects or events for the purpose of sharing experiences. Children with autism may have difficulty with all of these components, particularly those children meeting the criteria for autistic disorder. Those children on the autism spectrum who meet the criteria for atypical autism (pervasive developmental disorder-not otherwise specified) are more likely to show some or all of the earlier emerging social skills—orienting to social stimuli, shifting gaze between people and objects, and sharing positive affect—but may not communicate for joint attention. The children who do communicate for joint attention show a much greater degree of sociability. Because a deficit in joint attention is intimately related to communication and language development, it is critical to better characterize the nature and extent of such a deficit in this population and to outline the design of related interventions.

Capacity for Symbol Use

Children with autism have difficulty acquiring conventional and symbolic aspects of communication. They have been found to use fewer vocalizations to express intentions in the early stages of language development compared with children with language disorders, mental retardation, or typical development who are at the same language stage (McHale et al., 1980; Wetherby et al., 1998; Wetherby & Prutting, 1984; Wetherby et al., 1989). The quantity and quality of gestural use, however, is also limited. Children with autism predominantly use primitive presymbolic motoric gestures (i.e., contact gesture of leading, pulling or manipulating another's hand) to communicate. They lack the use of many conventional gestures, such as showing, waving, and pointing, and the use of symbolic gestures, including nodding one's head and depicting actions (Loveland & Landry, 1986; McHale et al., 1980; Stone & Caro-Martinez, 1990; Wetherby et al., 1998; Wetherby et al., 1989). Unlike children with language impairments or hearing impairments, children with autism do not compensate for their lack of speech by using other modalities, such as gestures.

Although deficits in gestural communication are characteristic of children with autism, there is much variability in the use of vocal and verbal communication. Some children with autism have been found to use a limited consonant inventory and less complex syllabic structure, whereas others show adequate complexity of vocalizations (McHale et al., 1980; Stone & Caro-Martinez, 1990; Wetherby & Prutting, 1984; Wetherby et al., 1989). The vast majority of those who do learn to talk go through a period of using echolalia, or the literal repetition of others' speech either immediately (i.e., immediate echolalia) or later (i.e., delayed echolalia; Prizant, Schuler, Wetherby, & Rydell, 1997; Schuler, 1979). An echolalic utterance may be equivalent to a single word or may serve as a label for a situation or event. Differentiating between echolalia and more typical forms of repetition or imitation is not easy. Echolalia is often described as being longer, more exact, and having a monotonous prosody, as compared with imitation of typically developing children (Schuler & Prizant, 1985). Echolalia may serve a variety of communicative and cognitive functions (Prizant & Rydell, 1993), and, not unlike imitation for typically developing children, it may be a productive language learning strategy for many children with autism. The way children who use echolalia learn to talk is by initially repeating phrases associated with situations or emotional states and subsequently learning the meanings of these phrases by finding out how they work. Over time, many children learn to use these "gestalt forms" purposefully in communicative interactions and eventually are able to break down the echolalic chunks into smaller meaningful units as part of the process of transitioning to a rule-governed, generative language system. Pronoun reversals are a byproduct of echolalia because the child repeats the pronoun heard, making the pronouns used in reference to self and other reversed. For example, a child may use the echolalic utterance "Do you want a piece of candy?" as a way to request the candy, although it sounds as though the child is offering the candy because the request is in the form of a question.

In light of evidence that immediate and delayed echolalia may be used for many different communicative functions (e.g., request, protest, affirmation, declarative, calling, rehearsal, self-regulation) (Prizant & Duchan, 1981; Prizant & Rydell, 1984), echolalia should no longer be dismissed as deviant or nonfunctional but rather should be considered relative to its use in communicative exchange. The emergence of echolalia may be a moment of celebration in a child's development, and efforts should be made to determine the boundaries of the gestalt forms that are meaningful to the child. By providing proper contextual support and matching language input, the child can be helped to acquire more creative language (see Prizant & Rydell, 1993). Children with autism who progress beyond echolalia acquire more advanced aspects of grammar; that is, they do well with language form. They develop grammatical skills in the same general progression as children developing typically but show persisting problems in following the social rules and shifting speaker/listener roles of conversation (Baltaxe, 1977; Fay & Schuler, 1980; Tager-Flusberg, 1996; see also Chapter 10), which are pragmatic aspects of language.

The use of echolalia may reflect a strategy that is similar to the primitive presymbolic gestures used by children with autism in the face of an impairment in symbolic communication. We have previously suggested that a reenactment strategy underlies the use of echolalia as well as the reliance on primitive presymbolic motoric gestures (Prizant & Wetherby, 1987; Schuler & Prizant, 1985; Wetherby, 1986). A reenactment involves the linear repetition of a single event or sequence of events in anticipation of an associated outcome. Examples of such strategies are the placement of an adult's hand on the door handle as a request to be let out, getting the car keys to request a car ride, making sounds or movements associated with a tickling game to request being tickled, or repeating a memorized portion of a song as a request to have someone sing the song. These most linear and literal modes of representation occur at early stages of typical communication development and are regarded as *indexical* communication rather than symbolic communication (McLean & Snyder-McLean, 1978). In symbolic communication, the symbol stands for and is separate from its referent. Repeating an action or phrase that is part of the referent or goal is indexical rather than symbolic because it is an index of or associated with the goal (Werner & Kaplan, 1963). An example may serve to clarify this point: A 4-year-old boy with ASD repeatedly approached his preschool teacher and stated, "Do ahh," while opening his mouth. It was clear by his nonverbal behavior that he was trying to communicate something, but his teacher was at a loss to understand his meaning. After school, the teacher called the boy's mother and explained the dilemma. Without hesitation, his mother explained that when her son is not feeling well, she tells her son to open his mouth and "Do ahh" so that she can observe whether his throat is inflamed. Recently, he had begun to initiate interactions with her using this same phrase to "tell" her that he wasn't feeling well. Thus, he used this rather unconventional gestalt language form that he had come to associate with feeling ill.

The communicative repertoire for a child with autism may be restricted to only reenactment strategies. The child's communicative intention may not be easily understood if the partner does not know how the behavior involved relates to a previous event or is not familiar with prior events, as in the example just stated. Reenactments are indicative of some level of anticipation and may be a necessary first step on the way toward symbolic communication for children with autism. These children may need to acquire a large set of communicative behaviors at a reenactment level before they become symbol users. Wetherby (1986) gave the example of a child's learning to call another's attention by first physically pulling her chin toward the child or holding her hand until she focused attention on the child, then later by using the echolalic utterance, "Are you ready?" to gain attention. Although these behaviors may not be conventional or symbolic, they do reflect some level of anticipation, which reflects the emergence of communicative intent.

In lieu of conventional means of communicating, children with autism may develop idiosyncratic, unconventional, or undesirable behaviors to communicate, such as self-injurious behavior, aggression, or tantrums. Despite the fact that at least 50% of individuals with autism display some functional speech and language skills (Lord & Paul, 1997), challenging behaviors often are used to procure attention, to escape from a task or situation, to protest against changes of schedule and routine, or to regulate social interactions in a predictable manner. For example, Carr and Durand (1985) reported that aggression, tantrums, and self-injury were more likely to occur in situations with a high level of task difficulty and a low level of adult attention (see Chapter 13 for strategies to teach replacement skills for challenging behaviors). The use of challenging behavior needs to be considered relative to the repertoire of other verbal and nonverbal communicative behaviors and may reflect limitations in symbolic capacity. Wetherby (1986) gave the example of a child progressing from slapping her face as a protest to using the delayed echolalic utterance, "Will you stop it?" and finally simply using the word, "No," illustrating the shift from reenactment to symbolic communication.

Further evidence of a deficit in the symbolic capacity in autism is the limited ability to develop symbolic or pretend play. Although play is a social-cognitive skill, it is noteworthy that a lack of varied, spontaneous make-believe play is one of the four possible features of impairment in communication in the DSM-IV (APA, 1994). Children with autism show significant deficits in symbolic or make-believe play (i.e., using pretend actions with objects) and limited abilities in functional play (i.e., using objects functionally) (Dawson & Adams, 1984; Sigman & Ungerer, 1984; Wetherby & Prutting, 1984; Wing, Gould, Yeates, & Brierley, 1977). Functional and symbolic play skills have been found to be significantly correlated with receptive and expressive language (Mundy, Sigman, Ungerer, & Sherman, 1987).

The relationship between symbolic play and language acquisition has been emphasized in developmental literature. Both play and language are symbol systems that require the knowledge and capacity to make one thing stand for and represent something else and that are acquired within a social context of sharing attention on objects (Bates, 1979). Typically developing children construct schematic representations of their world through play and exploration. In fact, Westby (1988) suggested that not only does play facilitate effective communication but also that it requires it, underscoring the developmental interaction between language and play (see Chapter 11).

In contrast to deficits in functional object use and symbolic play, children with autism perform at similar or higher levels on constructive play (e.g., using objects in combination to create a product, such as stacking blocks, nesting cups, or putting puzzles together) compared with typically developing children or children with language delays at the same language stage (Wetherby & Prutting, 1984; Wetherby et al., 1998). Bates (1979) suggested that symbolic play is acquired through observational learning and that constructive or combinatorial play can be acquired either through observational learning or trial-and-error problem solving. Children with autism seem to excel at behaviors that do not depend on social interaction and imitation of others but can be learned through trial and error. Many of the reenactment gestures used by children with autism (e.g., taking another's hand and leading the person to a goal) are contextually restricted and can be explained through trial-and-error learning strategies and body exploration. Similarly, constructive play can be learned through trial and error. Observational learning is required to learn more conventional gestures, word meanings, and object use, which entails observing and imitating others within a social context, and must be decontextualized, which involves using conventional behaviors in new contexts to become a functional, symbolic system. Learning shared meanings, using conventional behaviors, and decontextualizing meaning from the context compose the symbolic deficits in children with autism (see Chapter 3 for a discussion of observational and cultural learning).

Distinct Profile of Communicative, Social-Affective, and Symbolic Abilities

Exploring developmental patterns in communicative and symbolic abilities can contribute to better understanding of the nature of these problems in autism to design more effective interventions and predict which children will benefit from specific intervention approaches. Greenspan and Wieder (1997) reviewed 200 children with autism who received treatment and were followed for at least 2 years. The children were diagnosed between 22 months and 4 years of age. On the basis of chart reviews of these 200 children, they reported that 95% of these children evidenced some capacity for emotional relating, which included engagement based on need fulfillment in 30% of this population, some intermittent capacity to engage with reciprocal gestures and imitation in 40%, and the use of some symbolic actions and words in addition to intermittent engaging in the remaining 24%. They found that 96% of these children showed significant receptive language deficits, which included no receptive language understanding in 55% of this population and intermittent ability to understand single words and follow simple directions in 41%. They also reported that prior to 2 years of age, 68% of these children did not evidence complex gestures involving chains of reciprocal interactions (e.g., taking a caregiver to the door and motioning to go outside). The authors suggested that the children who made the most progress in their intervention program were the ones who displayed some ability to use complex gestural interactions. There are obvious limitations of a chart review of developmental patterns and outcomes including a sample that is not representative of the population and a lack of specificity of measures. This chart review of a large number of individuals, however, elucidated clinical patterns of this group of children and provided directions for future research.

Wetherby and colleagues (1998) examined the developmental profiles of children with ASD compared with children with delayed language (DL) who were at the same language stage. They used the Communication and Symbolic Behavior Scales (CSBS; Wetherby & Prizant, 1993) to measure sociocommunicative and symbolic abilities. The CSBS utilizes behavior sampling procedures that include adult-imposed structured and relatively unstructured activities. The context created resembles natural adult–child interactions and allows for the documentation of a child's use of a variety of communicative and symbolic behaviors. Behaviors collected in the sample are rated along a number of parameters and are converted to scores on 22 five-point rating scales of communication and symbolic behaviors. Seven cluster scores are derived from the 22 scales, the first six contributing to the child's profile of communication and the last one to the child's profile of symbolic behaviors:

1. *Communicative Functions* measures the use of gestures, sounds, or words for behavior regulation and for joint attention and measures the proportion of communication used for social functions.
2. *Gestural Communicative Means* measures the variety of conventional gestures (e.g., giving, showing, pointing, reaching), use of distal gestures (e.g., pointing at a distance), and coordination of gestures and vocalizations.
3. *Vocal Communicative Means* measures the use of vocalizations without gestures, inventory of different consonants, and syllabic structure.

4. *Verbal Communicative Means* measures the number of different words and different word combinations produced.
5. *Reciprocity* measures the use of communication in response to the adult's conventional gestures or speech, rate of communicating, and ability to repair communicative breakdowns by repeating and/or modifying previous communication when a goal is not achieved.
6. *Social/Affective Signaling* measures the use of gaze shifts between person and object, expression of positive affect with directed eye gaze, and episodes of negative affect.
7. *Symbolic Behavior* measures comprehension of contextual cues, single words and multiword utterances, the number of different action schemes and complexity of actions schemes in symbolic play, and the level of constructive play.

The CSBS cluster scores indicated distinct profiles of relative strengths and weaknesses for the two groups of children in the study by Wetherby and colleagues (1998). For the children with DL, the cluster scores illustrated a profile of relative strengths in communicative functions, reciprocity, social-affective signaling, and symbolic behavior and relative weaknesses in vocal and verbal means. This pattern is consistent with other research on young children with slow expressive language development (e.g., Paul, 1991; Paul, Looney, & Dahm, 1991; Wetherby et al., 1989) and indicates strengths in sociocommunicative foundation skills for learning to talk in the face of weaknesses in using sounds and words. Compared with the DL group, the children with ASD displayed substantially poorer scores in communicative functions, gestural communicative means, reciprocity, social-affective signaling, and symbolic behavior but displayed comparable scores in vocal and verbal communicative means. More specifically, the children with ASD displayed relative weaknesses in joint attention, sociability of function, gaze shift, and symbolic play and relative strengths in behavior regulation and constructive play. These findings suggest that the profile of children with ASD is characterized by a distinct constellation of strengths and weaknesses in parameters of communication.

Correlational findings from this study showed that there appear to be three clusters of impairments that characterize these young children with ASD: one in joint attention; one in symbolic play; and one in social-affective signaling. The intercorrelations among individual scales help to clarify these relationships. The deficits in joint attention and symbolic play displayed by these children with ASD were not found to be associated with performance on other scales. This finding is consistent with the previous research of Mundy and colleagues (1987) and supports their contention that deficits in joint attention and symbolic play are two independent sources of variation in children with ASD. The scaled scores on gaze shifts and shared positive affect were significantly correlated with numerous other scales, suggesting that the social-affective signaling deficit is associated with other aspects of the communicative and symbolic impairments in these children with ASD. In other words, children who displayed a greater capacity to coordinate attention and affect were more likely to communicate for more social reasons, use a larger repertoire of conventional gestures, use a higher rate of communicating, and use better repair strategies. These findings support the suggestion of Greenspan and Wieder that the difficulty in affect is associated with the capacity to engage in sequences of reciprocal interaction, or what they refer to as "circles of communication" (1997, p. 108).

The children studied by Wetherby and colleagues (1998) ranged from 17 to 60 months of age. The older group with ASD consisted primarily of 3- and 4-year-olds (mean age of 45 months, range from 35 to 60 months) and the younger group consisted primarily of 2-year-olds (mean age of 27 months, range from 17 to 34 months). When results were compared for the older and younger children with ASD, the most pronounced finding was that the 2-year-olds with ASD showed profiles that were very similar to the 3- and 4-year-olds on all clusters except two—vocal and verbal communicative means (Wetherby et al., 1998). The 3- and 4-year-olds with ASD used more consonants and words than did the 2-year-olds with ASD but did not display better performance on any of the other clusters. This finding is in contrast to the performance of the younger and older children with DL. The older children with DL showed substantially better scores than the younger children with DL on the majority of the clusters but showed the least difference on vocal communicative means. Longitudinal research is needed to examine growth curves of these different clusters. The findings of this cross-sectional study predict that growth curves for vocal and verbal communicative means would be very different from growth curves of other clusters of communication and symbolic behaviors for both of these populations. These findings also underscore the importance of documenting changes in communicative and social-affective parameters in addition to vocal/verbal gains, to determine the success of intervention for children with autism.

In summary, research efforts since the 1980s have served to clarify the nature of the communication and language impairments. Core deficits in joint attention, shared affect, conventional and symbolic aspects of communication, and symbolic play are strongly associated with language abilities. These findings provide a challenge for professionals designing intervention programs for individuals with autism and suggest that effective intervention programs should address and document progress in these core deficits. In other words, the efficacy of communication intervention should be determined by meaningful outcome measures in sociocommunicative parameters rather than just by the acquisition of verbal behaviors.

DEVELOPMENTAL FRAMEWORK FOR UNDERSTANDING COMMUNICATION AND LANGUAGE IMPAIRMENTS IN AUTISM

This section explores theoretical perspectives that may better elucidate the social communication problems of children with ASD. We first examine profiles of strengths and weaknesses that characterize the learning styles of children with ASD. Then we explore how developmental theory can contribute to a better understanding of the communication patterns in this population. Finally, we consider the influence of motor impairments on communication and language abilities.

Understanding Communication Patterns in Relation to Social-Cognitive Learning Styles

Aspects of developmental discontinuity in children with autism have intrigued caregivers as well as professionals ever since the publication of Kanner's first case studies (1943), in which he referred to his subjects as cognitively "well endowed" on the basis of observations of isolated specific ability. Approximately two thirds of all individuals with autism have subsequently been described as having intellectual impairments on the basis of their performance on standard IQ tests (DeMyer, 1975). (Of course, the discrepancies across different domains of ability in children with ASD, which range from significant to extreme, call into question the validity and value of distilling "intelligence" into one or two numbers.) Although some of the commonly observed areas of relative ability have been discarded as "splinter skills," the true nature of the cognitive differences and cognitive impairments continues to challenge researchers and practitioners. The often striking contradictions between significant limitations in communicative and adaptive skills and apparent intellectual potential based on observation of specific skills are a source of great frustration for those closely involved with people with ASD and are of great interest and promise as well.

Patterns of relative strengths and weaknesses identified in the literature provide some insight into this matter. Commonly cited abilities of people with autism include an excellent rote memory for both visual and auditory information and proficiencies in tasks demanding visuospatial judgment and pattern recognition (Grandin, 1995; Prior, 1979; Prizant; 1983; Schuler, 1995). Specific skills related to these abilities include memorization, recognition, and reproduction of melodic patterns and lists or series of facts; construction of visuospatial arrays from samples (e.g., elaborate arrangements of blocks); and solution of jigsaw puzzles, form boards, block design tasks, and so forth.

Information processing research, capitalizing on a now classic series of experiments conducted by Frith (1971) and Hermelin and O'Connor (1970), has further clarified the cognitive traits of individuals with autism. These experiments have demonstrated that these individuals perform well on tasks that rely on spatial location and simultaneous information processing but have difficulty with the coding and categorization of sequential information. Furthermore, children with autism performed equally well in the recall of nonsensical (not arranged or presented in a meaningful manner) as opposed to meaningful series of information, when visual as well as auditory stimulus input was presented (Hermelin, 1976). This finding is in contrast to control groups of typically developing children who did better in the recall of meaningful series because meaning was used to support processing. In other words, children with autism employed a rote memorization strategy that was not aided by meaningful stimuli. This has been interpreted by Hermelin and O'Connor as reflecting an impairment with the coding and categorization of information.

Frequently cited characteristics of language and communicative behavior in ASDs may be understood in reference to analogous differences in cognitive and language styles of typically developing children. A differentiation between gestalt versus analytic forms has been made in reference to differences in styles of language acquisition (i.e., gestalt versus analytic styles) (Peters, 1983; Prizant, 1983). Gestalt language forms are multiword utterances that are memorized and produced as single units or chunks, with little analysis of their internal linguistic structure and with little or no comprehension of the utterances themselves. Analytic forms, on the other hand, are generated on the basis of the application of previously acquired linguistic rules and greater comprehension of constituent structure and of the specific meanings encoded by those utterances and their component parts. These two different forms of language have been noted to be used by some typically developing children as well and appear to be of great relevance to understanding language acquisition strategies in populations with various disabilities (Prizant, 1983; Schuler & Prizant, 1985; Wills, 1979).

Prizant (1983) proposed that children with autism use a gestalt strategy in early language learning by repeating unanalyzed chunks or multiword units of speech and subsequently breaking down these units into meaningful segments. Repetition of language "chunks" may occur immediately (as in the case of immediate echolalia) or later (as in the case of delayed echolalia). It appears that most verbal individuals with autism demonstrate a gestalt style of language acquisition in that early utterances are typically rigidly echolalic (Ricks & Wing, 1975), and early communicative functions expressed through speech tend to be served by immediate and delayed echolalia (Prizant, 1983, 1987; Schuler & Prizant, 1985). This cognitive style is a relatively inflexible mode of information processing that results in the memorization of unanalyzed "chunks" of information including speech as well as visual stimulus input. In contrast, a more analytic style allows for the decoding of the specific meanings of the component parts of a sequence in relation to each other. This is based on the extraction of the meaning, or gist, of experiences by interrelating the relevant pieces of information with reference to previous experiences and not by simply storing information to be later reproduced in an identical fashion (Fay & Schuler, 1980; Prizant, 1983). Prizant suggested that for many verbal children with autism, language acquisition progresses from the predominant use of echolalia with little evidence of comprehension or communicative intent to the use of echolalia for a variety of communicative functions, later followed by a decrease in echolalia co-occurring with an increase in creative, spontaneously generated utterances. Pronoun reversals, stereotypic utterances, and insistence on certain verbal routines, all common characteristics of language use of verbal individuals, may also reflect a gestalt strategy in acquisition and use. The prevalence of gestalt forms can thus be conceptualized as variation at the extreme end of the typical continuum, which apparently corresponds with differences in cognitive style.

On the basis of extensive nonverbal investigations of the conceptual and representational abilities of a mute adolescent with autism, and on larger-scale follow-up studies, Schuler (1979, 1995) and Schuler and Bormann (1983) suggested that individuals with autism seem to perform considerably better with nontransient than with transient stimulus input and when only judgment of object, material properties, and spatial orientation is required rather than when judgment about the impact of one's own and others' action is required. An understanding of social causality requires processing of temporally organized, sequential cues. An understanding of object properties and spatial relations is acquired more readily by individuals with ASD because of the nontransient nature of the discriminations involved. It may be speculated that, at least in part, specific weaknesses are noted in social-communicative domains because signals that regulate social interactions are largely transient, as are the interactions themselves.

Weaknesses in processing transient signals may also contribute to gestalt patterns. Processing of transient signals is critical when it comes to comprehending the constituent structure of utterances and constructing a generative grammatical system. Construction of a linguistic rule system requires rapid processing of both auditory and visual transient information (speech as well as nonverbal cues) with the ability to focus on consistencies and variation within speech and nonverbal behavior as they occur relative to objects and social or nonsocial environmental events. A gestalt mode of processing is ill-suited to the apprehension of transient signals and clearly is counterproductive when it comes to unraveling the temporally coded segmental structure of spoken language as well as the temporal structure of social interaction (Prizant, 1983). Common reports on precocious written word skills, or even on so-called hyperlexia (Aram & Healy, 1988), are of relevance in this context. A major difference between written and spoken language lies within the coding mechanisms involved—that is, in the utilization of nontransient versus transient signals. Because the processing of written language is not as dependent on sequential analyses, superior written-word skills in individuals with autism are readily explained.

It may thus be that the preference for nontransient signals and the associated information processing style impedes the acquisition of the more flexible rule-governed systems of linguistic and social knowledge. Or, it also could be argued that the prevalent cognitive style in ASDs results from impaired social interaction, if early social experience is viewed as a primary determinant of more flexible social and linguistic rule systems and the modes of processing associated therewith. In other words, social interaction limitations can be explained partially on the basis of cognitive style differences, or cognitive style differences can be explained on the basis of early and pervasive limitations in joint attention and social interaction. Whatever the case, approaches to communication enhancement that address the cognitive discrepancies (taking into account both strengths and weaknesses) and the gestalt style of language acquisition and use would seem to be interventions of "best fit" considering the distinctly different learning style of children with autism (Grandin, 1995; Prizant & Rydell, 1993; Prizant & Wetherby, 1989; Schuler, 1995). Commonly cited challenges, including lack of flexibility in communication and language, development of unconventional verbal behavior including echolalia, insistence on preservation of sameness, and an overreliance on social routines and rituals, need to be approached and understood as a result of these cognitive differences, as opposed to simply as a related list of deficits (Prizant, 1983).

Another conceptualization of social-cognitive processing differences was offered by Frith (1989). She suggested that the extremely literal ways in which people with autism process information is indicative of a reduced awareness of how one's own state of mind may be similar to or different from the thoughts of others. Children with autism have been found to have difficulty understanding the beliefs and desires of others in experiments designed to measure the construct of theory of mind (ToM; Baron-Cohen, Leslie, & Frith, 1985, 1986). On the basis of ToM research findings, Baron-Cohen (1988) proposed that the primary deficit in autism is cognitive in nature, involving a selective impairment in the capacity for *metarepresentation* or beliefs about other people's mental states. Baron-Cohen accounted for the deficits in joint attention and other pragmatic skills, as well as in symbolic play and ToM, by an impaired metarepresentational capacity and urged for an integration of the cognitive and affective theories. In consideration of the relatively early emergence of joint attention, it is plausible and even likely that the impairment in joint attention, which precedes the emergence of metarepresentational skills, is primary and underlies subsequent impairments in ToM and intentionality at large. These interrelations speak to the close relationship between attention, cognition, and affect (Sigman & Kasari, 1995; Sigman et al., 1999; Chapter 4).

Understanding Communication Patterns from a Transactional Developmental Perspective

The literature on development of children without disabilities provides a rich theoretical foundation for both understanding communication problems and for guiding effective and developmentally appropriate interventions. The dramatic changes in language abilities that occur during the first 2 years of life are reflected in three major transitions: first, the transition to *intentional communication,* marked by the systematic use of conventional behaviors to deliberately affect another person; second, the transition to *symbolic communication,* marked initially by a period of slow acquisition of *first words* followed by a period of sudden acceleration in the rate of new word acquisition, which is known as the *vocabulary burst;* and third, the transition to *linguistic communication,* marked by the semantic basis of language development, the construction of multiword combinations, and the onset of grammar (see Wetherby, Reichle, & Pierce, 1998). Understanding how children proceed through these transitions in typical development offers a road map to guide clinicians and educators working with children with autism in their efforts to enhance communication and language abilities.

There is no evidence to suggest that children with ASD do not proceed through these major transitions in an order similar to that of typical children (Lord & Paul, 1997). Although many children with autism eventually acquire language, most have difficulties initially acquiring aspects of intentional communication and making the transition to symbolic communication. What differs in children with autism is the combination of skills that are available at each of these major developmental shifts. For example, children who first use echolalia may have the articulation and memory skills to produce "sentences" but may be functioning at the "first words" stage, which represents the transition between intentional and symbolic communication. That is, it appears as though they are talking in sentences, but their true language level is at the one word stage. Just like first words in typical development, early-appearing echolalic utterances may be tied to emotional states or specific contexts or situations.

Language learning is an active process in which children "construct" knowledge and shared meanings based on interactions with people and experiences in their environment (Bates, 1979; Bloom, 1993; Lifter & Bloom, 1998). It is interesting to reflect on the acquisition process and consider how and why children learn to talk. What is the impetus for moving through the transition to intentional, symbolic, and, ultimately, linguistic communication? What are implications of this for children with ASD?

Stern (1985) described three achievements that contribute to a child's sense of self and capacity to use language to share experiences about events and things and thus provide the foundation for socioemotional and communication development—sharing of focus of attention ("interattentionality"), sharing of intentions ("interintentionality"), and sharing of affective states ("interaffectivity"). These three achievements lead to the developmental leap of "intersubjective relatedness" as the infant discovers that he or she has a mind, that other people have minds, and that inner subjective experiences can be shared. Stern suggested that emotional regulation of different internal states promotes different senses of the self (see Chapter 9 for a discussion of the important role of emotional regulation in enhancing communication skills of children with ASD). Children with ASD may have grave difficulty sharing attention, intention, and affect. Deficits in these core socioemotional achievements may disrupt the transactional process required for communication and language acquisition.

Tomasello and colleagues (Tomasello, 1992; Tomasello, Kruger, & Ratner, 1993; see also Chapter 3) presented a theory of human cultural learning to account for the precision with which humans can transmit information and learn from one another that is not evident in nonhuman species. Building on Vygotsky's (1934/1962) view of language learning as a social enterprise, Tomasello (1992) suggested that two components are essential for a child to develop language—development within a cultural context that structures events for the child and the child's special capacity to learn from this cultural structuring. The structuring for language acquisition entails routine cultural activities that employ coordinated attention and delineated social roles. The child's social-cognitive skills of being able to attribute intentions to others and to adopt others' perspectives allows for these cultural forms of learning.

Bloom (1993) posited that the "child's intentionality drives the acquisition of language." Children acquire language in order to share their ideas, thoughts, and feelings. When children begin to talk, they use words to communicate the same meanings for the same purposes as they did through preverbal communicative means (Bates, 1976; Lahey, 1988). As their ideas and needs become more complex, a more explicit system of communicating is required. The emergence of ritualized, context-bound first words sets into motion the development of a symbolic, referential language system. A developmental perspective suggests that the most basic joint attention difficulties in children with ASD may underlie their difficulty acquiring contextually flexible use of language.

Bloom (1993) suggested that children are guided in their efforts to learn to talk by three principles of word learning: relevance, discrepancy, and elaboration. These three principles provide a developmental framework for targeting first words and lexicon at the vocabulary burst. First, the principle of relevance states that a child learns words when they are relevant to what the child has in mind. Therefore, the selection of words for an initial lexicon should reflect what captivates the child's attention and the important meanings that a child wants to share. The critical role of joint attention episodes in language learning supports this principle (Adamson & Chance, 1998). For children with ASD, the intention to communicate must drive the acquisition of language, and, therefore, emphasis should be placed on the child's intention to communicate not just on teaching language forms devoid of intention. Second, the principle of discrepancy states that what a child has in mind goes beyond that information known to others or anticipated from the context. Young children have an impressive ability to consider what information is needed by the listener and to provide just that. When children first use words, they are likely to talk about things that are evident from the context. As children approach the vocabulary burst, they talk more about events that they anticipate but that are not evident to someone else. Thus, for children with ASD, it is critical to design language learning contexts in which there is a real communicative need to share information, particularly as they approach the vocabulary burst, so that they can develop the ability to consider the listener's needs. Third, the principle of elaboration states that as a child's mental representations expand, the child must learn more words to express these ideas. Efforts to expand a child's vocabulary would be well placed on building a child's knowledge about objects, actions, agents, and recipients of actions. During the transition from symbolic communication to linguistic communication, a child's conceptual and emotional development promote the capacity and need for language learning. For children with autism, efforts to enhance language should be integrated with play and socioemotional development.

Many patterns of development in children with ASD are similar to typical development, although the timing of acquisition is different and, therefore, the combination of skills (i.e., discrepancies across social, cognitive, and linguistic domains) that a child with ASD has at any one point in time is unlikely to be seen in typical development. These rich developmental theories and the research that they have generated offer a framework for understanding a child's developing competencies in relationship to the social context and how these patterns change over developmental stages, which can offer intervention approaches that are developmentally appropriate (Wetherby et al., 1997; see Chapter 9).

Role of Motor Functioning in Communication Development for Children with Autism Spectrum Disorder

The role of motor functioning in communication and language development is widely recognized, yet little information has been reported on either fine motor development or the incidence of motor disorders in children with autism (Seal & Bonvillian, 1997). Children with ASD often are described as well coordinated or as having good motor skills; however, anecdotal observations and firsthand accounts as well as the limited research reported on motor functioning have revealed motor difficulties in the vast majority of children and adults with ASD (Hill & Leary, 1993). Although a thorough coverage of motor functioning is beyond the scope of this chapter, we briefly examine research on apraxia, dyskinesia, and motor imitation in autism (see Chapter 8 for a discussion of apraxia and Chapter 5 for a discussion of the role of imitation and apraxia in ASDs).

The difficulties children with autism have with learning to speak or using sign language may be compounded by apraxia, in addition to sociocommunicative and symbolic impairments. Apraxia is a neurogenic impairment involving difficulty planning, executing, and sequencing movements (LaPointe & Katz, 1998). Apraxia may involve oral, hand, and/or whole body movements and is not due to muscle weakness. The co-existence of apraxia in individuals with autism received much attention during the facilitated communication movement in the early 1990s (see Calculator, Fabry, Glennen, Prizant, & Schubert, 1995, and Shane, 1994, for a comprehensive consideration of research and practice in facilitated communication). Despite the controversy surrounding facilitated communication, the role of apraxia in speech and language acquisition of children with ASD is frequently observed by clinicians and merits attention and consideration, but little research is available. Seal and Bonvillian (1997) analyzed sign language formation of 14 low-functioning students with autism for accuracy of sign location, hand shape, and movement production and found that location aspects of signs were produced more accurately than either hand shape or movement aspects. The size of the sign vocabulary and accuracy of sign formation were highly correlated with measures of fine motor abilities and tests of apraxia. These findings support the role of a motor impairment in the competence attained in sign language acquisition and indicate the need for further research in this area.

Damasio and Maurer have formulated a theory of the neurological basis of autism based on commonalities between motor disturbances in autism and conditions found in adult neurology (Damasio & Maurer, 1978; Maurer, 1999; Maurer & Damasio, 1982). Vilensky, Damasio, and Maurer (1981) documented movement disturbances in individuals with autism that resemble dyskinesias in patients with Parkinson's disease. They conducted movement analyses on 21 individuals with autism and 15 typical children moving from a sitting to a standing position, walking barefoot, and jumping. They found that virtually all of the children with autism moved their limbs more slowly with diminished angular motion at three joints (hip, knee, and ankle) and displayed abnormalities of postural fixation comparable to patients with parkinsonism. More recently, Teitelbaum, Teitelbaum, Nye, Fryman, and Maurer (1998) studied movement disturbances from infant videotapes of 17 children later diagnosed with autism. They found differences in the age of acquisition and quality of lying, righting, sitting, crawling, and walking and noted an atypical mouth shape in some of the children. They reported that these abnormalities in movement were evident in children as young as 4–6 months of age and suggested that movement disturbances may play an important role in early diagnosis. Caution should be taken in drawing strong conclusions from these findings because no control groups of children with other developmental disabilities were reported with these techniques and therefore it is not known whether these motor differences distinguish children with ASD from children with other developmental disabilities.

Another line of research that supports the central role of motor impairments in autism is the study of imitation. Numerous studies have documented that children with autism have difficulty on tasks of body imitation involving simple motor movements and facial expressions as well as symbolic pantomimes and actions with objects, compared with chronological and mental age matched control groups (see Rogers & Pennington, 1991, and Chapter 5 for a thorough review of this research). Rogers and Pennington (1991) and Rogers and Bennetto (see Chapter 5) have proposed a developmental model of autism involving an imitation/praxis deficit very early in life that is related to the affective system and could disrupt the coordination of movement in social exchanges. As suggested in Chapter 5, it is critically important to consider the motor impairments in autism when making intervention decisions. For example, speech-language pathologists and occupational therapists may make important contributions in evaluating and treating motor speech impairments or more generalized motor impairments in children with ASD thanks to their training and expertise in working with patients who have neurogenic motor disorders.

In summary, a greater affinity for the world of objects and their physical attributes than for the world of people and their intentions and states of mind makes communication with others a most challenging enterprise for children with ASD. Learning to talk is only a major stumbling block for about half of those diagnosed with ASD. Analogous to temporal processing constraints and compounded by more specific motor impairments in some people with ASD, the coordination of sequential movement in social situations may be impaired. Yet, for all people with ASD the transitions to intentional and symbolic communication provide the biggest obstacles to achieving communicative competence.

An increased understanding of language acquisition in typically developing children speaks not only to the power of intentionality as a driving force but also to the importance of participation in shared cultural events and the situational relevance of utterances. These considerations become even more critical for people with ASD, whose attention, affect, and intentions are so often out of sync with those of others. Rather than focus on the rote reproduction of language forms that may be irrelevant to the communicative contexts at hand, intervention efforts need to emphasize communicative function, contextual relevance, and cultural belonging.

CLINICAL AND EDUCATIONAL IMPLICATIONS

The information presented in this chapter has implications for many aspects of clinical and educational practice. The next sections focus on the following issues: potential for earlier diagnosis, meaningful measures of abilities and outcomes, and evaluating intervention outcomes.

Potential for Earlier Diagnosis of Autism Spectrum Disorders

The communication and language patterns of children with autism that have been characterized in this chapter should be evident in very young children because they affect abilities that typically develop in the first year of life. Little is known, however, about early symptomatology in infants and toddlers with ASD. Osterling and Dawson (1994) studied home videotapes of first-year birthday parties for 11 children with autism and 11 typically developing children. They found that the children with autism displayed significantly fewer social and communicative behaviors and significantly more symptoms of autism at this young age. Lack of the following four behaviors correctly classified 10 of the 11 children with autism: pointing, showing objects, looking at the face of another, and orienting to their own names. Osterling and Dawson (1999) added a group with mental retardation and found that the children with autism looked at and oriented to their names less than did the children with mental retardation and that both groups used higher rates of repetitive motor actions and fewer nonverbal communication behaviors. Also using a retrospective video study, Baranek (1999) found that sensory motor functions in addition to social responses distinguished children with autism from children with developmental delays and typically developing children. These preliminary results suggest that impairments in these early social and communicative behaviors may contribute to earlier detection of autism/ASDs.

Baron-Cohen, Allen, and Gillberg (1992) administered the Checklist for Autism in Toddlers (CHAT; Baron-Cohen et al., 1996) to 41 children 18 months of age who were at genetic risk for developing autism. The CHAT consists of nine items reported by parents and five items observed by a health professional. Baron-Cohen and colleagues identified four children who failed three key items, protodeclarative pointing, gaze monitoring, and pretend play, and at 12-month follow-up were diagnosed with autism. Baron-Cohen and colleagues (1996) screened 16,000 children in southeast England using the CHAT during 18-month developmental checkups. They identified 12 children who failed the three key items. Of those 12 children, 10 received a diagnosis of autism by the time they were 3½ years old. They also identified 22 children (none of whom received a diagnosis of autism) who either failed protodeclarative pointing and/or pretend play but did not fail at gaze monitoring. Of those 22 children, 15 received a diagnosis of language delay.

These efforts to identify indicators for the early diagnosis of ASD are promising. The careful documentation of profiles of sociocommunicative and symbolic behaviors appears to be a critical component of the diagnosis of ASD in very young children. It is our contention that speech-language pathologists can play a critical role in identifying profiles of communicative and symbolic abilities in young children that are characteristic of ASDs. Practitioners should be aware of this profile to make appropriate referrals for diagnosis of young children who may be at risk for ASD because they may be among the first professionals to come in contact with a young child who has ASD. The literature reviewed in this chapter suggests that particular constellations of deficits in joint attention and symbolic communication (see Chapter 2) may serve as important early indicators of ASDs. Furthermore, when such deficits are accompanied by strengths in the communicative function of behavior regulation and constructive play, children with ASD may be distinguished more readily from children with other developmental disabilities (Wetherby et al., 1998).

Meaningful Measures of Abilities and Outcomes

Traditional formal language assessment instruments focus primarily on the structure of language in reference to identification of isolated milestones and often rely on eliciting specific responses that require a child's cooperation. Because language impairments associated with autism are most apparent in social or pragmatic aspects of language, formal assessment instruments have limited utility (Prizant et al., 1997; Schuler, Peck, Willard, & Thiemer, 1989; Schuler, Prizant, & Wetherby, 1997; Wetherby & Prizant, 1992). The assessment process, as we view it, is guided by some core questions, which are continuously redefined on the basis of overall developmental level, environmental needs, and preliminary assessment outcome. These core assessment questions pertain to the sociocommunicative, cognitive, and linguistic domains and the interrelations between domains so that areas of greatest needs as well as strengths are identified. Table 6.1 delineates these assessment domains based on our understanding of the sociocommunicative impairments in ASDs. Because assessment is viewed as a process for gathering information rather than as an end in itself, many different assessment approaches may be used: observational as well as experimental, formal as well as informal, structured as well as less structured, and so forth. A useful initial method for gathering information about a child's communication and language abilities is to interview significant others familiar with the subtle nuances of the child's communicative behaviors (Schuler et al., 1989; Schuler et al., 1997). The natural variation in behavior across contexts and interactants necessitates the use of multiple assessment tools and strategies in different contexts (for further discussion of these issues, see Prizant et al., 1997, and Schuler et al., 1997). Assessment, therefore, should not be limited to the evaluation of child variables only; it should be extended to contextual and interactional variables. The challenge that practitioners face is how to gather meaningful measures of a child's abilities to guide intervention decisions and determine whether intervention goals are being achieved.

Table 6.1. Core assessment domains

Language and communication domains

Expressive language and communication

- Gestural means (contact/distal, conventional, symbolic)
- Vocal means (consonant inventory, syllable structure)
- Verbal means (words, sentences, conversation)
- Modality strengths and preferences (speech, gesture, picture, written word)

Receptive language and communication

- Nonlinguistic response strategies
- Understanding of conventional meanings
- Comprehension of vocabulary, sentences, and discourse

Sociocommunicative and socioemotional domains

Range of communicative functions expressed

Reciprocity of interaction (rate of communicating, use of repair strategies)

Social-affective signals for social referencing and to regulate interaction

Comprehension of and expression of emotion in language and play

Self- and mutual regulatory strategies to modulate arousal and emotional state

Language-related cognitive domains

Attention in social and nonsocial contexts

Symbolic representation in symbolic and constructive play

Imitation strategies

Anticipation of routines and event knowledge

Evaluating Intervention Outcomes

Little empirical research is available to guide clinical decisions about how to enhance social communication skills. Dawson and Osterling (1997) reviewed eight model early intervention programs for preschool children with autism, ranging from intensive, one-to-one discrete trial approaches, which are generally carried out at home, to programs in inclusive settings using pragmatically oriented procedures and peer interactions in real-life environments. They concluded that the level of success achieved across these programs was promising and was fairly similar. On the basis of average changes in IQ score and percentage of children placed in regular classrooms, these programs generally were found to be effective for about half of the children. The issue of whether a program is effective, however, needs to be explored more carefully because this determination is directly related to the outcome measures selected for study. Dawson and Osterling noted that few of these programs documented progress on goals addressing social relatedness, joint attention, shared affect, or communicative intent. The literature reviewed in this chapter suggests that intervention programs for children with ASD need to be individualized based on the child's capacity for joint attention and symbol use. The findings of Wetherby and colleagues (1998) comparing younger and older children during communication samples with adults indicated that higher scores in vocal and verbal behavior are not necessarily accompanied by higher scores on other parameters, such as joint attention, gaze shifts, and symbolic play. In other words, enhancing communication skills for children with ASD entails not only increasing vocal and verbal repertoires but also increasing many aspects of social communication so that children will know how to initiate interactions with the words they have or will have other ways to communicate if they do not have words.

The strengths that children with ASD may have in communicating for the function of behavior regulation (e.g., requesting objects, actions, protesting) may be used to bootstrap weaknesses in other areas. Wetherby (1986) suggested that the easiest and first-emerging communicative function for children with autism is behavior regulation and the most difficult is joint attention, presumably because of the differing social underpinnings. Communicating for social interaction to draw attention to oneself may be viewed as a transition between communicating for behavior regulation to achieve an environmental end and joint attention to draw attention to an object or event. The findings of Stone and Caro-Martinez (1990) supported this ontogeny of functions and demonstrated significant correlations between motoric communication and behavior regulation and between symbolic communication and joint attention. The results of Wetherby and colleagues (1998) further support this ontogeny in even younger children. Most of the children with ASD did readily communicate for behavior regulation but did not communicate for joint attention. Many of the children did communicate for social interaction, which includes social goals such as requesting social routine, requesting comfort, calling, and greeting. Other strengths may also be used to compensate for weaknesses. Most children with ASD communicate primarily with contact gestures for behavior regulation (Stone & Caro-Martinez, 1990; Wetherby et al., 1998). Intervention is needed to build on these strengths and enhance the repertoire of conventional gestures and the capacity to use distal gestures, as well as to communicate for more social functions. Similarly, strengths in constructive play may be used as a basis to build understanding of language and functional use of objects as well as a context to target social-communicative goals. See Chapter 9 for intervention strategies that incorporate these and other related developmental principles.

Given that unconventional forms of behavior often come to serve communicative purposes, efforts to manage behavioral problems need to acknowledge the functions such behavior might serve. Long-term solutions to many behavioral problems ultimately involve the development of communicative skills, both to replace challenging behaviors used to communicate intent and to prevent the further development of behavioral problems. Positive, nonaversive, and respectful approaches to the management of challenging behaviors are becoming widely accepted as *recommended practice* for individuals with severe disabilities (see Carr et al., 1994; Horner et al., 1990; Reichle & Wacker, 1993;

Wetherby & Prizant, 1999; and Chapter 13). A significant body of literature is available that demonstrates how functional communication training can lead to a reduction in challenging behavior, support generalization across people and social contexts, and maintain acquired skills over time (see Durand, Berotti, & Weiner, 1993, for a review). It has been demonstrated that the challenging behavior will only be reduced if the alternative communicative means serves the same function as the challenging behavior (Carr & Durand, 1985; see Chapter 13).

DIRECTIONS FOR FUTURE RESEARCH

Considering that even the "model" intervention programs reviewed by Dawson and Osterling (1997) were effective with only about half of the children, there is a critical need to 1) predict which children will benefit from which programs or specific procedures, 2) guide decision making in terms of which goals to target for which children, and 3) improve the overall effectiveness of intervention. Greenspan and Wieder (1997) suggested that the capacity to use complex gestures in interactions with shared positive affect was an important predictor of success in their intervention. To better refine decision making in intervention, future research should examine the predictive value of a child's capacity for joint attention and symbol use and provide a better understanding of the role of motor functioning in communication and language outcomes. As professionals continue to work with younger and younger children, targeting goals and documenting progress for communicative and social-affective parameters become even more essential because doing so allows for finer-grained analysis of the early underpinnings of later social and linguistic competence. Future research should compare the efficacy of various intervention strategies that may be used to promote social relatedness, functional use of communication, and the sharing of positive affect in young children with ASD.

It is illuminating to examine the state of the art of intervention research in the field of autism in relation to that in the broader field of early intervention. The field of early intervention has been grappling with questions about the efficacy of intervention programs and the long-term effects on children, families, and communities (Shonkoff, Hauser-Cram, Krauss, & Upshur, 1988). Two important themes emerge that have important implications for the field of autism. First, outcome measures need to go beyond child outcomes to include family-oriented outcomes (Shonkoff et al., 1988, 1992). Early intervention research has demonstrated that family characteristics (e.g., socioeconomic conditions, stress, supports available) and parent involvement in the child's development are strong predictors of a child's outcome. Second, professionals need to go beyond traditional measures of psychomotor, cognitive, and language skills to include "ecologically compelling child characteristics" by measuring broader characteristics, such as emotional development, motivation, social competence, peer relationships, and the child's competence in natural environments (Shonkoff et al., 1988).

Intervention research on children with ASD has been negligent in documenting meaningful outcome measures. Therefore, extreme caution should be taken in drawing conclusions about the efficacy of a particular intervention approach, particularly when making decisions that have a dramatic impact on the cost of services to families and schools districts and the related time commitment of all parties involved. Future research should strive to document meaningful changes that reflect the core domains associated with autism, such as the capacity for joint attention and symbolic use, as well as measures of family functioning. Intervention research is needed to document the relation between specific treatment procedures, overall intervention models, and short-term as well as long-term outcomes. That will enable families and practitioners to determine which goals and which intervention strategies are most suitable for whom.

CONCLUSIONS

To effectively work with children with ASD, it is critical for professionals to have a thorough understanding of these children's unique communicative challenges and how they are compounded by cognitive and developmental differences and associated behavioral problems. Much of what professionals hope that children with ASD will learn about language and communication, such as greater flexibility in language production and language use and the ability to adjust communicative behavior to situational contexts, may be particularly difficult for these children to learn because of the social and communicative complexities involved. Progress in communication and language development must be conceptualized in reference to 1) the flexible use of multiple communicative means for an ever-diversifying range of functions and 2) how far a child has come in the acquisition of flexible, conventional communicative abilities rather than in reference to progress on targeted language forms produced in response to adult commands or in reference to typical age norms. Demonstrable or even quantifiable changes on standardized measurement instruments, which are defined by their insensitivity to contexts, are lacking in ecological validity because they fail to document progress in communication used in natural environments.

In evaluating the effectiveness of interventions, it is important that progress is measured in terms of meaningful outcomes, such as improvements in the quality of the lives of the children and their families involved in the intervention and the ability of children to experience a greater sense of efficacy by engaging in social interactions in a more mutually satisfactory way. To accomplish such gains it is important that intervention efforts do not solely target deficits within the child but target daily living and learning environments as well as communication partners, including parents, siblings, and peers, to create the types of contexts that are more responsive and conducive to communicative initiations. By creating contexts for joint action and joint attention (e.g., in sociodramatic play) and by coaching peers and adults in how to sustain interactions, a greater sense of communicative efficacy is established. In other words, intervention should be more ecologically referenced and should be sensitive to the surrounding peer and family culture. Such an emphasis will reduce the transactional secondary effects of more primary disabilities, which may be more devastating in the long run than the initial limitations exhibited by the child. It is difficult to establish a sense of communicative efficacy without ample opportunities for the child to practice success. Ultimately, the individual's competence in social interaction, in developing relationships, and in the capacity to cope with stress using flexible communicative strategies will determine the level of independence that can he or she can have beyond early childhood.

REFERENCES

Adamson, L.B., & Chance, S.E. (1998). Coordinating attention to people, objects, and language. In S.F. Warren & J. Reichle (Series Eds.) & A.M. Wetherby, S.F. Warren, & J. Reichle (Vol. Eds.), *Communication and language intervention series: Vol. 7. Transitions in prelinguistic communication* (pp. 15–37). Baltimore: Paul H. Brookes Publishing Co.

American Psychiatric Association. (1994). *Diagnostic and statistical manual of mental disorders* (4th ed.). Washington, DC: Author.

Aram, D.M., & Healy, J.F. (1988). Hyperlexia: A review of extraordinary word recognition. In L.K. Obler & D. Fein (Eds.), *The exceptional brain: Neuropsychology of talent and special abilities* (pp. 70–102). New York: Guilford Press.

Baltaxe, C. (1977). Pragmatic deficits in the language of autistic adolescents. *Journal of Pediatric Psychology, 2,* 176–180.

Baranek, G. (1999). Autism during infancy: A retrospective video analysis of sensory-motor and social behaviors at 9–12 months of age. *Journal of Autism and Developmental Disorders, 29,* 213–224.

Baron-Cohen, S. (1988). Social and pragmatic deficits in autism: Cognitive or affective? *Journal of Autism and Developmental Disorders, 18,* 379–402.

Baron-Cohen, S., Allen, J., & Gillberg, C. (1992). Can autism be detected at 18 months? The needle, the haystack, and the CHAT. *British Journal of Psychiatry, 161,* 839–843.

Baron-Cohen, S., Cox, A., Baird, G., Swettenham, J., Nightingale, N., Morgan, K., Drew, A., & Charman, T. (1996). Psychological markers in the detection of autism in infancy in a large population. *British Journal of Psychiatry, 168,* 158–163.

Baron-Cohen, S., Leslie, A.M., & Frith, U. (1985). Does the autistic child have a "theory of mind"? *Cognition, 21,* 37–46.

Baron-Cohen, S., Leslie, A.M., & Frith, U. (1986). Mechanical, behavioral and intentional understanding of picture stories in autistic children. *British Journal of Developmental Psychology, 4,* 113–115.

Bates, E. (1976). *Language and context: The acquisition of pragmatics.* San Diego: Academic Press.

Bates, E. (1979). *The emergence of symbols: Cognition and communication in infancy.* San Diego: Academic Press.
Bloom, L. (1993). *The transition from infancy to language.* New York: Cambridge University Press.
Bristol, M.M. (1984). Family resources and successful adaptation to autistic children. In E. Schopler & G.B. Mesibov (Eds.), *The effects of autism on the family* (pp. 289–310). New York: Plenum.
Bryson, S. (1996). Brief report: Epidemiology of autism. *Journal of Autism and Developmental Disorders, 26,* 165–168.
Calculator, S., Fabry, D., Glennen, S., Prizant, B.M., & Schubert, A. (1995). *Technical report on standards of practice for facilitated communication.* Rockville, MD: American Speech-Language-Hearing Association.
Carr, E.G., & Durand, V.M. (1985). Reducing behavior problems through functional communication training. *Journal of Applied Behavior Analysis, 18,* 111–126.
Carr, E.G., Levin, L., McConnachie, G., Carlson, J.I., Kemp, D.C., & Smith, C.E. (1994). *Communication-based intervention for problem behavior: A user's guide for producing positive change.* Baltimore: Paul H. Brookes Publishing Co.
Curcio, F. (1978). Sensorimotor functioning and communication in mute autistic children. *Journal of Autism and Childhood Schizophrenia, 8,* 281–292.
Damasio, A., & Maurer, R. (1978). A neurological model for childhood autism. *Archives of Neurology, 35,* 777–786.
Dawson, G., & Adams, A. (1984). Imitation and social responsiveness in autistic children. *Journal of Abnormal Child Psychology, 12,* 209–225.
Dawson, G., Hill, D., Spencer, A., Galpert, L., & Watson, L. (1990). Affective exchanges between young autistic children and their mothers. *Journal of Abnormal Child Psychology, 18,* 335–345.
Dawson, G., Meltzoff, A., Osterling, J., Rinaldi, J., & Brown, E. (1998). Children with autism fail to orient to naturally occurring social stimuli. *Journal of Autism and Developmental Disorders, 28,* 479–485.
Dawson, G., & Osterling, J. (1997). Early intervention in autism. In M.J. Guralnick (Ed.), *The effectiveness of early intervention* (pp. 307–326). Baltimore: Paul H. Brookes Publishing Co.
DeMyer, M.K. (1975). The nature of neuropsychological disability in autistic children. *Journal of Autism and Childhood Schizophrenia, 8,* 109–128.
Durand, V.M., Berotti, D., & Weiner, J. (1993). Functional communication training: Factors affecting effectiveness, generalization and maintenance. In S.F. Warren & J. Reichle (Series Eds.) & J. Reichle & D.P. Wacker (Vol. Eds.), *Communication and language intervention series: Vol. 3. Communicative alternatives to challenging behavior: Integrating functional assessment and intervention strategies* (pp. 317–340). Baltimore: Paul H. Brookes Publishing Co.
Fay, W.H., & Schuler, A.L. (Vol. Eds.). (1980). *Emerging language in autistic children.* In R.L. Schiefelbusch (Series Ed.), *Language intervention series* (Vol. 5). Baltimore: University Park Press.
Frith, U. (1971). Spontaneous patterns produced by autistic, normal, and subnormal children. In M. Rutter (Ed.), *Infantile autism: Concepts, characteristics, and treatment* (pp. 113–133). London: Churchill Livingstone.
Frith, U. (1989). *Autism: Explaining the enigma.* Oxford, England: Blackwell.
Garfin, D., & Lord, C. (1986). Communication as a social problem in autism. In E. Schopler & G. Mesibov (Eds.), *Social behavior in autism* (pp. 237–261). New York: Plenum.

Grandin, T. (1995). The learning style of people with autism: An autobiography. In K. Quill (Ed.), *Teaching children with autism: Methods to enhance communication and socialization* (pp. 33–52). Albany, NY: Delmar.

Greenspan, S.I., & Wieder, S. (1997). Developmental patterns and outcomes in infants and children with disorders in relating and communicating: A chart review of 200 cases of children with autistic spectrum diagnoses. *Journal of Developmental and Learning Disorders, 1,* 87–141.

Hermelin, B. (1976). Coding and the sense modalities. In L. Wing (Ed.), *Early childhood autism.* London: Pergamon.

Hermelin, B., & O'Connor, N. (1970). *Psychological experiments with autistic children.* Oxford: Pergamon.

Hill, D., & Leary, M. (1993). *Movement disturbance: A clue to hidden competencies in persons diagnosed with autism and other developmental disabilities.* Madison, WI: DRI Press.

Horner, R., Dunlap, G., Koegel, R., Carr, E., Sailor, W., Anderson, J., Albin, R., & O'Neill, R. (1990). Toward a technology of "nonaversive" behavioral support. *Journal of The Association for Persons with Severe Handicaps, 15,* 125–147.

Kanner, L. (1943). Autistic disturbances of affective contact. *Nervous Child, 2,* 217–250.

Kasari, C., Sigman, M., Mundy, P., & Yirmiya, N. (1990). Affective sharing in the context of joint attention. *Journal of Autism and Developmental Disorders, 20,* 87–100.

Lahey, M. (1988). *Language disorders and language development.* New York: Macmillan.

LaPointe, L., & Katz, R. (1998). Neurogenic disorders of speech. In G. Shames, E. Wiig, & W. Secord (Eds.), *Human communication disorders* (pp. 434–471). Needham Heights, MA: Allyn & Bacon.

Lifter, K., & Bloom, L. (1998). Intentionality and the role of play in the transition to language. In S.F. Warren & J. Reichle (Series Eds.) & A.M. Wetherby, S.F. Warren, & J. Reichle (Vol. Eds.), *Communication and language intervention series: Vol. 7. Transitions in prelinguistic communication* (pp. 161–195). Baltimore: Paul H. Brookes Publishing Co.

Lord, C., & Paul, R. (1997). Language and communication in autism. In D. Cohen & F. Volkmar (Eds.), *Handbook of autism and pervasive developmental disorders* (2nd ed., pp. 195–225). New York: John Wiley & Sons.

Loveland, K.A., & Landry, S.H. (1986). Joint attention and language in autism and developmental language delay. *Journal of Autism and Developmental Disorders, 16,* 335–349.

Maurer, R. (1999). Autism. In B. Maria (Ed.), *Current management in child neurology* (pp. 204–208). Hamilton, Ontario, Canada: B.C. Decker.

Maurer, R., & Damasio, A. (1982). Childhood autism from the point of view of behavioral neurology. *Journal of Autism and Developmental Disorders, 12,* 211–221.

McArthur, D., & Adamson, L.B. (1996). Joint attention in preverbal children: Autism and developmental language disorders. *Journal of Autism and Developmental Disorders, 26,* 481–496.

McEachin, J.J., Smith, T., & Lovaas, O.I. (1993). Long-term outcome for children with autism who received early intensive behavioral treatment. *American Journal on Mental Retardation, 97,* 359–372.

McHale, S., Simeonsson, R., Marcus, L., & Olley, J. (1980). The social and symbolic quality of autistic children's communication. *Journal of Autism and Developmental Disorders, 10,* 299–310.

McLean, J., & Snyder-McLean, L. (1978). *A transactional approach to early language training: Derivation of a model system.* Columbus, OH: Charles E. Merrill.

Mundy, P., Sigman, M., & Kasari, C. (1990). A longitudinal study of joint attention and language development in autistic children. *Journal of Autism and Developmental Disorders, 20,* 115–128.

Mundy, P., Sigman, M., Ungerer, J., & Sherman, T. (1987). Nonverbal communication and play correlates of language development in autistic children. *Journal of Autism and Developmental Disorders, 17,* 349–364.

Osterling, J., & Dawson, G. (1994). Early recognition of children with autism: A study of first birthday home videotapes. *Journal of Autism and Developmental Disorders, 24,* 247–257.

Osterling, J., & Dawson, G. (1999, April). *Early recognition of infants with autism versus mental retardation.* Poster presented at the meeting of the Society for Research in Child Development, Albuquerque, New Mexico.

Paul, R. (1991). Profiles of toddlers with slow expressive language development. *Topics in Language Disorders, 11,* 1–13.

Paul, R., Looney, S., & Dahm, P. (1991). Communication and socialization skills at ages 2 and 3 in "late-talking" young children. *Journal of Speech and Hearing Research, 34,* 858–865.

Peters, A. (1983). *The units of language acquisition.* London: Cambridge University Press.

Prior, M. (1979). Cognitive abilities and disabilities in autism: A review. *Journal of Abnormal Child Psychology, 2,* 357–380.

Prizant, B. (1983). Language acquisition and communicative behavior in autism: Toward an understanding of the "whole" of it. *Journal of Speech and Hearing Disorders, 48,* 296–307.

Prizant, B.M. (1987). Theoretical and clinical implications of echolalic behavior in autism. In T. Layton (Ed.), *Language and treatment of autistic and developmentally disordered children* (pp. 65–88). Springfield, IL: Charles C Thomas.

Prizant, B.M., & Duchan, J. (1981). The functions of immediate echolalia in autistic children. *Journal of Speech and Hearing Disorders, 46,* 241–249.

Prizant, B.M., & Rydell, P. (1984). Analysis of the functions of delayed echolalia in autistic children. *Journal of Speech and Hearing Research, 27,* 183–192.

Prizant, B.M., & Rydell, P.J. (1993). Assessment and intervention considerations for unconventional verbal behavior. In S.F. Warren & J. Reichle (Series Eds.) & J. Reichle & D. Wacker (Vol. Eds.), *Communication and language intervention series: Vol. 3. Communicative alternatives to challenging behavior: Integrating functional assessment and intervention strategies* (pp. 263–297). Baltimore: Paul H. Brookes Publishing Co.

Prizant, B.M., Schuler, A.L., Wetherby, A.M., & Rydell, P.R. (1997). Enhancing language and communication: Language approaches. In D. Cohen & F. Volkmar (Eds.), *Handbook of autism and pervasive developmental disorders* (2nd ed., pp. 572–605). New York: John Wiley & Sons.

Prizant, B.M., & Wetherby, A.M. (1987). Communicative intent: A framework for understanding social-communicative behavior in autism. *Journal of the American Academy of Child Psychiatry, 26,* 472–479.

Prizant, B., & Wetherby, A. (1989). Enhancing language and communication in autism: From theory to practice. In G. Dawson (Ed.), *Autism: Nature, diagnosis, and treatment* (pp. 282–309). New York: Guilford Press.

Prizant, B.M., & Wetherby, A.M. (1990). Toward an integrated view of early communication, language and socioemotional development. *Topics in Language Disorders, 10,* 1–16.

Reichle, J., & Wacker, D.P. (Vol. Eds.). (1993). *Communicative alternatives to challenging behavior: Integrating functional assessment and intervention strategies.* In S.F. Warren & J. Reichle (Series Eds.), *Communication and language intervention series: Vol. 3.* Baltimore: Paul H. Brookes Publishing Co.

Ricks, D., & Wing, L. (1975). Language, communication and the use of symbols in normal autistic children. *Journal of Autism and Childhood Schizophrenia, 5,* 191–221.

Rogers, S.J., & Pennington, B.F. (1991). A theoretical approach to the deficits in infantile autism. *Development and Psychopathology, 3,* 137–162.

Schuler, A.L. (1979). *An experimental analysis of conceptual and representational abilities in a mute autistic adolescent: A serial vs. a simultaneous mode of processing.* Unpublished doctoral dissertation, University of California, Santa Barbara.

Schuler, A.L. (1995). Thinking in autism: Differences in learning and development. In K. Quill (Ed.), *Teaching children with autism: Methods to enhance communication and socialization* (pp. 11–32). Albany, NY: Delmar.

Schuler, A.L., & Bormann, C. (1983). The interrelations between cognitive and communicative development; some implications of the study of a mute autistic adolescent. In C.L. Thew & C.E. Johnson (Eds.), *Proceedings of the Second International Congress on the Study of Child Language* (Vol. 2, pp. 269–282). Washington, DC: University Press of America.

Schuler, A., Peck, C., Willard, C., & Thiemer, K. (1989). Assessment of communicative means and functions through interview: Assessing the communicative capabilities of individuals with limited language. *Seminars in Speech and Language, 10,* 51–62.

Schuler, A.L., & Prizant, B. (1985). Echolalia. In E. Schopler & G. Mesibov (Eds.), *Communication problems in autism* (p. 163–184). New York: Plenum.

Schuler, A.L., Prizant, B., & Wetherby, A. (1997). Enhancing language and communication development: Prelinguistic approaches. In D. Cohen & F. Volkmar (Eds.), *Handbook of autism and pervasive developmental disorders* (2nd ed., pp. 539–571). New York: John Wiley & Sons.

Seal, B., & Bonvillian, J. (1997). Sign language and motor functioning in students with autistic disorder. *Journal of Autism and Developmental Disorders, 27,* 437–466.

Shane, H. (Ed.). (1994). *Facilitated communication: The clinical and social phenomenon.* San Diego: Singular Publishing Group.

Shonkoff, J., Hauser-Cram, P., Krauss, M., & Upshur, C. (1988). Early intervention efficacy research: What have we learned and where do we go from here? *Topics in Early Childhood Special Education, 8,* 81–93.

Shonkoff, J., Hauser-Cram, P., Krauss, M., & Upshur, C. (1992). Development of infants with disabilities and their families: Implications for theory and service delivery. *Monographs of the Society for Research in Child Development, 57*(6, Serial No. 230).

Sigman, M., & Kasari, C. (1995). Joint attention across contexts in normal and autistic children. In C. Moore & P. Dunham (Eds.), *Joint attention: Its origins and role in development* (pp. 189–203). Mahwah, NJ: Lawrence Erlbaum Associates.

Sigman, M., Mundy, P., Sherman, T., & Ungerer, J. (1986). Social interactions of autistic, mentally retarded, and normal children and their caregivers. *Journal of Child Psychology and Psychiatry and Allied Disciplines, 27,* 647–656.

Sigman, M., Ruskin, E., Arbelle, S., Corona, R., Dissanayake, C., Espinosa, M., Kim, N., Littleford, C., & Lopez, A. (1999). Social competence in children with autism, Down syndrome, and other developmental delays: A longitudinal study. *Monographs of the Society for Research in Child Development, 64.*

Sigman, M., & Ungerer, J. (1984). Cognitive and language skills in autistic, mentally retarded and normal children. *Developmental Psychology, 20,* 293–302.

Snow, M.E., Hertzig, M.E., & Shapiro, T. (1987). Expressions of emotion in young autistic children. *Journal of the American Academy of Child and Adolescent Psychiatry, 27,* 647–655.

Stern, D. (1985). *The interpersonal world of the infant.* New York: Basic Books.

Stone, W.L., & Caro-Martinez, L.M. (1990). Naturalistic observations of spontaneous communication in autistic children. *Journal of Autism and Developmental Disorders, 20,* 437–454.

Tager-Flusberg, H. (1996). Brief report: Current theory and research on language and communication in autism. *Journal of Autism and Developmental Disorders, 26,* 169–178.

Teitelbaum, P., Teitelbaum, O., Nye, J., Fryman, J., & Maurer, R. (1998). Movement analysis in infancy may be useful for early diagnosis of autism. *Proceedings of the National Academy of Sciences, 95,* 1–6.

Tomasello, M. (1992). *First verbs: A case study of early grammatical development.* New York: Cambridge University Press.

Tomasello, M., Kruger, A.C., & Ratner, H.H. (1993). Cultural learning. *Behavioral and Brain Sciences, 16,* 495–552.

Vilensky, J., Damasio, A., & Maurer, R. (1981). Disturbances of motility in patients with autistic behavior: A preliminary study. *Archives of Neurology, 38,* 646–649.

Vygotsky, L.S. (1962). *Thought and language* (F. Hanfmann & G. Valar, Trans.). Cambridge, MA: MIT Press. (Original work published 1934)

Werner, H., & Kaplan, B. (1963). *Symbol formation: An organismic-developmental approach to language and the expression of thought.* New York: John Wiley & Sons.

Westby, C. (1988). Children's play: Reflections of social competence. *Seminars in Speech and Hearing, 9,* 1–14.

Wetherby, A. (1986). Ontogeny of communicative functions in autism. *Journal of Autism and Developmental Disorders, 16,* 295–316.

Wetherby, A.M., & Prizant, B.M. (1992). Profiling young children's communicative competence. In S.F. Warren & J. Reichle (Series & Vol. Eds.), *Communication and language intervention series: Vol. 1. Causes and effects in communication and language intervention* (pp. 217–253). Baltimore: Paul H. Brookes Publishing Co.

Wetherby, A.M., & Prizant, B.M. (1993). *Communication and Symbolic Behavior Scales–Normed Edition.* Chicago: Applied Symbolix. (Available from Paul H. Brookes Publishing Co., Post Office Box 10624, Baltimore, MD 21285-0624; 800-638-3775)

Wetherby, A., & Prizant, B. (1999). Enhancing language and communication development in autism: Assessment and intervention guidelines. In D. Berkell Zager (Ed.), *Autism: Identification, education, and treatment* (2nd. ed., pp. 141–174). Mahwah, NJ: Lawrence Erlbaum Associates.

Wetherby, A.M., Prizant, B.M., & Hutchinson, T. (1998). Communicative, social-affective, and symbolic profiles of young children with autism and pervasive developmental disorder. *American Journal of Speech-Language Pathology, 7,* 79–91.

Wetherby, A.M., & Prutting, C.A. (1984). Profiles of communicative and cognitive-social abilities in autistic children. *Journal of Speech and Hearing Research, 27,* 364–377.

Wetherby, A., Schuler, A., & Prizant, B. (1997). Enhancing language and communication: Theoretical foundations. In D. Cohen & F. Volkmar (Eds.), *Handbook of autism and pervasive developmental disorders* (2nd ed., pp. 513–538). New York: John Wiley & Sons.

Wetherby, A., Yonclas, D., & Bryan, A. (1989). Communicative profiles of handicapped preschool children: Implications for early identification. *Journal of Speech and Hearing Disorders, 54,* 148–158.

Wills, D.M. (1979). Early speech development in blind children. *Psychoanalytic Studies of the Child, 34,* 85–117.

Wing, L., Gould, J., Yeates, R.R., & Brierley, L.M. (1977). Symbolic play in severely mentally retarded and in autistic children. *Journal of Child Psychology and Psychiatry and Allied Disciplines, 18,* 167–178.

7

Sensory Processing and Motor Performance in Autism Spectrum Disorders

Marie E. Anzalone and G. Gordon Williamson

The presence of sensory disturbances in children with autism is well documented in the basic science literature (Ornitz, 1989; Yeung-Courchesne & Courchesne, 1997), in the clinical literature (Baranek, 1999; Kientz & Dunn, 1997), and in first-person or case study accounts of living with autism (Grandin & Scariano, 1986; Williams, 1992). Many children with autism have problems in modulating their response to sensory input (i.e., over- or undersensitivity) and maintaining optimal arousal and focused attention (Courchesne, Townsend, Akshoomoff, & Saitoh, 1994; Ornitz, 1974, 1988). These deficits have been attributed to neuropathology of the limbic and cerebellar systems (Gillberg & Coleman, 1992; Haas, Townsend, Courchesne, & Lincoln, 1996; Kemper & Bauman, 1993; see also Chapter 8). First-person accounts describe problems in over- or underreactivity or distorted sensory perception leading to affective unavailability and fear reactions (Grandin, 1995). The initial appearance of sensory-related symptoms often predates diagnosis by as much as 2 years according to anecdotal report and retrospective analyses of home videotapes (Adrien et al., 1993; Baranek, 1999; Williams, 1994). Some authors have suggested that the sensory disturbance is a primary deficit underlying autism and not simply an associated problem (Grandin, 1995; Ornitz, 1989; Williams, 1992; ZERO TO THREE/National Center for Clinical Infant Programs, 1994).

Although documentation of the presence of sensorimotor deficits is important, more relevant from the family's and clinician's perspective is how these deficits can be managed and remediated. One approach that has been found to be helpful in conceptualizing and addressing these deficits is sensory integration (Ayres, 1972; Ayres & Tickle, 1980; Fisher, Murray, & Bundy, 1991). This chapter provides a theoretical overview of sensory integration, a description of sensorimotor profiles in children with autism, assessment guidelines, and principles of intervention.

Sensory integration is a process that involves organizing sensation from the body and the environment for adaptive purposes (Ayres, 1979; Kimball, 1993). Three aspects of this relatively simple definition are important. First, sensory integration refers to the dynamic processing or organization of information from multiple sensory modalities. It involves the initial registration of the input as something novel or meaningful, the modulation of that sensation as it is centrally processed, and the grading of the response. Much of the literature in autism focuses on the functioning of visual and auditory modalities (e.g., Cohen & Volkmar, 1997). In contrast, sensory integration also views the more proximal senses of touch, proprioception, and vestibular input as critically important. Proprioception is sensation from the muscles and joints that provides information about the posture and movement of the body. Vestibular receptors in the inner ear are responsive to movement of the body in relation to gravity.

Second, although sensory input is usually studied or discussed in terms of a single modality, in reality the central nervous system does not perceive or register sensation as an isolated modality (Gibson, 1988; Kandel, Schwartz, & Jessell, 1991; Lewkowicz & Lickliter, 1994). Within sensory integration theory, the mutual influences between the sensory modalities are used therapeutically to promote modulation and reinforce skilled performance (e.g., the visual, proprioceptive, and vestibular systems work together to stabilize the visual field while walking). The integration and convergence of input from several modalities are essential to learning and performance. Finally, sensory integration involves the *active* use of sensory input as the basis for an adaptive response. Sensory integration intervention is not synonymous with passive sensory stimulation.

In understanding sensory integration, the following attributes of a stimulus should be considered: intensity, location, and duration. These characteristics are properties of the *stimulus;* the *response* to the stimulus varies within and among individuals. Even within a single modality, there is variability of intensity. For example, light touch is more intense than firm touch with pressure and tends to be more alerting and arousing to most individuals. Similarly, rotary vestibular input has a high intensity, whereas slow rocking is generally more calming. One of the factors that contributes to intensity is the location of the stimulus. This is particularly true of tactile input in which touch to the face and ventral surface of the body is more arousing and potentially threatening than touch to the back or limbs (Brazelton, 1984; Royeen & Lane, 1991). Location is also a factor when considering the distal modalities of vision or hearing. A sound from a recognized source within one's visual field is less threatening than an unexpected sound from behind the body. Finally, one must also consider the duration of a stimulus and the duration of the effect of that stimulus in the central nervous system. Some sensory input is phasic (e.g., a visual image), whereas other input may be of longer duration both in terms of the absolute duration of the stimulus as well as the lasting effects (e.g., rapid spinning resulting in motion sickness or a prolonged increase in activity level).

SENSORY INTEGRATION AND THE 4 A'S OF BEHAVIOR

Psychologist Barry Lester and his colleagues (Lester, Freier, & LaGasse, 1995) discussed human behavior in the context of the "4 A's"—arousal, attention, affect, and action. The 4 A's serve as a key to understanding how infants and young children understand and interact with their environment. Each of these processes has a mutual regulatory influence on the other processes (e.g., the ability to maintain attention is dependent on the ability to maintain an alert state and, in turn, influences the ability to accomplish an action successfully). This framework is a useful way of describing the outcomes of the sensory integrative process (Williamson & Anzalone, 1997).

Arousal refers to the ability to maintain alertness and transition between different sleep and wake states. The child's current state of arousal influences the registration and interpretation of sensory input and conversely is influenced by sensory input (e.g., touch may be acceptable or even pleasant during a drowsy or quiet alert state but may be interpreted as aversive during active, alert, stressed, or crying states). Variability of response to sensory input is frequently linked to the child's state of arousal and previous sensory experiences. Children with autism may have problems in arousal that are related to their impairments in sensory registration and interpretation (Kientz, 1996). For example, a child who is hyperreactive may be very active, fearful, or aggressive when in a high state of arousal. Another child who is equally stressed by sensory input and in a high state of arousal may not show it behaviorally. The latter child essentially shuts down and has a flat and unresponsive affect (Baranek, 1998; Porges, McCabe, & Yongue, 1982; Williams, 1994).

Attention is the ability to focus selectively on a desired stimulus or task. There are two components to attention: selection (choosing what to attend to and shifting between several foci) and allocation (the amount of time a child can attend to a stimulus and the amount of effort inherent in maintaining that focus). Both selection and allocation of attention are influenced by sensory integrative dysfunction in children with autism (Cermak, 1988; Ornitz, 1988; Williamson & Anzalone, 1997). Poor sensory registration undermines the child's ability to attend. Children who are easily overstimulated by the environment may be hypervigilant as a protective mechanism to enable them to avoid threatening sensory input. Most children have a sensory preference in attention. For example, one child may learn better through kinesthetic or proprioceptive input, whereas another individual may learn better through visual input. Children with autism tend to have particular difficulty attending to auditory and tactile input and may prefer visual and vestibular channels (Baranek, Foster, & Berkson, 1997a; Kientz & Dunn, 1997). They also tend to avoid eye contact and joint attention and generally favor attending to inanimate objects (Sigman & Capps, 1997; Sigman, Mundy, & Yirmiya, 1990).

Some children have an excessively narrowed focus of attention in which they attend to minute detail and are oblivious to the rest of the environment (Burack, 1994; Casey, Gordon, Mannheim, & Rumsey, 1993; Cermak, 1988; Kinsbourne, 1983). Other children may have particular problems shifting attention either within or among modalities (Townsend, Harris, & Courchesne, 1996; see also Chapter 8). Another problem can be inattentiveness, in which the child is either inner directed or completely unfocused on environmental stimuli. Stereotypies may provide the focus of attention for many children with autism. For example, these children may engage in repetitive behaviors such as tapping, spinning, or hand flapping to provide a focus that enables them to exclude disorganizing or threatening environmental input (Baranek, Foster, & Berkson, 1997b; Carr, 1994).

Affect, the emotional component of behavior, is one of the primary areas of dysfunction in children with autism (American Psychiatric Association, 1994; Dawson & Lewy, 1989; Greenspan, 1992; see also Chapter 12). Instead of full coverage of this broad topic, this chapter focuses on the sensory contribution to deficits in emotional regulation. The hypersensitivity of many children with autism causes them to react with fear and negativity to situations that are not necessarily threatening (Kientz & Dunn, 1997; ZERO TO THREE/National Center for Clinical Infant Programs, 1994). This fear may be in response to the physical or social environments. Because people are a source of strong and unpredictable sensation, the children may particularly avoid social contact. A deficit in sensory modulation also influences the intensity and amplitude of a child's emotional reactivity (Dunn, 1997). A high sensory threshold (i.e., requiring a lot of sensory input before registration) results in a low level of arousal that may manifest as a dampened or constrained range of affect. In contrast, a low sensory threshold may lead to a high level of arousal, which may cause exaggerated, labile, or negative emotions or a withdrawn pattern of internal focus and affective unavailability (Baranek, 1998). The emotional expression of some children with autism spectrum disorders (ASDs) tends to be flat and restricted (Freeman, 1993; Sigman et al., 1990). An exception to this flatness is often observed when children are engaged in high-intensity vestibular activities; in these circumstances they appear excited and happy.

Action, the last of the 4 A's, is the ability to engage in adaptive goal-directed behavior. Motor abilities are involved in action, but action is more complex than just motor function. Action also involves perceptual and cognitive contributions to purposeful behavior (Anzalone, 1993; Losche, 1990). Some children with autism are proficient in their motor skills, particularly in the fine manipulation of objects (Rapin, 1997). Other children have delayed development in their gross or fine motor skills (Leary & Hill, 1996; Manjiviona & Prior, 1995; Mauk, 1993) and difficulties in coordination or clumsiness (Mailloux, Parham, & Roley, 1998). Still others have problems in the neuromotor processes underlying motor performance and executive functions. Problems with neuromotor processes include such factors as low muscle tone and decreased strength (Greenspan, 1992; Leary & Hill, 1996; ZERO TO THREE/National Center for Clinical Infant Programs, 1994).

An important aspect of action is praxis, the ability to plan and sequence unfamiliar purposeful behaviors (Ayres, 1985). Children with autism may have primary problems in goal formulation (Williamson & Anzalone, 1997). As a result they may be very repetitive or rigid in their interactions with objects or may engage in very simplistic sensory-seeking behaviors. Some children also have problems in motor planning and imitation of movements or postures because of poor sensorimotor awareness of their bodies (Mailloux et al., 1998).

At times the goal of the action is to regulate the other A's (arousal, attention, and affect). For example, children may be quite intentional in the use of their visual gaze (action) to modulate the level of excitement (arousal) and interaction (attention and affect). Stereotypies, although not optimally adaptive, may also serve this function (Carr, 1994; Freeman, 1993). Twirling, body rocking, and other sensory-based stereotypic behaviors may help children with autism to manage arousal and sensory modulation. In addition, repetitive sensory-based actions may be used to foster organization of the child's behavior and emotions (e.g., spinning in a circle, opening and closing a door, holding a vibrating vacuum cleaner, rhythmically tapping on one's arm) (Schreibman, 1988; Williams, 1994).

It is difficult for the child with autism and sensory deficits to engage in social transactions because of poor self- and mutual regulation of the 4 A's. Social transactions require flexible, responsive modulation and clear communication on the part of all participants. Adults may have difficulty in reading the child's cues, understanding the cause of the behavior, knowing reliable strategies for helping the child to regulate, and managing emotions that result from mismatched communication with the child. For instance, Joey is a child who is hypersensitive to touch, sound, and movement. When Joey is upset, his self-regulation is poor (i.e., his arousal is heightened, attention is focused inward, affect is negative and fearful, and actions are avoidant and disorganized). In response to this behavior pattern, Joey's mother tries a wide variety of interventions to help him to self-comfort (i.e., she talks to him, carries him around the room, pats his back, wipes his face, and introduces a bottle). These actions sensorially overload Joey and escalate his response. Although it is counterintuitive to regular caregiving practices, the mother needs to do less, not more, to assist Joey to regulate his 4 A's. For example, the mother could hold or pat Joey but not talk or move him around. When Joey is upset, there is a breakdown in social reciprocity. Although motivated to help, the mother misreads the situation, overstimulates her son, and does not understand why her actions do not get desired results. Over time this mismatch may lead to Joey's feeling avoidant and fearful due to expectations of being overstimulated when interacting with his mother. In contrast, Joey's mother may interpret his anxiety in terms of rejection of her instead of an inability to tolerate the sensory input that she provides.

CLINICAL PROFILES

Three profiles of sensory integration dysfunction are commonly seen in children with autism—two involve problems in sensory modulation (hyperreactive and hyporeactive patterns); the third is dyspraxia. These clinical profiles are discussed in terms of their sensory contributions to the regulation of the 4 A's. These profiles are based on the emerging clinical literature and require empirical validation (Baranek, 1998; Williamson & Anzalone, 1997; ZERO TO THREE/National Center for Clinical Infant Programs, 1994). In addition, they should not be interpreted as defining discrete and mutually exclusive categories of behavior along a unitary dimension. The profiles, however, provide a helpful framework for appreciating the behavioral patterns of these children. It is recognized that a specific child may have a combination of symptoms and may not fit clearly into any one category.

Hyperreactivity

Children with hyperreactivity tend to have a low sensory threshold and a bias toward a sympathetic nervous system reaction. (Sympathetic responses are those that indicate activation of the central nervous system such as increased blood pressure, heart rate, and respiration.) In terms of the 4 A's, these children have a restricted range of optimal arousal. Their arousal level tends to be high with a narrow, rigid control of sensory input. It is important to note that the observable behavioral arousal is not always the same as physiological arousal as reflected by measures such as heart rate and respiration (Miller & McIntosh, 1998; Porges et al., 1982; Wilbarger & Wilbarger, 1991). Some hyperreactive children may appear to have a flat affect or to be underaroused when they are in fact physiologically overaroused (e.g., they have either a high level of cortisol or an elevated heart rate) (Miller, 1996). In a few children this sensory overload becomes so threatening that they respond with an involuntary behavioral and physiological shutdown.

Attention of hyperreactive children may be overly focused on detail (Kinsbourne, 1983). This phenomenon serves as a gatekeeping or screening function, excluding a more generalized sensory awareness of the environment. Affective range is usually limited, varying from disconnection from sensory input to negative withdrawal. An exception is the positive affect often associated with spinning of self or objects. Action in children with hyperreactivity tends to be narrowly focused, with limited elaboration and inflexibility of behavior. Some children show little or no initiation of engagement. Others engage in repetitive actions; still others display surprising competence in very specific skills. Hyperreactive children are very concerned about becoming disorganized and develop rigid routines, compulsions, and stereotypic patterns that help them to keep themselves in control. All of these behaviors can be seen as adaptive at some level—as ways in which children are trying to monitor and manage their registration and interpretation of sensory input so that they can maintain a level of comfort. These behaviors, however, often interfere with interaction rather than foster it. Certain types of everyday sensation (e.g., school bells, the texture of a new shirt) actually are painful for these children. The sound of a door slamming, unexpected laughter on a television soundtrack, or thunder can be so uncomfortable that the children will do everything they can to avoid experiencing that sensation again. Their rigid, controlling behaviors and rituals are understandable attempts to limit noxious sensory input or at least to make the input predictable.

Although most of the preceding discussion has focused on the body senses, it is also important to think of auditory processing as a sensory-based precursor of language (Lincoln, Courchesne, Harms, & Allen, 1995). It is critical to address the child's registration of sounds before one can assess the ability to process language. Dysfunction may be noted in the registration and perception of the volume, frequency, and pitch of sounds.

Hyporeactivity

Children with hyporeactivity tend to have a high sensory threshold; that is, they require a lot of sensory input to achieve registration and activation of the 4 A's. Often these children have not registered novel sensory input and therefore have minimal information on which to base any interpretation. They do not learn from the environment because they have not noticed it. Their state of arousal is usually low or unmodulated. Attention is unfocused or narrowly targeted to a specific type of sensory input to meet inner needs. Affect may be flat or uninvested but may brighten with vestibular input. Action tends to be passive, aimless, and wandering. Some hyporeactive children, however, may have an insatiable craving for a preferred type of sensory input and may seek it out in order to be "fueled up." Spinning (rotary vestibular activity) is a favorite type of stimulation. One frequently sees children with bland, disconnected affects become delighted once they start to spin. It should be noted that the sensory input that is the most arousing for these children is not necessarily the most organizing.

There are two caveats in understanding the sensory modulation profiles of children with ASD. First, one cannot assume that a child who has a flat affect and appears unavailable is hyporeactive. As previously mentioned some of these children are actually physiologically hyperreactive, and the behavioral shutdown reflects the opposite of their internal state. In assessment, one can differentiate between these two profiles by systematically decreasing sensory input, providing organizing activity, and observing behavioral responses over time. With decreased sensory input the child who is truly hyperreactive will become calmer and more attentive, whereas the child who is truly hyporeactive may become more lethargic. Second, it is important to remember that not all sensory-seeking behaviors are associated with hyporeactivity. Some children with hyperreactivity or sensory defensiveness may engage in sensory seeking as a way of modulating their reactions to sensation (i.e., discharging tension or refocusing attention to organize themselves).

Mixed Patterns

A child can have a mixed pattern of being hypersensitive in certain modalities (often auditory or tactile) and hyposensitive in others (frequently proprioceptive or vestibular). Likewise, a child may have variability of responses within a single sensory modality (e.g., a child may be hyperreactive to high-frequency sounds and hyporeactive to low-frequency sounds). A child can also be inconsistent in responding to the same stimulus over time. Both types of variability frequently are linked to the child's shifting state of arousal, attention, and previous sensory experiences.

Some children have jumbling or distortion of sensory input and do not fit into the described clinical profiles. There is an erratic fluctuation in the registration of sensory input, somewhat like a volume switch being turned up and down repeatedly. For example, these children may hear only parts of words (the first part, the last part, or no consonants) or find that auditory or visual signals are intermeshed. Some adults with autism report seeing vibrations around a television set when it is on (Grandin, 1995).

Dyspraxia

Praxis can be conceptualized as encompassing three different steps: 1) ideation (formulating the goal), 2) motor planning (figuring out specifically how to accomplish the goal; this step involves problem solving based on a sensorimotor awareness of the body), and 3) execution (the actual carrying out of the planned action) (Ayres, 1985; Parham & Mailloux, 1996). As discussed previously, many children with autism have special problems in ideation, the first component of praxis. They tend to have difficulty thinking about the multiple ways that toys, objects, or one's body can be used in play and learning situations (Ayres, 1985; Restall & Magill-Evans, 1994). As a result they may tend either to be inactive or to play with limited perseverative schemas. This component of praxis has a strong cognitive basis. Children with autism displaying deficits in ideation do not demonstrate complex, developmentally appropriate play or exploration even in the presence of age-appropriate motor competence.

They may attempt to decrease novelty by creating order (e.g., horizontally arranging items against the wall), performing the same actions with all objects (e.g., twirling different toys regardless of their intended play potential), or perseverating on familiar routines or rituals.

Problems can also occur in the next step of praxis, motor planning. This step involves the sensorimotor planning and sequencing of motor tasks based on a body scheme (Mailloux et al., 1998). It is the most sensory-dependent component of praxis. Adults with autism report having distorted or inadequate body awareness that does not adequately prepare them for new motor challenges (Williams, 1994). A body scheme is normally acquired through past movement experiences and provides the sensory basis for the anticipatory, or feedforward, control of movement (Ayres, 1972, 1985; Cermak, 1991; Ghez, Gordon, Ghilardi, & Sainburg, 1995). For example, to walk up stairs, one relies on proprioceptive information from previous stair climbing to provide the feedforward motor program for current stair climbing. Children with a poor body scheme fail to develop an integrated awareness of how their body parts fit together and move through space. The final step of praxis is the actual motor component—the execution of the task based on the previously established goal and plan. Execution is influenced by the child's motor development, skill, and coordination.

To contrast performance deficits in children with these three different components of dyspraxia, one can envision a child with a problem in ideation who may look at a carpeted tunnel and not have the concept that he or she can crawl through it. There is little idea of a goal for action. A child with a deficit in motor planning knows that he or she wants to go through the tunnel but does not know how to accomplish the task. This child does not have the ability to problem solve and sequence the necessary actions or to know how his or her body can fit into the tunnel. Finally, the child with problems in execution has difficulty in the motor control required to move through the tunnel. He or she may have gross or fine motor delays with associated incoordination.

This section has focused on developmental dyspraxia, which relates to gross and fine motor performance and serves as a foundation for sensorimotor exploration, play, and functional tasks. It is important to note, however, the associated prevalence of oral/verbal dyspraxia in children with autism. These difficulties in motor planning interfere with the proper development of speech and feeding skills (see Chapters 5 and 6).

GUIDELINES FOR ASSESSMENT

There are a variety of ways to gather information about a child's capacity to process sensory information. The most effective methods are talking with parents and observing the child within the natural context of relationships, play, and daily activities (Cook, 1991; Dunn & Oetter, 1991; Greenspan & Meisels,

1996). Observation of the following situations is particularly generative in understanding a child's sensorimotor processing: independent free play in both novel and familiar environments, parent–child interaction, peer group experiences, mealtimes, and transitions between activities. Sensory integrative functions serve as the basis for these flexible interactions with a changing social and physical environment. A child who is unable to modulate sensory input, understand that input, and organize an adaptive motor response will be unable to engage successfully in social relationships. Table 7.1 provides guidelines for observing sensory-based self-regulation related to the 4 A's and the environmental contexts in which the behaviors occur.

In assessment it is important to look at the child in context and not in isolation. The relationship between the child and environmental challenges and supports is the critical issue. It is an error to assume that a specific child with autism has a sensory integrative disorder. One needs to recognize that functional difficulties can arise from a poor fit between the child's needs and available resources. For instance, a child may demonstrate aversive responses when presented with various tactile experiences. One cannot assume that this behavior necessarily implies a problem with tactile defensiveness. Alternative possibilities are that the child is having an avoidant response to 1) the novelty of the activity, 2) the difficulty of the cognitive and sequential task demands, 3) the adult-imposed structure, or 4) a lack of motivation to accomplish the task. The determination of the existence of a sensory-based problem is achieved through ongoing observation of the child over time and discussion of the behaviors with the parents.

Questions to parents about activities of daily living can often yield relevant information about the child's sensory tolerances and preferences. What is

Table 7.1. Observation of sensory-based self-regulation

- Does the child's state of arousal and sensory modulation support attention, affect, and action (e.g., organized state, hyperarousal, hypoarousal, state lability)?
- Is the child able to self-regulate behavior and emotional tone?
- Does the child have a sensory preference in attention and learning?
- Is there a predictable time of day or type of activity (sensory diet) when the child is most and least organized?
- Does the child express an appropriate range of affect in response to sensory input?
- Is the child playful during social interaction?
- What types of social situations facilitate the child's sensory integration and optimal performance (e.g., adult–child interaction, peer interaction, small-group peer interaction)?
- What is the stylistic pattern of the child's independent or peer play (e.g., preferences, energy, intensity, tempo, pacing)?
- Does the child initiate exploration of novel as well as familiar situations?
- How does the child manage transitions and changes in daily routines?
- What motivates and interests the child?
- Are the child's activities of daily living and self-care tasks limited by sensory or motor problems?

a typical Saturday or weekday like? How does the child manage feeding, bathing, and other routines? What are your nighttime and morning routines? Are certain sensory systems areas of strength or vulnerability? What are your child's favorite activities? Does the child consistently avoid any activities? How does the child act around other children or during holiday celebrations? Through this type of inquiry one is constructing a clinical picture reflecting how the flow of sensory input, environmental demands, and behavioral state fit together in each child's daily routine (Kientz, 1996; Wilbarger & Wilbarger, 1991; Williams & Shellenberger, 1996).

This flow can be considered a sensory "diet" analogous to a nutritional diet. It is the ongoing mix of sensory input obtained through the experiences of daily activities that modulate arousal, attention, affect, and action. There are wide individual differences in this sensory diet among children as well as within a specific child over time. The practitioner looks for patterns of stimulating and quiet activities within the child's day and the presence of adaptive or nonadaptive behaviors (Hanft & Place, 1996; Williams & Shellenberger, 1996).

The assessment protocol needs to provide an organized sensory environment to allow observation of how the child responds to different stimuli. A well-designed environment can "open up" some children with severe difficulties in relating and communicating and allow them to achieve their best performance. For example, a sensory-enriched environment may give a young child the opportunity to crawl over a large furry pillow, through a rocking barrel, and down a ramp to attain a favorite toy. Another child may do better in a quiet, soft "nest" in the corner. The practitioner observes the child's responses and the environmental opportunities as they influence arousal, attention, affect, and action.

Some standardized procedures and tools can help to structure the evaluation. One approach is to gain information about the child's tolerances and preferences for sensory stimulation in the context of activities of daily living. This approach involves a parent interview or questionnaire regarding the child's sensory or self-regulatory performance. For instance, the Infant and Toddler Symptom Checklist (DeGangi, 1995) addresses such areas as self-regulation, attention, sleeping, eating, dressing, bathing, movement, language, vision, and emotional functioning in children between 7 and 30 months of age. The Sensory Profile (Dunn, 1997) is a parent questionnaire appropriate for assessing sensory processing of school-age children. This questionnaire was used to contrast parental reports of children with autism with those of typically developing children (Dunn & Brown, 1997; Kientz & Dunn, 1997). Children with autism were found to have particular problems in sensory modulation in the tactile, auditory, and vestibular systems. They tended to be hyperreactive to touch (i.e., tactilely defensive), to be hypo- or hyperreactive to sounds, and to have a heightened craving and tolerance for rapid movement when compared with typically developing children.

Two norm-referenced tests that may also be helpful are the Miller Assessment for Preschoolers (Miller, 1988) and the Test of Sensory Functions in Infants (DeGangi & Greenspan, 1989). The Miller Assessment for Preschoolers is a general developmental screening instrument that captures some important abilities relating to sensory processing and motor planning in addition to more traditional language and cognitive skills. It also provides a useful guide for structuring observations relevant to the quality of sensory integrative performance. The Test of Sensory Functions in Infants measures sensory reactivity and adaptive motor behaviors in children between 4 and 18 months of age. Although not a sensory-based tool, the School Function Assessment (Coster, Deeney, Haltiwanger, & Haley, 1998) addresses categories of behavior (e.g., transitions, self-regulation) that may be problematic for children with autism who have sensory deficits. Likewise, the Early Coping Inventory (Zeitlin & Williamson, 1988) captures the coping style of young children according to their sensorimotor organization, reactivity, and self-initiation, which can be vulnerabilities for these children.

The key to assessment is to focus on *how* the child processes sensory information and manages environmental challenges and not on the specific skills or milestones the child displays. For instance one would observe how the child organizes attention and under what conditions and not merely the length of the attention span. Or, likewise, one would note what environmental conditions precede or follow engagement in repetitive rocking. The practitioner needs this kind of qualitative information to design intervention.

GENERAL GUIDELINES FOR INTERVENTION

Intervention with children who have autism and associated problems in sensory integration should target three different levels: 1) helping parents to understand their child's behavior and fostering relationships, 2) modifying the environment to facilitate a goodness-of-fit, and 3) direct intervention strategies designed to remediate identified problems. For some children with severe difficulties in relating and communicating, an occupational therapist trained in sensory integration needs to be involved to address these complex issues. The following general principles apply to most children with sensory integrative disorders.

Effective intervention must begin with understanding the child's specific clinical profile and how that sensory profile may relate to problematic behaviors (Wilbarger, 1995; Williams & Shellenberger, 1996). Parents become more effective when they understand the sensory-based reasons for the child's difficult behavior. One needs to know the extent to which naturally occurring activities and the child's daily routine provide the sensory input required throughout the day to maintain the 4 A's—arousal, attention, affect, and action. Because there is variability of sensory diet and profile even within a given child's day, intervention should be based on sensitive observation of the child, not on a preestablished treatment protocol. Intervention does not always require provision of additional sensory input. Often what is necessary is a decrease in the sensory stimulation that the child is receiving.

One should consider how the child's sensory diet varies throughout the day and how this variation influences the child's arousal and ability to engage in functional activity (Wilbarger & Wilbarger, 1991). After recognizing a child's pattern, the adult tries to anticipate the child's needs and provides an appropriate sensory diet. The parent or practitioner does not wait until a child is sluggish to do something arousing or until a child is overloaded to do something calming. One way to assist the child to self-regulate is to provide a routine throughout the day that is reasonably consistent, predictable, and structured. Routines can help the child to predict what is about to happen and make adjustments for the inherent sensory changes (e.g., forecasting transitions, daytime routines, or nighttime routines). The ability to anticipate events enables one to move from a reactive mode to a purposeful, self-initiated mode. Therefore, the child is better able to cope flexibly with change and sensory perturbations. It is hypothesized that some behavioral rigidity of children with autism is related to sensory avoidance (Baranek et al., 1997b).

Providing an appropriate sensory diet in this way is likely to lead to a decrease in self-injurious, challenging, and stereotypic behavior. These are all behaviors that may meet some sensory need. If parents and practitioners provide sensory input in a more "typical," naturalistic way, unwanted behaviors are likely to decrease in frequency (Ornitz, 1989; Rankin, 1998; Williams & Shellenberger, 1996). A sensory diet allows the adult to respect the preferences and comfort level of the child and therefore enables the establishment of a more trusting and reciprocal relationship.

One may not see the influence of sensory input immediately because of the latency of response and cumulative effect. Because response to sensation builds up over time, a child may be more sensitive to touch at the end of a long day than in the morning. In contrast, the adult may tend to overload the hyporeactive child due to the child's tendency to have a delayed sensory response. Both of these situations make it essential that any changes in the amount or type of sensory input be provided slowly and conservatively.

The senses are functionally unified in that input from one modality can regulate another modality (Ayres, 1972; Grandin, 1992; Koomar & Bundy, 1991). Proprioception and pressure touch are often used to regulate light touch and vestibular stimulation. For instance, rubbing one's arm after being tickled "erases" the noxious light touch. Another example is having a child in a "nested" position in an inner tube placed on a platform swing. In this case, the position provides deep pressure, which has an inhibitory influence on the nervous system. The active swinging provides vestibular stimulation, which has an excitatory influence. The convergence of these two inputs may lead to maintenance of a balanced state of arousal and sustained attention to the activity.

Intervention is designed to encourage a goodness-of-fit (or the just-right challenge) between resources and the sensory-related demands and expectations on the child (Zeitlin & Williamson, 1994). Intervention may be geared toward changing the sensory properties of the physical environment. For example, a hyperreactive child may be easily overstimulated by an excessively animated teacher or a brightly lit classroom with mobiles and bulletin boards, whereas the same situation may assist the hyporeactive child to reach an appropriate threshold. Knowledge of the child's sensory profile provides insight into the environmental demands that best support interaction and self-regulation. Hyperreactive children may need calm settings with minimal distractions and controlled sensory "flow." In contrast the hyporeactive child may do better in a sensory-rich environment that provides many opportunities for active sensory-based exploration with adult facilitation.

Stereotypies and repetitive sensory-based behaviors serve different functions depending on the child's current sensory threshold. A child who is hyperreactive at a given moment (i.e., low threshold) may use hand flapping to gain selective focus and to screen out the rest of the visual surroundings. The outcome can be calming and organizing. The child who is hyporeactive (i.e., high threshold) may use this same behavior to increase arousal and activation. A third child may use hand flapping to discharge tension (Bonoclonna, 1981). Practitioners must use their knowledge of sensory processing and each child's unique sensory profile to understand these stereotypical mannerisms and rituals. Behavioral techniques that do not consider sensory needs may result in stereotypies that resurface in a different form. Inappropriate behavioral intervention would involve intrusive, highly adult-directed discrete trials when a child has major problems in sensory modulation. Likewise, it is a therapeutic error in such cases to interpret gaze avoidance or tactile defensiveness as noncompliant behavior.

The primary goal of intervention is to provide appropriate, graded sensory experiences as a means to help the child with autism to acquire more adaptive behavior (Ayres, 1972; Fisher et al., 1991; Greenspan, 1992). Intervention for sensory processing dysfunction is not the same as "sensory stimulation" (Kimball, 1993; Parham & Mailloux, 1996). Sensation should be a natural component of activities. All sensory-based activities (especially those that are new to the child) should be active and should require an organizing response from the child. Activities are made purposeful when they are linked to the child's affect, intentions, and intrinsic motivation. No matter how rich and stimulating the sensory input, if the activity is not purposeful there is little benefit. This is a great clinical challenge when working with some children with autism because of their inattention and limited motivation.

Child-directed activities should be emphasized, no matter how simple or purposeless they may initially seem. Imitation of the child's play can provide insight into the sensory properties of the activity and can support social reciprocity. Once the sensory basis of the child's behavior is understood, the practitioner then knows how to elaborate on the initial sensory experience and how to introduce alternative activities providing similar sensory input. A common therapeutic error is to make too many changes too quickly. Changes should be small and gradual. The child's behavioral response should be monitored to determine whether the activity changes are increasing behavioral complexity or causing the child to withdraw, become threatened, or become increasingly disorganized. One of the most difficult aspects of sensory integrative intervention is allowing the child to direct the activity and to engage in a task long enough for adequate practice and learning to occur.

Another aspect of child-directed intervention is that the practitioner determines the communicative intent of the child's behaviors. Children with autism frequently wish to express their sensory needs. Gestures, facial expressions, body postures, signs, or vocalizations suggest how they would like sensory input to be altered—slowed, sped up, discontinued, increased, or lessened. The communication that occurs during a treatment session utilizing sensory integration is often subtle and nonverbal. When these behaviors are responded to contingently, they may became the foundation of reciprocity. Engagement in appropriate and organizing sensory-based activities (especially vestibular) can also increase vocalizations (Fisher et al., 1991; Frick & Lawton-Shirley, 1994; Ray, King, & Grandin, 1988).

Guidelines for Intervention with Hyperreactivity

The following suggestions are designed to 1) decrease or prevent sensory overload and assist modulation of sensory reactivity, 2) achieve an optimal level of arousal and attention, and 3) create a safe and predictable social and physical environment to support more effective engagement. It is critical that the child have a sense of security and feel free of threat and anxiety in order to explore meaningfully. Early signs of distress need to be monitored. If there are signs of discomfort, one stops the activity and provides time for recovery. Slowing the pace rather than stopping the activity is sufficient for some children but not others. Autonomic signs of distress indicating overstimulation include sweating, rapid color change, pupillary dilation, nausea, and behavioral or state lability. Calming techniques can be effective when they are consistent in application. The practitioner needs to stay with one calming activity rather than jump from one to another. Inhibition can be achieved through the use of deep pressure touch and proprioceptive input that are rhythmically applied (Grandin, 1992; Zissermann, 1992). Some examples are downward pressure on the shoulders of the child; bear hugs with the child facing away from the practitioner; and engagement in tasks that involve pushing, lifting, and climbing.

The adult must consider the complexity of the sensory input during activities and interactions. Some children with autism may only be able to handle input from one sensory modality at a time (i.e., looking, listening, touching, or moving, but not two modalities together) (Ayres, 1972; Grandin, 1995). Other children may require specific multisensory combinations (e.g., rocking while being hugged or held). A particularly powerful source of sensory input is eye contact. Therefore, requiring eye contact during an auditory-based activity may be overstimulating for some children.

A child's irritability may tend to cause the adult to overreact emotionally. Clinicians should be aware of their response to the child's behavior and modulate their own 4 A's during intervention. The child's difficult behavioral pattern should not condition the adult to avoid presenting appropriate developmental challenges (e.g., making disciplinary demands, avoiding novelty or structure in the environment).

Hypersensitive responses to sensory input are often inconsistent. Sensory input is cumulative and an exaggerated response may be a result of the whole day's stimulation and not just a single touch or sensory experience. Breaks need to be scheduled to enable recovery and calming, even when the child has not shown intolerance. As discussed, hyperreactivity is not always expressed in overt behavior. Some children on sensory overload will shut down and appear inwardly directed, flat, and disconnected. Their physiological signs, however, are biased toward a sympathetic nervous system reaction (i.e., fight-or-flight reaction).

Guidelines for Intervention with Hyporeactivity

The following suggestions are designed to 1) provide adequate sensory experiences to achieve and maintain a desired sensory threshold, 2) achieve an optimal level of arousal and attention, and 3) support social and environmental interaction.

It is important to differentiate between a child who is truly hyporeactive and a child who is hyperreactive but avoids sensory input (has a low threshold and is sensory avoidant). The hyporeactive child will gradually become alert with tactile or self-controlled vestibular sensation, but the sensory avoidant child may withdraw even further with additional sensory input. One may want to try taking away input (e.g., decreasing auditory or visual stimuli) before adding stimulation to differentiate between the two states of reactivity (Williamson & Anzalone, 1997).

The hyporeactive child needs to be activated to engage in more effective exploration, social interaction, or manipulative play. The practitioner introduces a sensory-enriched environment to provide arousing input to "jump-start" the child. Sensory input should be provided in a slow, controlled, systematic manner that brings the child to threshold but not beyond. Too much input can cause the child to become disorganized and even appear hyperreactive. The most organizing sensory inputs are proprioception and pressure touch, which are low in intensity and have a prolonged influence on the nervous system. As such, these somatosensory inputs are incorporated both in direct intervention and in the activities that make up the child's sensory diet. The following arousing activities designed to foster sensorimotor readiness can be graded based on each child's unique response: walking on a mattress on the floor, crawling on and around couch cushions, swinging that is carefully graded, enjoying playground activities such as riding on a merry-go-round, and using a loofah sponge for the bath. All of these activities are child directed and not imposed by an adult. Some sensory input, such as light touch or rapid rotary vestibular stimulation, can be very powerful and cause an exaggerated response hours after it was provided (e.g., flushing, sweating, sleep disturbances, appetite changes).

Some children who have high thresholds may have slow reactions to sensory input. They will react but will do so gradually. Enough time needs to be provided for the child to plan and initiate a response before offering additional sensory input. The child needs to be engaged in activities of interest. When motivated, the child is better able to organize, integrate, and use sensory input. One should avoid passive stimulation of the hyporeactive child. The child's sensory-based needs and motivation must be what dictate the pacing of the treatment based on sensory integration theory. There is a tendency for the therapist to overstructure the sessions, to not allow for adequate practice and repetition, to introduce too many activities too quickly, and to overdirect the child with language.

Guidelines for Intervention with Dyspraxia

The following suggestions are designed to improve the performance of children with dyspraxia and autism. If the child has problems in ideation, then the practitioner works to improve sensory modulation and the ability to interact flexibly with the environment. If the child has problems with motor planning, then one works to improve body scheme by increasing tactile and proprioceptive feedback from movement and to expand the ability to initiate and sequence motor strategies. For the child with problems in the execution of motor acts, targeted practice of motor skills is integrated into activities. Intervention for the child with dyspraxia is complex and usually requires a specialized environment and a therapist with advanced training. A full discussion of intervention for dyspraxia is beyond the scope of this chapter. The following discussion, however, will introduce some of the major principles of this intervention (Kimball, 1993; Koomar & Bundy, 1991; Parham & Mailloux, 1996).

A major concern is to enhance body awareness and motor control by increasing somatosensory input (i.e., pressure touch and proprioception) through self-selected, resistive, gross motor activities. For example, the child's movements are resisted when he or she propels him- or herself on a swing or "helps" to move a heavy beanbag chair. The practitioner joins in child-directed play by using imitation of the child's activities without asking questions or initiating any demands. One follows the child's lead and allows time for the long latency of response found in some of these children. Rather than suggest solutions to a novel task during play, the adult provides time for independent problem solving and possibly asks questions about next steps. Gradually the clinician introduces a change in the environment that requires a modification in the child's play behavior. Repetition and practice need to be provided even if at times the behavior may appear perseverative. It usually takes the child with dyspraxia longer to learn motor activities.

The child needs to be involved in generating goals and planning activities. In this context, *planning* does not usually imply verbalization of a goal or planned sequence. Instead, the term refers to engagement in a meaningful and productive activity that emphasizes somatosensory input. There is no way to provide a list of practic activities that are meaningful and developmentally challenging for all children. Rather, a practic activity emerges from the child's motivation, the environmental opportunities, and the practitioner's clinical reasoning about the child's strengths and needs. As an example, searching for a partially hidden object is a practic task for a child with autism and minimal environmental interaction. The clinician's task is then to create challenges and novelty in the pathway to the object. One can hide it under a large pillow; in a container full of balls or rice; or across a room filled with ramps, pillows, and bridges. Another child may be motivated by swinging, so the practic activity is getting onto and moving the swing. Still another child may be able to participate in the more complex task of building an obstacle course for exploration. The key is modifying the environment to provide a motivating, sensory-enriched situation that requires repeated coordinated action. In this process the practitioner avoids the tendency of too much verbal or physical directiveness.

DIRECTIONS FOR FUTURE RESEARCH

Although some research has occurred in this important domain, there is clearly a need for continued investigations regarding the nature of sensory processing in children who have ASD. This research should validate the clinical profiles and the relationship between observable behavior and underlying physiological functioning using both cross-sectional and longitudinal designs. Descriptive research needs to study the regulation and dysregulation of arousal, attention, affect, and action as they relate to the sensory properties of activity and the environment. Of particular importance with this population is exploration of the link among sensory seeking, stereotypies, and other nonadaptive behaviors. It is also useful to investigate the contributions of deficits in sensory modulation and praxis to other domains such as social relatedness, affect, and communication.

Clinically relevant assessment procedures should be developed and refined because they relate to early identification of autism and sensory disorders. In addition, effectiveness studies need to be designed to examine intervention for different sensory integrative deficits. Outcome measures should focus on targeted behaviors that are functionally relevant and appropriate to specific clinical presentations and not to global diagnostic categories (e.g., operationally defining self-regulation of arousal in children with hyperreactivity to tactile stimuli or of flexibility of environmental interaction in children with dyspraxia). Finally, because sensory integrative treatment is rarely applied in isolation, some efficacy research should target the contributions of multiple intervention approaches within a treatment regime (e.g., contrasting progress in behavioral programs with and without sensory integration consultation and direct intervention).

CONCLUSIONS

Sensory integration deficits are present in many children with autism. Of particular concern are problems in sensory modulation. Children may exhibit hyperreactivity to input in one or more sensory modalities that results in fearfulness or avoidance. Conversely, other children may have an underreactivity to sensation resulting in either a lack of awareness of the environment or sensory-seeking behaviors designed to meet sensory needs. Problems in sensory modulation may underlie many of the perseverative stereotypic behaviors so typical of children with autism (Baranek et al., 1997b; Carr, 1994). Another clinical profile indicative of sensory integrative dysfunction is dyspraxia. Children with autism and dyspraxia have difficulty in formulating, planning, and executing unfamiliar activities and typically have a poor sensory-based body scheme.

Assessment of sensory integrative processes involves careful observation of how these children respond to the naturally occurring activities of daily living. Of special importance is observation of the goodness-of-fit between the child and the environment and how the fit changes throughout the course of the day. A parent interview provides information about the child's sensory tolerances and preferences and how they influence daily living, relationships, and learning. Intervention begins with an appreciation of the child's unique sensory profile. On the basis of this profile, the practitioner must 1) incorporate the use of a sensory diet to help the child self-regulate arousal, attention, affect, and action; 2) facilitate a good fit between the child and the physical and social environments; and 3) provide remediation through child-directed sensory experiences that produce purposeful adaptive behavior. The role of sensory integrative deficits in children with autism has been documented. Additional research, however, is required to describe the nature of sensory integrative dysfunction in children with autism, to validate the clinical profiles, and to refine intervention strategies.

REFERENCES

Adrien, J.L., Lenoir, P., Marineau, J., Perrot, A., Hameury, L., Larmande, C., & Sauvage, D. (1993). Blind ratings of early symptoms of autism based upon family home movies. *Journal of the American Academy of Child and Adolescent Psychiatry, 32,* 617–626.

American Psychiatric Association. (1994). *Diagnostic and statistical manual of mental disorders* (4th ed.). Washington, DC: Author.

Anzalone, M.E. (1993). Sensory contributions to action: A sensory integrative approach. *ZERO TO THREE Bulletin, 14*(2), 17–20.

Ayres, A.J. (1972). *Sensory integration and learning disabilities.* Los Angeles: Western Psychological Services.

Ayres, A.J. (1979). *Sensory integration and the child.* Los Angeles: Western Psychological Services.

Ayres, A.J. (1985). *Developmental dyspraxia and adult onset apraxia.* Torrance, CA: Sensory Integration International.

Ayres, A.J., & Tickle, L.S. (1980). Hyper-responsivity to touch and vestibular stimuli as a predictor of positive response to sensory integration procedures by autistic children. *American Journal of Occupational Therapy, 34,* 375–380.

Baranek, G.T. (1998). Sensory processing in persons with autism and developmental disabilities: Considerations for research and clinical practice. *American Occupational Therapy Association Sensory Integration Special Interest Section Quarterly, 21*(2), 1–4.

Baranek, G.T. (1999). Autism during infancy: A retrospective video analysis of sensory-motor and social behaviors at 9–12 months of age. *Journal of Autism and Developmental Disorders, 29*(3), 213–224.

Baranek, G.T., Foster, L.G., & Berkson, G. (1997a). Sensory defensiveness in persons with developmental disabilities. *Occupational Therapy Journal of Research, 17,* 173–185.

Baranek, G.T., Foster, L.G., & Berkson, G. (1997b). Tactile defensiveness and stereotyped behaviors. *American Journal of Occupational Therapy, 51,* 91–95.

Bonoclonna, P. (1981). Effects of a vestibular stimulation program on stereotypic rocking behavior. *American Journal of Occupational Therapy, 35,* 775–781.

Brazelton, T.B. (1984). *Neonatal Behavioral Assessment Scale: Clinics in developmental medicine.* (2nd ed.). Philadelphia: Lippincott-Raven.

Burack, J.A. (1994). Selective attention deficits in persons with autism. *Journal of Abnormal Psychology, 103,* 525–543.

Carr, E.G. (1994). Emerging themes in functional analysis of problem behavior. *Journal of Applied Behavior Analysis, 27,* 393–399.

Casey, B.J., Gordon, C.T., Mannheim, G.B., & Rumsey, J.M. (1993). Dysfunctional attention in autistic savants. *Journal of Clinical and Experimental Neuropsychology, 15,* 933–946.

Cermak, S.A. (1988). The relationship between attention deficit and sensory integration disorders (Part 1). *American Occupational Therapy Association Sensory Integration Special Interest Section Newsletter, 11*(9), 1–4.

Cermak, S.A. (1991). Somatodyspraxia. In A.G. Fisher, E.A. Murray, & A.C. Bundy (Eds.), *Sensory integration: Theory and practice* (pp. 137–171). Philadelphia: F.A. Davis.

Cohen, D.J., & Volkmar, F.R. (1997). *Handbook of autism and pervasive developmental disorders* (2nd ed). New York: John Wiley & Sons.

Cook, D.G. (1991). The assessment process. In W. Dunn (Ed.), *Pediatric occupational therapy: Facilitating effective service provision* (pp. 35–73). Thorofare, NJ: Slack.

Coster, W., Deeney, T., Haltiwanger, J., & Haley, S. (1998). *School Function Assessment.* San Antonio, TX: The Psychological Corporation.

Courchesne, E., Townsend, J., Akshoomoff, N.A., Saitoh, O., Yeung-Courchesne, R., Lincoln, A.J., James, H.E., Haas, R.H., Schreibman, L., & Lau, L. (1994). Impairment in shifting attention in autistic and cerebellar patients. *Behavioral Neuroscience, 108,* 848–865.

Dawson, G., & Lewy, A. (1989). Arousal attention and the socioemotional impairments of individuals with autism. In G. Dawson (Ed.), *Autism: Nature, diagnosis, and treatment* (pp. 49–74). New York: Guilford Press.

DeGangi, G.A. (1995). *Infant and Toddler Symptom Checklist.* San Antonio, TX: Therapy Skill Builders.

DeGangi, G.A., & Greenspan, S. (1989). *Test of Sensory Functions in Infants.* Los Angeles: Western Psychological Services.

Dunn, W. (1997). The impact of sensory processing abilities on the daily lives of young children and their families: A conceptual model. *Infants and Young Children, 9,* 23–35.

Dunn, W., & Brown, C. (1997). Factor analysis on a sensory profile from a national sample of children without disabilities. *American Journal of Occupational Therapy,* 51, 490–499.

Dunn, W., & Oetter, P. (1991). Application of assessment principles. In W. Dunn (Ed.), *Pediatric occupational therapy: Facilitating effective service provision* (pp. 75–123). Thorofare, NJ: Slack.

Fisher, A.G., Murray, E.A., & Bundy, A.C. (Eds.). (1991). *Sensory integration: Theory and practice.* Philadelphia: F.A. Davis.

Freeman, B.J. (1993). The syndrome of autism: Update and guidelines for diagnosis. *Infants and Young Children, 6,* 1–11.

Frick, S.M., & Lawton-Shirley, N. (1994). Auditory integrative training from a sensory integrative perspective. *American Occupational Therapy Association Sensory Integration Special Interest Section Newsletter, 17,* 1–3.

Ghez, C., Gordon, J., Ghilardi, M.F., & Sainburg, R. (1995). Contributions of vision and proprioception to accuracy in limb movements. In M.S. Gazzaniga (Ed.), *The cognitive neurosciences* (pp. 548–564). Cambridge, MA: MIT Press.

Gibson, E.J. (1988). Exploratory behavior in the development of perceiving, acting, and the acquiring of knowledge. *Annual Review of Psychology, 39,* 1–41.

Gillberg, C., & Coleman, M. (1992). *The biology of the autistic syndromes* (2nd ed.). New York: Cambridge University Press.

Grandin, T. (1992). Calming effects of deep touch pressure in patients with autistic disorder, college students, and animals. *Journal of Child and Adolescent Psychopharmacology, 2,* 63–72.

Grandin, T. (1995). *Thinking in pictures.* New York: Bantam Doubleday Dell.

Grandin, T., & Scariano, M.M. (1986). *Emergence: Labeled autistic.* New York: Warner Books.

Greenspan, S.I. (1992). Reconsidering the diagnosis and treatment of very young children with autistic spectrum or pervasive developmental disorder. *ZERO TO THREE Bulletin, 13*(2), 1–9.

Greenspan, S.I., & Meisels, S.J. (1996). Toward a new vision for the developmental assessment of infants and young children. In S.J. Meisels & E. Fenichel (Eds.), *New visions for the developmental assessment of infants and young children* (pp. 11–26). Washington, DC: ZERO TO THREE: National Center for Infants, Toddlers, and Families.

Haas, R.H., Townsend, J., Courchesne, E., & Lincoln, A.J. (1996). Neurologic abnormalities in infantile autism. *Journal of Child Neurology, 11,* 84–92.

Hanft, B.E., & Place, P.A. (1996). *The consulting therapist: A guide for OTs and PTs in schools.* San Antonio, TX: Therapy Skill Builders.

Kandel, E.R., Schwartz, J.H., & Jessell, T.M. (1991). *Principles of neural science* (3rd ed.). Norwalk, CT: Appleton & Lange.

Kemper, T.L., & Bauman, M.L. (1993). The contribution of neuropathological studies to the understanding of autism. *Neurologic Clinics, 11,* 175–187.

Kientz, M.A. (1996). Sensory based needs in children with autism: Motivation for behavior and suggestions for intervention. *American Occupational Therapy Association Developmental Disabilities Special Interest Section Newsletter, 19*(3), 1–3.

Kientz, M.A., & Dunn, W. (1997). A comparison of the performance of children with and without autism on the sensory profile. *American Journal of Occupational Therapy, 51,* 530–537.

Kimball, J.G. (1993). Sensory integrative frame of reference. In P. Kramer & J. Hinojosa (Eds.), *Frames of reference for pediatric occupational therapy* (pp. 87–167). Baltimore: Lippincott Williams & Wilkins.

Kinsbourne, M. (1983). Toward a model of attention deficit disorder. In M. Perlmutter (Ed.), *The Minnesota Symposium on Child Psychology: Vol. 16. Development and policy concerning children with special needs.* Mahwah, NJ: Lawrence Erlbaum Associates.

Koomar, J.A., & Bundy, A.C. (1991). The art and science of creating direct intervention from theory. In A.G. Fisher, E.A. Murray, & A.C. Bundy (Eds.), *Sensory integration theory and practice* (pp. 251–314). Philadelphia: F.A. Davis.

Leary, M.R., & Hill, D.A. (1996). Moving on: Autism and movement disturbance. *Mental Retardation, 34,* 39–59.

Lester, B.M., Freier, K., & LaGasse, L. (1995). Prenatal cocaine exposure and child outcome: What do we really know? In M. Lewis & M. Bendersky (Eds.), *Mothers, babies, and cocaine: The role of toxins in development* (pp. 19–40). Mahwah, NJ: Lawrence Erlbaum Associates.

Lewkowicz, D.J., & Lickliter, R. (1994). *The development of intersensory perception: Comparative perspectives.* Mahwah, NJ: Lawrence Erlbaum Associates.

Lincoln, A.J., Courchesne, E., Harms, L., & Allen, M. (1995). Sensory modulation of auditory stimuli in children with autism and receptive developmental language disorder: Event-related brain potential evidence. *Journal of Autism and Developmental Disorders, 25,* 521–539.

Losche, G. (1990). Sensorimotor and action development in autistic children from infancy to early childhood. *Journal of Child Psychology and Psychiatry and Allied Disciplines, 31,* 749–761.

Mailloux, Z., Parham, L.D., & Roley, S.S. (1998, June). Sensory processing and praxis in high functioning children with autism. *Proceedings of the World Federation of Occupational Therapy,* 1160. Montréal, Québec, Canada.

Manjiviona, J., & Prior, M. (1995). Comparison of Asperger syndrome and high-functioning autistic children on a test of motor impairment. *Journal of Autism and Developmental Disorders, 25,* 23–40.

Mauk, J.E. (1993). Autism and developmental disorders. *Pediatric Clinics of North America, 40,* 567–578.

Miller, H. (1996). Eye contact and gaze aversion: Implications for persons with autism. *American Occupational Therapy Association Sensory Integration Special Interest Section Newsletter, 19*(2), 1–3.

Miller, L.J. (1988). *Miller Assessment for Preschoolers* (Rev. manual). San Antonio, TX: Psychological Corporation.

Miller, L.J., & McIntosh, D.N. (1998). The diagnosis, treatment and etiology of sensory modulation disorder. *American Occupational Therapy Association Sensory Integration Special Interest Section Quarterly, 21,* 1–3.

Ornitz, E.M. (1974). The modulation of sensory input and motor output in autistic children. *Journal of Autism and Developmental Disorders, 4,* 197–215.

Ornitz, E.M. (1988). Autism: A disorder of directed attention. *Brain Dysfunction, 1,* 309–322.

Ornitz, E.M. (1989). Autism at the interface between sensory processing and information processing. In G. Dawson (Ed.), *Autism: Nature, diagnosis, and treatment* (pp. 174–207). New York: Guilford Press.

Parham, L.D., & Mailloux, Z. (1996). Sensory integration. In J. Case-Smith, A.S. Allen, & P.N. Pratt (Eds.), *Occupational therapy for children* (3rd ed., pp. 307–356). St. Louis, MO: C.V. Mosby.

Porges, S.W., McCabe, P.M., & Yongue, B.G. (1982). Respiratory-heart rate interactions: Psychophysiological implications for pathophysiology and behavior. In J. Cacioppo & R. Petty (Eds.), *Perspectives in cardiovascular psychophysiology* (pp. 223–264). New York: Guilford Press.

Rankin, V. (1998). *The effects of supplementary consultation based on sensory integration on the incidence of self stimulatory behaviors in autistic children.* Unpublished master's thesis, Columbia University, New York.

Rapin, I. (1997). Autism. *New England Journal of Medicine, 337,* 97–104.

Ray, T., King, L.J., & Grandin, T. (1988). The effectiveness of self initiated vestibular stimulation in producing speech sounds in an autistic child. *Occupational Therapy Journal of Research, 8,* 186–190.

Restall, G., & Magill-Evans, J. (1994). Play and preschool children with autism. *American Journal of Occupational Therapy, 48,* 113–120.

Royeen, C.B., & Lane, S.J. (1991). Tactile processing and sensory defensiveness. In A.G. Fisher, E.A. Murray, & A.C. Bundy (Eds.), *Sensory integration: Theory and practice* (pp. 108–131). Philadelphia: F.A. Davis.

Schreibman, L. (1988). Diagnostic features of autism. *Journal of Child Neurology, 3* (Suppl.), S57–S64.

Sigman, M., & Capps, L. (1997). *Children with autism: A developmental perspective.* Cambridge, MA: Harvard University Press.

Sigman, M., Mundy, P., & Yirmiya, N. (1990). Affect sharing in the context of joint attention interactions of normal, autistic, and mentally retarded children. *Journal of Autism and Developmental Disorders, 20,* 87–100.

Townsend, J., Harris, N.S., & Courchesne, E. (1996). Visual attention abnormalities in autism: Delayed orienting to location. *Journal of the International Neuropsychological Society, 2,* 541–550.

Wilbarger, P. (1995). The sensory diet: Activity programs based on sensory processing theory. *American Occupational Therapy Association Sensory Integration Special Interest Section Quarterly, 18*(2), 1–4.

Wilbarger, P., & Wilbarger, J.L. (1991). *Sensory defensiveness in children aged 2–12: An intervention guide for parents and other caretakers.* Santa Barbara, CA: Avanti Education Programs.

Williams, D. (1992). *Nobody nowhere.* New York: Avon.

Williams, D. (1994). *Somebody somewhere.* New York: Times Books.

Williams, M.S., & Shellenberger, S. (1996). *How does your engine run?: A leaders guide to the Alert Program for Self-Regulation.* Albuquerque, NM: Therapy Works, Inc.

Williamson, G.G., & Anzalone, M.E. (1997). Sensory integration: A key component of the evaluation and treatment of young children with severe difficulties in relating and communicating. *ZERO TO THREE Bulletin, 17,* 29–36.

Yeung-Courchesne, R., & Courchesne, E. (1997). From impasse to insight in autism research: From behavioral symptoms to biological explanations. *Development and Psychopathology, 9,* 389–419.

Zeitlin, S., & Williamson, G.G. (1988). *The Early Coping Inventory.* Bensonville, IL: Scholastic Testing Service.

Zeitlin, S., & Williamson, G.G. (1994). *Coping in young children: Early intervention practices to enhance adaptive behavior and resilience.* Baltimore: Paul H. Brookes Publishing Co.

ZERO TO THREE/National Center for Clinical Infant Programs. (1994). *Diagnostic Classification: 0–3 diagnostic classification of mental health and developmental disorders of infancy and early childhood.* Arlington, VA: Author.

Zissermann, L. (1992). The effects of deep pressure on self stimulatory behaviors in a child with autism and other disabilities. *American Journal of Occupational Therapy, 46,* 547–557.

8

Neurological Underpinnings of Autism

Natacha Akshoomoff

This chapter reviews the most recent empirical findings and theoretical positions in the literature on the neural basis of autism that may lead to hypothesis-driven empirical investigations. Although many investigators have described the behavioral deficits present in most individuals with autism, it is a more difficult task to determine the neural abnormalities that may be responsible for these behavioral deficits. There is a limited understanding of the normal brain systems involved in the development of these functions. With a developmental disorder, one must also tackle the difficult task of determining the etiology and ontogenetic path that leads to the common neurological and behavioral outcome at a much later point in brain development.

NEUROANATOMICAL ABNORMALITIES

On the basis of diagnostic and related features observed in individuals with autism, theories of the neuroanatomical basis of autism have included nearly every part of the association cortex as well as the brain stem, cerebellum, and other subcortical regions of the brain. There are several reasons for the diverse hypotheses regarding the underlying neurological mechanisms. Some researchers have hypothesized that the behavioral and neuropsychological differences observed in individuals with autism are similar to those observed in people with damage to the prefrontal cortex. Others have suggested that the early deficits observed in this disorder and the pervasiveness of these symptoms are more consistent with damage to subcortical systems that would, in turn, affect the development of some but perhaps not all neocortical systems. Until recently, brain–behavior relationships were difficult to address in this type of developmental disorder. The advent of in vivo neuroimaging techniques has allowed researchers to analyze structural and functional data about specific brain regions from well-defined individuals with autism and compare them with matched control subjects. Technical complications continue to make it difficult to measure reliably all neural regions, but improvements continue in this area (Courchesne & Plante, 1996). Results from autopsy studies have also been limited, but cases continue to be added to the literature with improved subject descriptions and more extensive quantitative and microscopic analyses.

The vermis of the cerebellum was the first structure that was quantitatively analyzed in autism using magnetic resonance imaging (MRI). The human cerebellum includes the medial region, or the vermis, which connects the two lateral lobes or hemispheres. The evolutionarily newest and largest portion of the cerebellum is the neocerebellum, which comprises lobules VI and VII of the vermis as well as the posterior lobe of the cerebellar hemispheres. The vermis has become the focus of many different investigations, not only to test a hypothesis that early damage to this area was a factor in autism (Courchesne, 1987) but also because it is technically easier to quantitatively measure using MRI (Courchesne & Plante, 1996). Because the cerebellar abnormality in autism is developmental, it is possible that maldevelopment of the cerebellum will result in additional structural abnormality of later-developing brain systems such as the cerebral cortex (Courchesne, Press, & Yeung-Courchesne, 1993; Courchesne, Townsend, & Saitoh, 1994).

Results from Neuroimaging Studies

The majority of neuroimaging studies have focused on the cerebellum. Some studies, however, have also included quantitative analyses of the cerebral cortex, whole brain volume, midbrain structures, and the hippocampus.

Hypoplasia of the Neocerebellar Vermis

In 1987 Courchesne introduced the hypothesis that developmental damage to the cerebellum might be a common feature in autism. Two subsequent studies reported hypoplasia (reduced growth) of the neocerebellar vermis (lobules VI and VII) in individuals with autism (Courchesne, Hesselink, Jernigan, & Yeung-Courchesne, 1987; Courchesne, Yeung-Courchesne, Press, Hesselink, & Jernigan, 1988). In the years that have followed, a number of investigations have focused on measuring the cerebellar vermis and hemispheres in an attempt to determine whether this hypothesis is indeed correct. In fact, abnormality of the neocerebellum is the most consistent neuroanatomical abnormality in autism (for reviews see Courchesne, Townsend, & Saitoh, 1994; Yeung-Courchesne & Courchesne, 1997).

Regarding the role of the cerebellum in autism, reviews (Filipek, 1995; Minshew & Dombrowski, 1994; Minshew, Sweeney, & Bauman, 1997; Waterhouse, Fein, & Modahl, 1996) have focused on five published quantitative MRI studies in which the authors reported that they were unable to detect hypoplasia of vermal lobules VI and VII. The authors of these reviews have interpreted the results of these five studies as a "failure to replicate" the results of Courchesne and colleagues (1988) and have suggested there is not enough available evidence for "specific" cerebellar pathology in autism. As discussed elsewhere in the literature (Courchesne, Townsend, Akshoomoff, Yeung-Courchesne, et al., 1994; Courchesne, Yeung-Courchesne, & Egaas, 1994), all five MRI studies used small sample sizes. To accurately measure the cerebellar vermis, a mid-line structure that is relatively narrow, a mid-sagittal MRI is crucial. Three of the studies that reported no vermis abnormality in autism, however, used anatomical landmarks outside the cerebellum for selecting mid-sagittal coordinates rather than the more accurate landmarks within the cerebellar vermis (Garber & Ritvo, 1992; Garber et al., 1989; Holttum, Minshew, Sanders, & Phillips, 1992).

Courchesne, Townsend, and Saitoh (1994) statistically reanalyzed MRI data from 78 children with autism obtained from the other two studies that reported no vermis abnormality in autism (Kleiman, Neff, & Rosman, 1992; Piven et al., 1992). They combined these data with data from their own published studies (Courchesne et al., 1988; Courchesne, Saitoh, et al., 1994) as well as with data from 91 typical children. These analyses revealed that when data from independent samples of individuals with autism were analyzed together, there was significant and *strong* evidence of hypoplasia of vermal lobules VI and VII. This large data set also extended Courchesne, Saitoh, and colleagues' (1994) study, in which the authors reported that a subset of individuals with autism (approximately 12%) had abnormally enlarged cerebellar lobules VI and VII (hyperplasia). From an embryological standpoint, injuries to the developing brain are sometimes followed by increased neurogenesis, and, thus, it appears reasonable that the cerebellum could be abnormally large or small in autism following a (presumed) early insult (Rodier, Ingram, Tisdale, Nelson, & Romano, 1996).

Hyperplasia among individuals with autism may also help to explain why the authors of two of the studies (Kleiman et al., 1992; Piven et al., 1992) reported that they found no evidence of hypoplasia in their samples of people with autism. Given the small sample sizes (13 and 15 children, respectively), the presence of individuals with hyperplasia appears to have skewed the mean of the mid-sagittal area measurements for the groups, masking the difference between the control subjects and the individuals with autism (Courchesne, 1997). Despite these considerations, the consistency of the findings across the majority of published studies is compelling.

It appears that individuals with autism who have the lowest verbal IQ scores tend to have the most deviant vermis measures, whereas those with higher verbal IQ scores tend to have less deviant measures. All individuals with autism with hyperplasia in one study had verbal IQ scores of 70 or less (Courchesne, Saitoh, et al., 1994). Despite the argument that the hypoplasia result simply reflects an IQ-score effect (Piven et al., 1992), few investigators have reported the correlation between vermis area measurements and IQ scores. One should consider using the verbal IQ scores rather than nonverbal

IQ scores as an indicator of clinical impairment in autism because the latter may be relatively spared (Courchesne, Townsend, & Saitoh, 1994). The range of IQ scores in study groups should also be considered. The group used in some of Piven's studies (Piven, Arndt, Bailey, & Andreasen, 1996; Piven et al., 1995; Piven, Bailey, Ranson, & Arndt, 1997) had nonverbal IQ scores ranging from 52 to 136, and the group included in an earlier study (Piven et al., 1992) had nonverbal IQ scores ranging from 60 to 130. No mention is made of screening individuals for fragile X syndrome or excluding those who met criteria for Asperger syndrome. The latter point is important because a quantitative MRI study of seven individuals with Asperger syndrome suggested that there are distinct differences in the size of the cerebellar vermis and the corpus callosum between Asperger syndrome and autism (Lincoln, Courchesne, Allen, Hanson, & Ene, 1998). Inclusion of high-functioning individuals who may meet criteria for Asperger syndrome may therefore also mask the differences between control subjects and individuals with autistic disorder.

It is difficult to quantify "autism severity," particularly with regard to social skills, and it appears that intelligence is partially independent from social skill level (Waterhouse, 1994). Individuals with IQ scores below 70, however, tend to have poorer prognosis in adulthood, a higher incidence of epilepsy, and more neurodevelopmental abnormalities (for a review, see Wing, 1997). If there is some neuroanatomical abnormality that is correlated with or causally related to the severity of autism (e.g., amount of vermal hypoplasia, neuron loss, degree of reduced axon or dendritic growth, degree of cell-packing density), then this abnormality may also be related to IQ score. It may be, for instance, that the degree of abnormality within a certain structure is correlated with certain aspects of language processing, which in turn is related to the overall IQ score. When comparing children with autism with typical children, controlling for IQ scores may thus reduce or eliminate the possibility of finding a group difference in terms of the brain abnormality.

Hypoplasia of vermal lobules VI and VII may also be found in other types of neurogenetic syndromes, including those without autism-like behaviors (e.g., Schaefer et al., 1996). This suggests that damage to the neocerebellum may be a factor in a number of neurodevelopmental conditions. It is interesting to note that the cerebellar vermis is abnormally large in Williams syndrome, with a significantly greater ratio of lobules VI–VII compared with lobules I–V (Jernigan & Bellugi, 1990; Jernigan, Bellugi, Sowell, Doherty, & Hesselink, 1993). Individuals with Williams syndrome and those with autism certainly differ in many aspects of behavior. This may indicate a differential outcome of early cerebellar abnormality on cognitive and social development.

If one takes a narrow view of brain–behavior development, one may wonder how two disorders could share a common biological characteristic (cerebellar vermis hyperplasia in children with Williams syndrome and in a subset of individuals with autism) yet have different behavioral phenotypes. If one uses a specificity criterion, then clearly hypoplasia of the neocerebellum does not fit as a core deficit in autism (Yeung-Courchesne & Courchesne, 1997). There are many ways, however, to produce neural growth abnormalities or atrophy, and the neural distinctions all reside at the sub-MRI level of visualization. Although individuals with different developmental disorders may have hypoplasia of the cerebellum, this could be a result of different types of neuropathology that could have different effects on subsequent brain and behavioral development. The discovery that most individuals with autism have hypoplasia of the neocerebellar vermis is just one piece of the puzzle. Researchers must now determine the other neural abnormalities commonly found among individuals with autism and how these abnormalities may fit together to explain the developmental consequences on brain, behavioral, and cognitive development.

Abnormalities in Other Brain Regions

Although the most consistent neuroimaging finding in autism has been hypoplasia of the neocerebellar vermis, there is sufficient evidence to suggest this is not the only neural abnormality present in autism. Two MRI studies found no significant differences in measurements of the pons (a brain stem structure) between control subjects and individuals with autism (Hsu, Yeung-Courchesne, Courchesne, & Press, 1991; Piven et al., 1992). Two studies, however, including one that used a prospective, longitudinal design, reported hypoplasia of brain stem structures in autism (Gaffney, Tsai, Kuperman, & Minchin, 1988; Hashimoto et al., 1995). Quantitative MRI studies of the hippocampus have not found any evidence for abnormalities in autism (Piven, Bailey, & Arndt, 1998; Saitoh, Courchesne, Egaas, Lincoln, & Schreibman, 1995).

Piven and colleagues (1995) reported they found enlarged brain size among children with autism. In another study, they suggested that brain enlargement may be more restricted to the temporal, parietal, and occipital lobes (Piven et al., 1996). Careful MRI techniques and analysis of individual cases, however, suggest that although some individuals with autism do appear to have macroencephaly, this does not appear to be the norm (Courchesne et al., 1999).

In the first quantitative MRI study of frontal lobe volume in autism, the volume of the frontal lobes in a group of 23 young children with autism was not significantly different from a group of age-matched control subjects (Carper, Courchesne, & Chisum, 1997). Differences in metabolism or functional activation of the frontal cortex (during a resting state), however, have been reported in single photon emission computerized tomography and positron emission tomography (PET) studies of autism (e.g., Rumsey et al., 1985; Zilbovicius et al., 1995). These findings suggest that although the structural appearance of the frontal lobes may appear normal in size on the MRI, abnormal connections may still be present. It is also possible that abnormal functioning of the frontal lobes is a result of faulty input from other affected structures (e.g., cerebellum, medial temporal lobe, other areas of association cortex; see also Waterhouse et al., 1996). This possibility was supported by a significant inverse correlation between the size of cerebellar vermis lobules VI–VII and frontal lobe volume (Carper et al., 1997).

In a qualitative review of MRI scans from groups of adolescents and adults with autism, a subset of individuals (43%) were identified with bilateral sulcal widening of the parietal lobe region, posterior callosal thinning, and white matter volume loss (Courchesne et al., 1993). It is difficult to determine the developmental timing of these abnormalities, but given the characteristics of this pattern of tissue abnormality, the authors suggested that it may have occurred prior to age 5. Longitudinal studies are needed to determine whether this type of abnormality, when present, changes with age. In a study of 28 children with autism (6–18 years of age), Haas and colleagues (1996) found that these individuals demonstrated significantly more abnormalities than age-matched control subjects on four of five standard neurological tests of cerebellar function (gait, alternating movements, sequential movements, and balance but not hypotonia) and two of three tests of parietal lobe function (graphesthesia and stereognosis but not somatosensory localization). No significant group differences were found on tests of mixed motor function or tests of the cranial nerves. Two quantitative MRI studies reported reduced size of the posterior regions of the corpus callosum (Egaas, Courchesne, & Saitoh, 1995; Piven et al., 1997). This is the area of the corpus callosum where parietal lobe fibers are known to project and therefore may also reflect abnormalities in the parietal lobes in autism.

One study also suggested that some individuals with autism may have cell migration abnormalities in the cerebral cortex. Developmental cortical malformations were found in the MRI scans of 7 of 13 children with autism using blind ratings from two neurologists (Piven et al., 1990). The individuals were relatively high-functioning without fragile X and without a history of major neurological abnormalities (including seizures) or medical abnormalities. The gyral malformations (polymicrogyria, schizencephaly, macrogyria) were not confined to one particular lobe or hemisphere. The prevalence of these cortical malformations is not known but may represent a "subgroup phenomenon" rather than an explanation for the symptoms in the majority of people with autism. These types of cortical abnormalities are consistent with other pieces of evidence (e.g., abnormal cell migration in the cerebellum) that suggest that the onset of the neurological disorder in autism occurs within the first 6 months of gestation.

Results from Autopsy Studies

Autopsy studies provide structural data that are not available from MRI scans. The number of cases reported in the literature to date, however, is limited. Studies vary in terms of the number and extent of different brain regions that have been analyzed. For example, some studies have been limited to analysis of the cerebellum with no information about other structures, whereas others have not consistently reported brain weights. Analysis of samples in some cases includes qualitative descriptions of neuronal appearance but not cell counts. Finally, studies also vary in terms of diagnostic and clinical information available on the individuals. Some individuals are reported to have experienced potential confounding factors, such as serious seizure disorders, associated disorders (e.g., phenylketonuria, mental retardation requiring pervasive supports), or even a questionable diagnosis of autistic disorder (e.g., probable Rett syndrome).

A significant reduction of Purkinje cells and, to a lesser extent, granule cell loss in the cerebellum have been reported in autopsy studies from different laboratories (Bauman, Filipek, & Kemper, 1997; Ritvo et al., 1986; Williams, Hauser, Purpura, DeLong, & Swisher, 1980). The neurons of the deep cerebellar nuclei and inferior olive (a group of neurons in the medulla that sends projections to the cerebellum) were enlarged and plentiful in the brains of two children, but neurons were decreased in both size and number in the deep cerebellar nuclei and smaller in the inferior olive in the brains of three adults (Bauman et al., 1997). Although it is difficult to reach conclusions at this point on such a restricted sample, the neurons in the deep cerebellar nuclei and inferior olive may change with age in autism. These changes may signify that these regions are responding to abnormalities in their target cells or their input. That is, primary damage to the cerebellar cortex may lead to changes in the nuclei that send out efferent projections from the cerebellum, or damage to the inferior olive, deep cerebellar nuclei, and cerebellar cortex may be secondary to damage that occurred even earlier in development (Rodier et al., 1996). Bauman and her colleagues have suggested that because there was an absence of glial cell hyperplasia, which commonly co-occurs with cell loss as a result of disease or injury, and an absence of retrograde cell loss in the inferior olive, the abnormal development of the cerebellum occurred at or before 30 weeks of gestation.

Reduced neuronal size and increased cell-packing density in the hippocampus, amygdala, mammillary body, anterior cingulate cortex, and septum were also found in six individuals with autism compared with the brains of individuals in a control group (Bauman & Kemper, 1985, 1994). Neuronal counts were not available in most of these cases.

A study of the motor nuclei in the brain stem of one individual with autism revealed near-complete absence of the facial nucleus and superior olive, and the region normally surrounding the facial nucleus was shortened (Rodier et al., 1996). An unusual cluster of neurons was also present within the hypoglossal nucleus. The authors discussed these results in conjunction with reports of autism following prenatal thalidomide exposure as evidence for the initiation of damage in autism occurring around the time of neural tube closure. Because the formation of Purkinje neurons quickly follows the embryonic formation of the cranial motor nerve neurons, Rodier and colleagues hypothesized that motor neuron damage could have consequences for the cerebellum or that early injury to the developing nervous system could affect both areas directly.

Megalencephaly was reported for two of four autism postmortem cases (Bailey, Luthert, Bolton, LeCouteur, & Rutter, 1993). Courchesne, Müller, and Saitoh (1999) included these 4 cases in a study of 5 new postmortem cases along with 12 previously published cases. Compared with normative brain weight data, the results of this study suggest that brain weight is normal in most individuals with autism with some rare instances of megalencephaly and possibly micrencephaly.

An extensive follow-up autopsy study of the four cases from the Bailey et al. (1993) study was conducted that included two additional individuals (Bailey et al., 1998). All individuals were described as "mentally handicapped." The purpose of this study was to evaluate previous claims of cerebellar and temporal lobe abnormalities by autopsy and to determine whether there are more extensive brain abnormalities in individuals with autism. Decreased number of Purkinje neurons in the cerebellum were reported in six of six cases. Five of the six cases had Purkinje neuron loss in both vermis and cerebellar hemispheres, consistent with a previous study (Ritvo et al., 1986). In the absence of significant cerebellar atrophy, this neuron loss and the presumed changes in neural growth consequent to that neuron loss are reasonable explanations for the reported hypoplasia of hemispheres and vermis seen in vivo.

In terms of regions outside the cerebellum, no consistent hippocampal abnormalities were identified, although neuronal density was relatively high across all fields of the hippocampus in one case (Bailey et al., 1998). The authors concluded that they failed to replicate the claim of Bauman and her colleagues (1997) of consistently elevated neuronal density in the hippocampus. Frontal cortical neuronal density appeared to be increased in three cases. Morphometry was limited, but the presence of cortical dysgenetic lesions suggests that there may have been abnormalities in cortical neuronal proliferation, migration, and programmed cell death. The investigators have not completed their examination of the other structures discussed in previous autopsy studies (amygdala, medial septal nuclei, mammillary bodies, facial nuclei). Macroscopic abnormalities in the development of the brain stem (e.g., olive, cerebellar peduncles), however, were present in five of five cases examined.

On the basis of their findings, Bailey and colleagues (1998) concluded that there is no evidence for highly localized pathology in autism. They also discussed the implications of their results in terms of the timing of the pathology. Although it is difficult to determine whether a single event led to the abnormalities in each case, they agreed with Bauman and colleagues' (1997) conclusion that abnormal development occurred before the time of olivary cell migration (before the end of the third month gestation). In reviewing findings from autopsy and MRI studies, it appears that a combination of diverse but related neurodevelopmental abnormalities give rise to the characteristic symptoms of autism. It has been a challenge to researchers, however, to determine how these symptoms are related to early damage to structures such as the cerebellum and brain stem.

BRAIN–BEHAVIOR RELATIONSHIPS IN AUTISM

Identification of some of the neural abnormalities in people with autism has allowed investigation of the association of these brain abnormalities with the behavioral deficits that characterize this disorder. Although great advances have been made in identifying neurological abnormalities that are fairly consistent across individuals with autism, this disorder remains one that is heterogeneous in terms of etiology, neurobiology, and behavioral abnormalities. Researchers who attempt to link neuropathology with behavioral and cognitive development face a tremendous challenge.

Two theories about how early damage to different sites within the nervous system leads to the complex disorder of autism are reviewed in the following sections. The primary diagnostic symptoms of autism have not yielded to models suggesting that there is a unitary psychological or neurological deficit (for reviews, see Waterhouse & Fein, 1997, and Waterhouse et al., 1996; see also Yeung-Courchesne & Courchesne, 1997). To evaluate any model that attempts to account for the symptoms and neuropathology of autism, one must first consider the interaction among neural development, behavioral and cognitive development, and early insult to the developing nervous system. These factors are briefly discussed next, with reference to more complete discussions of these topics.

Neural Basis of Language, Communication, and Social Development

There is currently a great deal of interest in the fields of cognitive neuroscience, cognitive science, and developmental science in understanding how the mind is built from the developing brain (Elman et al., 1996; Quartz & Sejnowski, 1997). As many studies have demonstrated, the regional specialization of functions observed in human adults, such as language and higher cognitive functions, is not present at the time of birth. Instead, development involves a process of competition and recruitment that takes advantage of regional differences in "computing style" that are in place early in development (Elman et al., 1996). Neurobiological evidence indicates that the development of the cerebral cortex depends on interaction with the environment. In other words, the process of learning may induce large changes in the structures that are involved in learning (Quartz & Sejnowski, 1997).

One cannot simply take an adult neuropsychological model and assume that damage to certain brain regions leads to the same types of cognitive and behavioral deficits in the developing child as it does in adults. Longitudinal data from animal studies have shown that the degree and even the nature of deficits can change over the course of development (e.g., Goldman, 1971,

1974; Goldman-Rakic, Isseroff, Schwartz, & Bugbee, 1983; Rosenzweig, Bennett, & Alberti, 1984). Lesions early in life can lead to altered anatomical connections and remote loss of cells. Changes in connections may thus support functions early in development but may not be adequate for more complex functions that develop later.

Studies have found that the neural structures involved in the process of language acquisition are not limited to the traditional "language areas" of the left cerebral hemisphere. For example, event-related brain potentials (ERPs) were recorded from typical infants while they listened to words (Mills, Coffey-Corina, & Neville, 1997). Within 200 milliseconds after word onset, ERP differences were noted between comprehended words and unknown words. For infants between 13 and 17 months of age, these responses were bilateral and broadly distributed over anterior and posterior regions of the scalp. At 20 months of age, these effects were restricted to electrodes over temporal and parietal regions of the left hemisphere. Comparisons between same-age children with differing language skills indicated that increasing language abilities contributed to further specialization. More studies are needed to determine how these changes relate to the typical "vocabulary burst" observed at around this time in development. It is also not certain to what extent subcortical regions may be involved in language acquisition.

In addition to functional neuroimaging techniques, studies of children with early brain injury provide another method for testing theories about the brain systems involved in cognitive development and for learning more about the effects of early brain injury. The findings from a longitudinal study of children with early unilateral brain injury (Bates et al., 1997) revealed that language outcome following early cortical damage not only differs markedly from that of damage acquired later in life but also differs with the effects of developmental disorders such as autism, Down syndrome, Williams syndrome, and developmental language disorder. The individuals in this study suffered a single unilateral lesion either prenatally or around the time of birth. The children with damage that involved the left temporal cortex (i.e., Wernicke's area) did not demonstrate delays in language comprehension but were more likely to exhibit delays in expressive language. Damage to either the left or the right frontal cortex (i.e., Broca's area), however, resulted in delays in vocabulary and grammar skills between the ages of 19 and 31 months. It is also interesting to note that after age 5 there were no detectable deficits in discourse between the children with early brain injury and a control group (Reilly, Bates, & Marchman, 1998). These children also perform much better on language tests than children with developmental language disorder, who show no evidence of neurological symptoms or cortical or subcortical lesions on MRI scans.

These results demonstrate that the neural structures involved in language acquisition are not necessarily restricted to the cortical areas that typically subserve different aspects of language later in life. This is in contrast to the development of spatial cognitive skills in these same individuals (Stiles & Thal,

1993; Stiles, Trauner, Engel, & Nass, 1997). The effects of unilateral brain injury on these skills are more similar to those observed in adults with acquired unilateral brain injury. The deficits are more subtle, however, and development or "recovery" does occur. The authors of these studies have concluded that there are strong computational constraints in the infant brain that normally lead to the pattern of left hemisphere specialization for language and right/left differences for certain aspects of spatial processing (Bates et al., 1997; Stiles, 1998; Stiles & Thal, 1993). Specific areas within the left temporal lobe appear to play an early role in extraction of perceptual detail, whereas analogous regions in the right temporal lobe play a role in integration of inputs. As a result of early injury to these areas, the typical cascade of events during development cannot take place. Therefore, the process of language and spatial cognitive development is delayed, and the final organization may not be optimal but most functions are supported within the normal range.

Individuals with autism who acquire language have a primary impairment in pragmatics, the form of communication used to accomplish certain social goals (Tager-Flusberg, 1997). The social use of language (e.g., gestures, sounds) to share information or request help comes well before the development of words and sentences (Bates, 1976). Social knowledge also plays a role in the acquisition of words and grammar. Compared with sounds, words, and grammar, however, pragmatics is difficult to study. There is some evidence that the right hemisphere plays an important role in some aspects of pragmatics. This may not be the case, however, in the developing child. In a study of children ages 6–12 who sustained a unilateral brain lesion before 6 months of age, children with a right hemisphere lesion did not differ in their performance on an idiom comprehension test from children with a left hemisphere lesion (Kempler, van Lancker, Marchman, & Bates, 1999). In autism, the impact of early deficits in pragmatics probably has a significant impact on other aspects of language development.

Waterhouse and colleagues (1996) proposed that impaired social interaction in autism results from atypical attachment and social affiliation. Animal studies have revealed that neuropeptides, including oxytocin and vasopressin, play an important role in attachment and social affiliation (Insel, 1997). The receptors for these neuropeptides are found in the limbic system, including the amygdala and hippocampus. In addition, the medial temporal lobes are thought to play a key role in affect and social communication (Bachevalier, 1994). Therefore, it may that development of the medial temporal lobe system not only leads to its important role in memory and cognitive functions but also an important role in social and emotional behavior.

Several researchers have suggested that damage to the limbic system accounts for the symptoms of autism. Little is known about the behavioral and cognitive effects of developmental damage to these areas, particularly in humans. Ablation of the amygdala and hippocampus in monkeys during the neonatal period resulted in behaviors similar to those in autism (Bachevalier,

1994). A study of four young children with early-onset bilateral hippocampal sclerosis also suggests hippocampal damage contributed to autism (DeLong & Heinz, 1997). Each of these children failed to develop language or lost the language they had attained with the onset of the hippocampal dysfunction. These children also exhibited poor social and adaptive skills, even after their epilepsy was controlled, but showed typical motor and sensory functions. MRI and PET results were indicative of isolated bilateral anterior temporal lobe hypometabolism. In a follow-up study of infants who had been evaluated for seizure surgery using PET, children with bitemporal glucose hypometabolism had a poor developmental outcome and 10 of the 14 met the *Diagnostic and Statistical Manual of Mental Disorders, Fourth Edition* (American Psychiatric Association, 1994), criteria for autism (Chugani, Silva, & Chugani, 1996).

Damage limited to the hippocampus alone, however, may not lead to the social deficits seen in autism (Bachevalier, 1994). For example, a study of three individuals with bilateral hippocampal damage (but not significant seizure disorder) provides an interesting contrast (Vargha-Khadem et al., 1997). Hippocampal damage for these individuals occurred at the time of birth, age 4, and age 9. Although these children suffered from pronounced amnesia for everyday memories, their language and academic skills were within the low average to average range. No social skill deficits for any individuals were noted in this study. It also appears that high-functioning individuals with autism do not display significant learning and memory deficits in the same way as individuals with hippocampal damage do (Bachevalier, 1994). In fact, the work of Bachevalier and Merjanian suggests that autism may primarily involve dysfunction of the amygdala rather than the hippocampus (Bachevalier, 1994).

Two Neurodevelopmental Models of Autism

Some theories of brain–behavior relationships in autism have focused on the higher-level difficulties that are fairly consistent across individuals. Alternatively, one can consider that the child with autism may suffer damage to "lower level" systems that are typically thought to regulate simpler functions. Neural regions that regulate higher-order behaviors and cognitive processes (e.g., the prefrontal cortex) mature later and are dependent on input from a variety of neural systems. Deficits in planning and organization and other higher-order skills are found in a variety of other developmental disorders for which there is also little evidence of frontal lobe "damage." Neocortical areas could therefore be essentially "normal," at least in early development, and yet the child may have extensive behavioral and cognitive deficits due to long-standing, faulty input from subcortical systems.

A Complex Neurodevelopmental Model

Waterhouse and colleagues (1996) proposed that there are four dysfunctional systems in autism: the hippocampus, the amygdala, the oxytocin-opiate system, and the temporal and parietal association cortices. They argued that damage to these systems leads to (respectively): 1) canalesthesia (abnormal fragmentation of the cross-modal information processing for an ongoing event and long-term memory for past events), 2) impaired assignment of the affective significance of stimuli, 3) asociality, and 4) extended selective attention. They proposed that the combined effects of damage to these systems and subsequent abnormalities in these functions lead to the primary diagnostic features in autism: social impairment, communication impairment, and aberrant activities.

This model is appealing because it is difficult to think of an explanation for autism that relies solely on damage to one brain region (e.g., hippocampus, amygdala, prefrontal cortex, cerebellum, brain stem). There is limited evidence, however, for abnormalities in the hippocampus and amygdala (Bailey et al., 1998; Minshew et al., 1997; Piven et al., 1998; Saitoh et al., 1995). Waterhouse and colleagues (1996) also proposed that the temporal and parietal polysensory association cortex is abnormally organized. As reviewed previously, some individuals with autism have cortical malformations in these areas or increased sulcal width in the parietal lobe. It is possible, however, that maldevelopment of the parietal lobe may be secondary to early damage in other areas that develop earlier, such as the cerebellum (Courchesne, 1995). Although it was proposed that damage to the hippocampus and amygdala would be sufficient to explain the attention and orienting deficits in autism (discussed later in this chapter), this hypothesis remains to be tested. Waterhouse and Fein (1997) criticized other researchers' hypotheses that suggest attention and arousal abnormalities are the primary (developmental) explanation for the social deficits in autism (e.g., Courchesne, 1995; Dawson & Lewy, 1989), stating that attention and arousal deficits are "key nondiagnostic deficits found in autism" (pp. 903–904). Waterhouse and colleagues (1996), however, used extended selective attention as part of their model to explain the diagnostic features of autism.

Although there is a great deal of neuroimaging and autopsy evidence to suggest that the cerebellum is associated with the neuropathological processes of autism, Waterhouse and colleagues (1996) omitted the cerebellum from their model. They concluded that "cerebellar dysfunction signals medial temporal lobe deficit, exacerbates information-processing deficits, and may contribute to associated motor abnormalities in autism" (p. 475). Waterhouse and Fein (1997) later acknowledged this potential limitation to their model but stated that they have "relegated cerebellar impairment to nonsyndromic status" (p. 910). Given that the cerebellum has connections with all of the neural systems in their model, it is possible that damage to the cerebellum in addition to damage to these areas may be necessary to produce the symptoms of autism. More research is needed to determine the extent and timing of damage in the cerebellum, amygdala, and hippocampus in autism and whether damage to temporal and parietal regions occurs after damage to these subcortical structures.

The Cerebellum and Attention Hypothesis

Since the 1980s, there has been a great deal of interest in the role of the cerebellum in cognition and behavior. Clinical reports, animal studies, neuropsychological experiments, and studies using functional neuroimaging techniques have revolutionized the view that the cerebellum participates solely in motor operations. PET and functional MRI (fMRI) studies have demonstrated that the cerebellum is activated during a range of cognitive operations, such as attention, learning novel skills, and complex problem solving, that are also deficient in people with autism (see Akshoomoff, Courchesne, & Townsend, 1997, for a review). It has also been demonstrated that the cerebellum has physioanatomical connections with many nonmotor brain systems.

The discovery that the cerebellum is affected in autism has added to the interest in uncovering the role of the cerebellum in cognition and behavior. Courchesne and his colleagues have proposed that the cerebellum may play a more fundamental role in a variety of operations (Akshoomoff et al., 1997; Courchesne & Allen, 1997). They have hypothesized that the cerebellum predicts the internal conditions needed for a particular motor or mental operation and prepares the neural systems necessary for upcoming events. The output of the cerebellum provides moment-to-moment, unconscious, very short timescale, anticipatory information.

Courchesne and his colleagues have developed a model that attempts to incorporate behavioral and cognitive findings in autism with neuroscientific discoveries about the systems that appear to be affected in autism (Courchesne, 1995; Courchesne, Townsend, Akshoomoff, Yeung-Courchesne, et al., 1994). In this model, attention is viewed as a critical deficit in autism. These attention deficits are hypothesized to be present from early development and thus contribute to the development of atypical social and cognitive deficits that characterize this disorder. In this model, the language problems in autism (i.e., pragmatics) are viewed as secondary to or the result of an inability to deal with social input. Joint social attention, which relies on the early ability to shift attention, is deficient in people with autism (e.g., Lewy & Dawson, 1992; Mundy, Sigman, & Kasari, 1990; see also Chapter 4). The typical development of joint social attention is also critical for the development of typical social and communication skills. If one considers the importance of emotion regulation in the early development of joint attention, it is easier to see how early deficits in motivation, modulation of affect, and attention contribute to the severe deficits children with autism have in initiating and maintaining joint attention and regulating emotion (Adamson & Russell, in press).

Courchesne (1995) has hypothesized that the attentional abnormalities that are so pervasive in autism are the result of early damage to subcortical systems, particularly the cerebellum. The cerebellum, however, is not viewed as the only possible site of abnormality in autism. One must consider the principles of convergence heterogeneity (many paths can lead to similar signs and symptoms) and divergence heterogeneity (the same initial state can lead to many different outcomes) in neurodevelopment. Genotype, prenatal injury, experience, and other factors have a powerful influence on the developing brain. Yeung-Courchesne and Courchesne have concluded, "No single biological defect can be the underlying initial cause of all cases of autism" (1997, p. 402).

Courchesne, Akshoomoff, and Townsend (1990) have attempted to test the hypothesis that the cerebellum plays a role in the behavioral and cognitive deficits reported in autism. Their preliminary study demonstrated that high-functioning adults with autism have difficulty rapidly shifting attention between sensory modalities. Their subsequent studies (e.g., Akshoomoff & Courchesne, 1992; Courchesne, Townsend, Akshoomoff, Saitoh, et al., 1994) have included younger individuals with autism, individuals with acquired damage to the cerebellum, and individuals with acquired damage to the cerebral cortex. These experiments have focused on attentional operations that were hypothesized to be atypical in autism, particularly attention shifting, orienting, and the distribution of attention.

The participants in two of Courchesne and colleagues' studies included children with focal cerebellar damage, a young adult with an idiopathic cerebellar degenerative disorder, adolescents diagnosed with autism, a control group of typical children, and a control group of typical adolescents (Akshoomoff & Courchesne, 1992; Courchesne, Townsend, Akshoomoff, Saitoh, et al., 1994). Each child participated in two tasks that consisted of visual and auditory stimuli: a focus-attention task and a shift-attention task. The focus-attention task tested the children's ability to continuously maintain a focus of attention and to detect a target that occurred infrequently in one sensory modality while ignoring all stimuli in the other modality. On the basis of a previous study (Ciesielski, Courchesne, & Elmasian, 1990), Courchesne and colleagues predicted that individuals with autism would not have significant difficulty maintaining their attention under these circumstances. The physiological responses from even the individuals with autism, however, indicated abnormalities in between- and within-channel stimulus selection. The shift-attention task used the same stimuli as the focus-attention task but required individuals to alternate attention between visual and auditory stimuli as signaled by the appearance of the target. Courchesne and colleagues predicted that individuals would have difficulty with this task, given the characteristic deficits in joint social attention and perseveration that are associated with autism.

Behavioral performance in the focus-attention task, which required continuous attention to only a single principal focus of information for a long period of time, was similar among participants. Behavioral performance on the shift-attention task differed between the groups, particularly with respect to time elapsed following cues to execute a shift of attention. Within 2.5 seconds of a cue to shift attention to the other modality, both individuals with cerebellar damage and individuals with autism performed significantly worse than typical control participants in correctly detecting target information in the new focus. It is important to note that the time-related deficit in the shift-attention task was not a result of slowed response times among the individuals. ERPs recorded during task performance also suggested that these individuals failed to respond to targets that followed a cue to shift attention because they had failed to shift their attention rapidly enough to the new focus of attention (i.e., the other sensory modality) to detect that information. Individuals with cerebellar damage were also shown to have difficulty rapidly shifting their attention during a shift-attention task that included only visual stimuli (Akshoomoff & Courchesne, 1994). Two fMRI studies of typical adults using this type of focus-attention and shift-attention task revealed that different regions of the cerebellum are activated during these two tasks and that these regions are different from those activated during a motor task (Allen, Buxton, Wong, & Courchesne, 1997; Le, Pardo, & Hu, 1998).

Townsend and colleagues have conducted several studies to investigate the orienting deficits in autism and the brain systems that underlie these operations (Townsend & Courchesne, 1994; Townsend et al., 1999; Townsend, Courchesne, & Egaas, 1996; Townsend, Singer-Harris, & Courchesne, 1996). These studies have demonstrated that damage to the cerebellum leads to extremely slowed attention orienting. That is, individuals with autism and individuals with acquired cerebellar damage were significantly slower to detect a target presented shortly after an attentional cue than were control participants but were as fast as control participants when given more time to orient their attention (Akshoomoff et al., 1997; Townsend, Courchesne, et al., 1996). Other researchers have also reported atypical orienting effects in this type of paradigm for individuals with autism (Bryson, Landry, & Wainwright, 1997; Casey, Gordon, Mannheim, & Rumsey, 1993).

To control for concerns about a potential motor speed explanation for these findings, Townsend and her colleagues (1996b) developed a task in which performance depended on speed of perceptual processing (target discrimination), not on speed of motor response (target detection). Just as in the previous task, individuals with autism were slow to orient attention to a cued location but significantly improved with a longer delay between cue and target. There was also a strong correlation ($r = .82$; $p < .01$) between neocerebellar vermis size (the area of vermal lobules VI–VII divided by total brain volume to control for overall brain size) and the degree of orienting deficit. Individuals with acquired cerebellar damage showed similar effects (Townsend et al., 1999). An fMRI study with typical individuals also revealed that both the cerebellum and areas of the parietal cortex are involved in covert attention (Townsend, McKeown, Covington, & Allen, 1997).

Stimulus overselectivity or overselective attention has been reported for many individuals with autism. In experiments that measured focused spatial attention, electrophysiological and behavioral data provided evidence for overselectivity in some individuals and broad, ungraded attention in other individuals (Townsend & Courchesne, 1994; Townsend, Courchesne, et al., 1996; Townsend, Singer-Harris, et al., 1996). It appears that overselective attention is found primarily in individuals with autism who have parietal cortex abnormalities (in addition to the cerebellar abnormalities previously described), whereas individuals with no parietal abnormality have atypically broad, unfocused attentional responses. Atypically long reaction times to invalidly cued targets were found only in individuals with parietal cortex abnormalities and were highly correlated with the degree of parietal lobe involvement. These findings provide evidence for the hypothesis that subgroups of individuals may have distinct causal neural deficits for the phenotype of autism.

These studies have all included older adolescents and young adults with autism. One study included 17 children (mean age 7.5 years) who had previously been (provisionally) diagnosed with autism and underwent MRI between 2.6 and 6.3 years of age (Harris, Courchesne, Carper, & Lord, 1999). These children participated in an attention orienting experiment similar to that used in studies with older individuals with autism (Townsend, Courchesne, et al., 1996). Degree of slowed orienting to visual cues was significantly correlated with degree of cerebellar abnormality but not frontal lobe volume. Following completion of this experiment, 11 of the 17 children were found to continue to meet diagnostic criteria for autism. The area of vermal lobules VI–VII was significantly smaller in this subgroup compared with the typical age-matched control group. This study provides further evidence that slowed attentional orienting in autism is related to cerebellar vermis abnormality.

CLINICAL AND EDUCATIONAL IMPLICATIONS

Autism is a neurological disorder that is probably caused by a number of biological defects. To some, this may send the message that there is relatively little that may be done to treat children with this disorder. Others may have the notion that one could design a medication to treat or even "cure" this biological disorder. Neither view is correct. It is known that brain development is driven by experience and thus that there is great potential for change in the developing brain. With a developmental disorder, intervention can potentially lead to modification of and compensation for early disruption. As in any developmental disorder, this would suggest that early identification and intervention are the keys to success. Researchers are attempting to devise valid, reliable methods for identifying infants and young children at risk for autism (see Chapter 2). Follow-up studies of these children will provide fascinating insights into issues surrounding typical variations in development, differential diagnostic issues regarding autism and pervasive developmental disorder, the effectiveness of early intervention programs, and prognostic indicators.

Given the theories on the "primary" deficits underlying the diagnostic criteria in autism, it is important to consider targeting early intervention efforts on these primary deficits rather than restricting them to social skills and language. Several types of intervention strategies that target attention deficits in autism have been evaluated in the literature. Given the neurological evidence, it appears that these intervention strategies should take individual differences (reflecting various neurological abnormalities) into consideration. Physiological data indicate that as children with autism mature, they may compensate for deficits in selective attention despite these neurological abnormalities. The younger child must (obviously) attend to the parent or therapist to build communication and social skills. More specifically, some individuals with autism have overselective, narrow attention, whereas others have diffuse, nonselective attention. In addition, individuals with autism have been shown to have deficits in rapidly orienting and shifting their attention. These skills appear to be crucial for cognitive and social information processing. Behavioral data indicate that some individuals are able to perform typically when given more time to respond to cues to shift their attention. Therefore, interventions that take speed of shifting attention as well as the size of the attentional "spotlight" into consideration will potentially lead to better outcomes.

DIRECTIONS FOR FUTURE RESEARCH

As discussed, cerebellar abnormality is the most consistent neuroanatomical finding in autism to date. Research has also shown that there are subgroups of individuals with abnormalities in other areas (parietal cortex, hippocampus, enlarged brain areas). As more information is obtained about neural abnormalities in autism, it will be necessary to modify existing theories. Some theories have taken into consideration that damage to brain systems that develop early can result in persistent abnormalities in basic functions (e.g., attention, affiliation) and can also result in the sending of faulty feedback to connected structures or can have an impact on the development of later-developing skills, thus leading to further dysfunction than initially present.

ASDs make up a heterogeneous group of disorders in terms of etiology and in terms of neuropsychological outcome. Although not discussed in this chapter, research has also made advances in determining the genetic abnormalities present in some individuals with autism and the effects of certain teratogens and viruses that lead to autism. Technological advances allow researchers to study brain–behavior relationships with a high degree of temporal and spatial resolution using safe, noninvasive techniques. This will allow researchers to determine the degree to which neural systems that appear to be anatomically abnormal in autism are contributing to specific cognitive, language, and social skill deficits and how intervention strategies may modify these systems at a physiological level.

CONCLUSIONS

In the field of developmental psychopathology, a great deal of research has been devoted to discovering the neurobiological underpinnings of autism. It is important to consider that the brain of a child with autism has developed differently throughout prenatal and postnatal development. Therefore, phenotypic differences are to be expected and make it challenging to trace the origins of these differences back to infancy. The cerebellum is the most consistent neuroanatomical site of abnormality identified by neuroimaging and autopsy studies of individuals with autism. Studies of attention have linked a variety of deficits in autism with variations in size of the neocerebellar vermis and posterior parietal cortex. Functional MRI studies of typical adults also have demonstrated that these brain areas usually participate in these cognitive skills. More studies are needed to determine how damage to these regions may help to explain the development of social and cognitive skills in autism. Studies have also identified other neural abnormalities in carefully selected individuals with autism. It appears likely that a combination of related and possible heterogeneous abnormalities contribute to this complex developmental disorder. From a neurodevelopmental perspective, it is not necessary that all cases share the same exact neuroanatomical abnormalities to explain the symptoms that they share.

REFERENCES

Adamson, L.B., & Russell, C.L. (1999). Emotion regulation and the emergence of joint attention. In P. Rochat (Ed.), *Early social cognition* (pp. 281–297). Mahwah, NJ: Lawrence Erlbaum Associates.

Akshoomoff, N.A., & Courchesne, E. (1992). A new role for the cerebellum in cognitive operations. *Behavioral Neuroscience, 106,* 731–738.

Akshoomoff, N.A., & Courchesne, E. (1994). ERP evidence for a shifting attention deficit in patients with damage to the cerebellum. *Journal of Cognitive Neuroscience, 6,* 388–399.

Akshoomoff, N.A., Courchesne, E., & Townsend, J. (1997). Attention coordination and anticipatory control. In J.D. Schmahmann (Ed.), *International review of neurobiology, Vol. 41. The cerebellum and cognition* (pp. 575–598). San Diego: Academic Press.

Allen, G., Buxton, R.B., Wong, E.C., & Courchesne, E. (1997). Attentional activation of the cerebellum independent of motor involvement. *Science, 275,* 1940–1943.

American Psychiatric Association. (1994). *Diagnostic and statistical manual of mental disorders* (4th ed.). Washington, DC: Author.

Bachevalier, J. (1994). Medial temporal lobe structures and autism: A review of clinical and experimental findings. *Neuropsychologia, 32,* 627–648.

Bailey, A., Luthert, P., Bolton, P., LeCouteur, A., & Rutter, M. (1993). Autism and megalencephaly. *Lancet, 341,* 1225–1226.
Bailey, A., Luthert, P., Dean, A., Harding, B., Janota, I., Montgomery, M., Rutter, M., & Lantos, P. (1998). A clinicopathological study of autism. *Brain, 121,* 889–905.
Bates, E. (1976). *Language and context: Studies in the acquisition of pragmatics.* San Diego: Academic Press.
Bates, E., Thal, D., Trauner, D., Fenson, J., Aram, D., Eisele, J., & Nass, R. (1997). From first words to grammar in children with focal brain injury. *Developmental Neuropsychology, 13,* 275–343.
Bauman, M.L., & Kemper, T.L. (1985). Histoanatomic observations of the brain in early infantile autism. *Neurology, 35,* 866–874.
Bauman, M.L., & Kemper, T.L. (1994). Neuroanatomic observations of the brain in autism. In M.L. Bauman & T.L. Kemper (Eds.), *The neurobiology of autism* (pp. 119–145). Baltimore: Johns Hopkins University Press.
Bauman, M.L., Filipek, P.A., & Kemper, T.L. (1997). Early infantile autism. In J.D. Schmahmann (Ed.), *International Review of Neurobiology: Vol. 41. The cerebellum and cognition* (pp. 367–386). San Diego: Academic Press.
Bryson, S.E., Landry, R., & Wainwright, J.A. (1997). A componential view of executive dysfunction in autism In J.A. Burack & J.T. Enns (Eds.), *Attention, development, and psychopathology* (pp. 232–259). New York: Guilford Press.
Carper, R.A., Courchesne, E., & Chisum, H.J. (1997). Frontal lobe volume correlates with hypoplasia of cerebellar vermis in young autistic patients. *Society for Neuroscience Abstracts, 23,* 1624.
Casey, B.J., Gordon, C.T., Mannheim, G.B., & Rumsey, J. (1993). Dysfunctional attention in autistic savants. *Journal of Clinical and Experimental Neuropsychology, 15,* 933–946.
Chugani, H.T., Silva, E.D., & Chugani, D.C. (1996). Infantile spasms: III. Prognostic implications of bitemporal hypometabolism on positron emission tomography. *Annals of Neurology, 39,* 643–649.
Ciesielski, K.T., Courchesne, E., & Elmasian, R. (1990). Effects of focused selective attention tasks on event-related potentials in autistic and normal individuals. *Electroencephalography and Clinical Neurophysiology, 75,* 207–220.
Courchesne, E. (1987). A neurophysiological view of autism. In E. Schopler & G.B. Mesibov (Eds.), *Neurobiological issues in autism* (pp. 258–324). New York: Plenum.
Courchesne, E. (1995). Infantile autism. Part 2: A new neurodevelopmental model. *International Pediatrics, 10,* 155–165.
Courchesne, E. (1997). Brainstem, cerebellar and limbic neuroanatomical abnormalities in autism. *Current Opinion in Neurobiology, 7,* 269–278.
Courchesne, E., Akshoomoff, N.A., & Townsend, J. (1990). Recent advances in autism. *Current Opinion in Pediatrics, 2,* 685–693.
Courchesne, E., & Allen, G. (1997). Prediction and preparation, fundamental functions of the cerebellum. *Learning and Memory, 4,* 1–35.
Courchesne, E., Carper, R., Davis, H., Tigue, Z., Chisum, H.J., Cowles, A., Worden, B., Karns, C., Zaccardi, R., Lord, C., Lincoln, A.J., Pizzo, S., Schreibman, L., Haas, R.H., & Courchesne, R.Y. (1999). *Unusual patterns of cerebral growth and cerebellar growth during early life in patients with autism as quantified by in vivo MRI.* Manuscript submitted for publication.
Courchesne, E., Hesselink, J.R., Jernigan, T.L., & Yeung-Courchesne, R. (1987). Abnormal neuroanatomy in a nonretarded person with autism: Unusual findings with magnetic resonance imaging. *Archives of Neurology, 44,* 335–341.

Courchesne, E., Müller, R.A., & Saitoh, O. (1999). Brain weight in autism: Normal in the majority of cases, megalencephalic in rare cases. *Neurology, 52,* 1057–1059.

Courchesne, E., & Plante, E. (1996). Measurement and analysis issues in neurodevelopmental magnetic resonance imaging. In R.W. Thatcher, G.R. Lyon, J. Rumsey, & N. Krasnegor (Eds.), *Developmental neuroimaging: Mapping the development of brain and behavior* (pp. 43–65). San Diego: Academic Press.

Courchesne, E., Press, G.A., & Yeung-Courchesne, R. (1993). Parietal lobe abnormalities detected on magnetic resonance images of patients with infantile autism. *American Journal of Roentgenology,* 160, 387–393.

Courchesne, E., Saitoh, O., Yeung-Courchesne, R., Press, G.A., Lincoln, A.J., Haas, R.H., & Schreibman, L. (1994). Abnormality of cerebellar vermian lobules VI and VII in patients with infantile autism: Identification of hypoplastic and hyperplastic subgroups with MR imaging. *American Journal of Roentgenology, 162,* 123–130.

Courchesne, E., Townsend, J., & Saitoh, O. (1994). The brain in infantile autism: Posterior fossa structures are abnormal. *Neurology, 44,* 214–223.

Courchesne, E., Townsend, J., Akshoomoff, N.A., Saitoh, O., Yeung-Courchesne, R., Lincoln, A., James, H., Haas, R.H., Schreibman, L., & Lau, L. (1994). Impairment in shifting attention in autistic and cerebellar patients. *Behavioral Neuroscience, 108,* 848–865.

Courchesne, E., Townsend, J.P., Akshoomoff, N.A., Yeung-Courchesne, R., Press, G.A., Murakami, J.W., Lincoln, A.J., James, H.E., Saitoh, O., Egaas, B., Haas, R.H., & Schreibman, L. (1994). A new finding: Impairment in shifting attention in autistic and cerebellar patients. In S.H. Broman & J. Grafman (Eds.), *Atypical cognitive deficits in developmental disorders: Implications for brain function* (pp. 101–137). Mahwah, NJ: Lawrence Erlbaum Associates.

Courchesne, E., Yeung-Courchesne, R., & Egaas, B. (1994). Methodology in neuroanatomic measurement. *Neurology, 44,* 203–208.

Courchesne, E., Yeung-Courchesne, R., Press, G., Hesselink, J.R., & Jernigan, T.L. (1988). Hypoplasia of cerebellar vermal lobules VI and VII in infantile autism. *New England Journal of Medicine, 318,* 1349–1354.

Dawson, G., & Lewy, A. (1989). Reciprocal subcortical-cortical influences in autism: The role of attentional mechanisms. In G. Dawson (Ed.), *Autism: Nature, diagnosis, and treatment* (pp. 144–173). New York: Guilford Press.

DeLong, G.R., & Heinz, E.R. (1997). The clinical syndrome of early-life bilateral hippocampal sclerosis. *Annals of Neurology, 42,* 11–17.

Egaas, B., Courchesne, E., & Saitoh, O. (1995). Reduced size of corpus callosum in autism. *Archives of Neurology, 52,* 794–801.

Elman, J.L., Bates, E.A., Johnson, M.H., Karmiloff-Smith, A., Parisi, D., & Plunkett, K. (1996). *Rethinking innateness: A connectionist perspective on development.* Cambridge, MA: MIT Press/Bradford Books.

Filipek, P.A. (1995). Quantitative magnetic resonance imaging in autism: The cerebellar vermis. *Current Opinion in Neurology, 8,* 134–138.

Gaffney, G.R., Tsai, L.Y., Kuperman, S., & Minchin, S. (1988). Morphological evidence of brainstem involvement in infantile autism. *Biological Psychiatry, 24,* 578–586.

Garber, H.J., & Ritvo, E.R. (1992). Magnetic resonance imaging of the posterior fossa in autistic adults. *American Journal of Psychiatry, 149,* 245–247.

Garber, H.J., Ritvo, E.R., Chui, L.C., Griswold, V.J., Kashian, A., & Oldendorf, W.H. (1989). A magnetic resonance imaging study of autism: Normal fourth ventricle size and absence of pathology. *American Journal of Psychiatry, 146,* 532–535.

Goldman, P. (1971). Functional development of the prefrontal cortex in early life and the problem of neuronal plasticity. *Experimental Neurology, 32,* 366–387.

Goldman, P. (1974). An alternative to developmental plasticity: Heterology of CNS structures in infants and adults. In D.G. Stein, J.J. Rosen, & N. Butters (Eds.), *Plasticity and recovery of function in the central nervous system* (pp. 149–174). New York: Academic Press.

Goldman-Rakic, P.S., Isseroff, A., Schwartz, M.L., & Bugbee, N.M. (1983). The neurobiology of cognitive development. In P. Mussen (Ed.), *Handbook of child psychology: Infancy and developmental psychobiology* (pp. 281–344). New York: John Wiley & Sons.

Haas, R.H., Townsend, J., Courchesne, E., Lincoln, A.J., Schreibman, L., & Yeung-Courchesne, R. (1996). Neurologic abnormalities in infantile autism. *Journal of Child Neurology, 11,* 84–92.

Harris, N.S., Courchesne, E., Carper, R., & Lord, C. (1999). Neuroanatomic contributions to slowed orienting of attention in children with autism. *Brain Research and Cognitive Brain Research, 8,* 61–71.

Hashimoto, T., Tayama, M., Murakawa, K., Yoshimoto, T., Miyazaki, M., Harada, M., & Kuroda, Y. (1995). Development of the brainstem and cerebellum in autistic patients. *Journal of Autism and Developmental Disorders, 25,* 1–18.

Holttum, J.R., Minshew, N.J., Sanders, R.S., & Phillips, N.E. (1992). Magnetic resonance imaging of the posterior fossa in autism. *Biological Psychiatry, 32,* 1091–1101.

Hsu, M., Yeung-Courchesne, R., Courchesne, E., & Press, G.A. (1991). Absence of pontine abnormality in infantile autism. *Archives of Neurology, 48,* 1160–1163.

Insel, T.R. (1997). A neurobiological basis of social attachment. *American Journal of Psychiatry, 154,* 726–735.

Jernigan, T., & Bellugi, U. (1990). Anomalous brain morphology on magnetic resonance images in Williams syndrome and Down syndrome. *Archives of Neurology, 47,* 429–533.

Jernigan, T.L., Bellugi, U., Sowell, E., Doherty, S., & Hesselink, J.R. (1993). Cerebral morphological distinctions between Williams and Down syndromes. *Archives of Neurology, 48,* 539–545.

Kempler, D., van Lancker, D., Marchman, V., & Bates, E. (1999). Idiom comprehension in children and adults with unilateral brain damage. *Developmental Neuropsychology, 15,* 327–349.

Kleiman, M.D., Neff, S., & Rosman, N.P. (1992). The brain in infantile autism: Are posterior fossa structures abnormal? *Neurology, 42,* 753–760.

Le, T.H., Pardo, J.V., & Hu, X. (1998). 4 T-fMRI study of nonspatial shifting of selective attention: Cerebellar and parietal contributions. *Journal of Neurophysiology, 79,* 1535–1548.

Lewy, A.L., & Dawson, G. (1992). Social stimulation and joint attention in young autistic children. *Journal of Abnormal Child Psychology, 20,* 555–566.

Lincoln, A., Courchesne, E., Allen, M., Hanson, E., & Ene, M. (1998). Neurobiology of Asperger syndrome: Seven case studies and quantitative magnetic resonance imaging findings. In E. Schopler, G.B. Mesibov, & L.J. Kunce (Eds.), *Asperger syndrome or high-functioning autism?* (pp. 145–163). New York: Plenum.

Mills, D.L., Coffey-Corina, S., & Neville, H.J. (1997). Language comprehension and cerebral specialization from 13 to 20 months. *Developmental Neuropsychology, 13,* 397–445.

Minshew, N.J., & Dombrowski, S.M. (1994). In vivo neuroanatomy of autism: Neuroimaging studies. In M.L. Bauman & T.L. Kemper (Eds.), *The neurobiology of autism* (pp. 66–85). Baltimore: Johns Hopkins University Press.

Minshew, N.J., Sweeney, J.A., & Bauman, M.L. (1997). Neurological aspects of autism. In D. Cohen & F. Volkmar (Eds.), *Handbook of autism and pervasive developmental disorders* (2nd ed., pp. 344–369). New York: John Wiley & Sons.

Mundy, P., Sigman, M., & Kasari, C. (1990). A longitudinal study of joint attention and language development in autistic children. *Journal of Autism and Developmental Disorders, 20,* 115–128.

Piven, J., Arndt, S., Bailey, J., & Andreasen, N. (1996). Regional brain enlargement in autism: A magnetic resonance imaging study. *Journal of the American Academy of Child and Adolescent Psychiatry, 35,* 530–536.

Piven, J., Arndt, S., Bailey, J., Havercamp, S., Andreasen, N.C., & Palmer, P. (1995). An MRI study of brain size in autism. *American Journal of Psychiatry, 152,* 1145–1149.

Piven, J., Bailey, J., & Arndt, S. (1998). No difference in hippocampus volume detected on magnetic resonance imaging in autistic individuals. *Journal of Autism and Developmental Disorders, 28,* 105–110.

Piven, J., Bailey, J., Ranson, B.J., & Arndt, S. (1997). An MRI study of the corpus callosum in autism. *American Journal of Psychiatry, 154,* 1051–1056.

Piven, J., Berthier, M.L., Starkstein, S.E., Nehme, E., Pearlson, G., & Folstein, S. (1990). Magnetic resonance imaging evidence for a defect of cerebral cortical development in autism. *American Journal of Psychiatry, 147,* 734–739.

Piven, J., Nehme, E., Simon, J., Barta, P., Pearlson, G., & Folstein, S.E. (1992). Magnetic resonance imaging in autism: Measurement of the cerebellum, pons, and fourth ventricle. *Biological Psychiatry, 31,* 491–504.

Quartz, S.R., & Sejnowski, T.J. (1997). The neural basis of cognitive development: A constructivist manifesto. *Behavioral and Brain Sciences, 20,* 537–596.

Reilly, J., Bates, E., & Marchman, V. (1998). Narrative discourse in children with early focal brain injury. *Brain and Language, 61,* 335–375.

Ritvo, E.R., Freeman, B.J., Scheibel, A.B., Duong, T., Robinson, H., Guthrie, D., & Ritvo, A. (1986). Lower Purkinje cell counts in the cerebella of four autistic subjects: Initial findings of the UCLA-NSAC autopsy research report. *American Journal of Psychiatry, 143,* 862–866.

Rodier, P.M., Ingram, J.L., Tisdale, B., Nelson, S., & Romano, J. (1996). Embryological origin for autism: Developmental anomalies of the cranial nerve motor nuclei. *Journal of Comparative Neurology, 370,* 247–261.

Rosenzweig, M.R., Bennett, E.L., & Alberti, M. (1984). Multiple effects of lesions on brain structure in young rats. In C.R. Almli & S. Finger (Eds.), *Early brain damage: Vol. 2. Neurobiology and behavior* (pp. 49–70). San Diego: Academic Press.

Rumsey, J.M., Duara, R., Grady, C., Rapoport, J.L., Margolin, R.A., Rapoport, S.I., & Cutler, N.R. (1985). Brain metabolism in autism: Resting cerebral glucose utilization rates as measured with positron emission tomography. *Archives of General Psychiatry, 42,* 448–455.

Saitoh, O., Courchesne, E., Egaas, B., Lincoln, A.J., & Schreibman, L. (1995). Cross-sectional area of the posterior hippocampus in autistic patients with cerebellar and corpus callosum abnormalities. *Neurology, 45,* 317–324.

Schaefer, G.B., Thompson, J.N., Bodensteiner, J.B., McConnell, J.M., Kimberling, W.J., Gay, C.T., Dutton, W.D., Hutchings, D.C., & Gray, S.B. (1996). Hypoplasia of the cerebellar vermis in neurogenetic syndromes. *Annals of Neurology, 39,* 382–385.

Stiles, J. (1998). The effects of early focal brain injury on lateralization of cognitive function. *Current Directions in Psychological Science, 7,* 21–26.

Stiles, J., & Thal, D. (1993) Linguistic and spatial cognitive development following early focal brain injury: Patterns of deficit and recovery. In M. Johnson (Ed.), *Brain development and cognition: A reader* (pp. 643–664). Oxford, England: Blackwell Publishers.

Stiles, J., Trauner, D., Engel, M., & Nass, R. (1997). The development of drawing in children with congenital focal brain injury: Evidence for limited functional recovery. *Neuropsychologia, 35,* 299–312.

Tager-Flusberg, H. (1997). Perspective on language and communication in autism. In D. Cohen & F. Volkmar (Eds.), *Handbook of autism and pervasive developmental disorders* (2nd ed., pp. 894–900). New York: John Wiley & Sons.

Townsend, J., & Courchesne, E. (1994). Parietal damage and narrow "spotlight" spatial attention. *Journal of Cognitive Neuroscience, 6,* 220–232.

Townsend, J., Courchesne, E., Covington, J., Westerfield, M., Harris, N.S., Lyden, P., Lowry, T.P., & Press, G.A. (1999). Spatial attention deficits in patients with acquired or developmental cerebellar abnormality. *Journal of Neuroscience, 19,* 5632–5643.

Townsend, J., Courchesne, E., & Egaas, B. (1996). Slowed orienting of covert visual-spatial attention in autism: Specific deficits associated with cerebellar and parietal abnormality. *Development and Psychopathology,* 8, 563–584.

Townsend, J., McKeown, M., Covington, J., & Allen, G. (1997). Cerebellar and parietal activation during orienting of spatial attention. *Society for Neuroscience Abstracts, 23*(2), 1588.

Townsend, J., Singer-Harris, N.S., & Courchesne, E. (1996). Visual attention abnormalities in autism: Delayed orienting to location. *Journal of the International Neuropsychological Society, 2,* 541–550.

Vargha-Khadem, F., Gadian, D.G., Watkins, K.E., Connelly, A., Van Paesschen, W., & Mishkin, M. (1997). Differential effect of hippocampal pathology on episodic and semantic memory. *Science, 277,* 376–380.

Waterhouse, L. (1994). Severity of impairment in autism. In S.H. Broman & J. Grafman (Eds.), *Atypical cognitive deficits in developmental disorders: Implications for brain function* (pp. 159–180). Mahwah, NJ: Lawrence Erlbaum Associates.

Waterhouse, L., & Fein, D. (1997). Perspectives on social impairment. In D. Cohen & F. Volkmar (Eds.), *Handbook of autism and pervasive developmental disorders* (2nd ed., pp. 901–919). New York: John Wiley & Sons.

Waterhouse, L., Fein, D., & Modahl, C. (1996). Neurofunctional mechanisms in autism. *Psychological Review, 103,* 457–489.

Williams, R.S., Hauser, S.L., Purpura, D.P., DeLong, R., & Swisher, C.N. (1980). Autism and mental retardation: Neuropathological studies performed in four retarded persons with autistic behavior. *Archives of Neurology, 37,* 749–753.

Wing, L. (1997). Syndromes of autism and atypical development. In D. Cohen & F. Volkmar (Eds.), *Handbook of autism and pervasive developmental disorders* (2nd ed., pp. 148–170). New York: John Wiley & Sons.

Yeung-Courchesne, R., & Courchesne, E. (1997). From impasse to insight in autism research: From behavioral symptoms to biological explanations. *Development and Psychopathology, 9,* 389–419.

Zilbovicius, M., Garreau, B., Samson, Y., Remy, P., Barthélémy, C., Syrota, A., & LeLord, G. (1995). Delayed maturation of the frontal cortex in childhood autism. *American Journal of Psychiatry, 152,* 248–252.

Part II

Assessment and Intervention Issues

9

Communication Intervention Issues for Children with Autism Spectrum Disorders

Barry M. Prizant, Amy M. Wetherby, and Patrick J. Rydell

In this chapter, we explore current issues in enhancing language and communication abilities in young children with autism spectrum disorders (ASDs) from a developmental and transactional orientation. This discussion is based on the significant contributions of researchers and clinical scholars from both developmental and contemporary behavioral orientations whose research and clinical practice are grounded in developmental and transactional theory and research on communication, language, and socioemotional development. First, the essential underpinnings of a developmental, social-pragmatic model are described. The contributions of developmental practice to contemporary behavioral methods for assessment and intervention are also noted. Developmental social-pragmatic models, which are consistent with transactional theory, are contrasted with traditional behavioral approaches, which rely primarily on discrete trial training conducted outside of social contexts, to clearly delineate aspects of practice that are seen as contributing to as well as potentially limiting initiated, spontaneous communication. We conclude with a discussion of an evolving model, which we refer to as the *SCERTS model of intervention,* which focuses on **s**ocial-**c**ommunication, **e**motional **r**egulation, and **t**ransactional **s**upport as the major components and priorities in enhancing communication and related abilities of young children with ASD.

CONTINUUM OF APPROACHES: DISCRETE TRIAL-TRADITIONAL BEHAVIORAL TO DEVELOPMENTAL SOCIAL-PRAGMATIC

We believe it is best to conceptualize approaches to enhancing language and communicative abilities along a continuum, with traditional behavioral approaches such as discrete trial-traditional behavioral (DT-TB) at one end

(Lovaas, 1977, 1981) and developmental social-pragmatic (DSP) approaches at the other end, which include "relationship-based" approaches that are individualized and grounded in a transactional model (Greenspan, 1992, 1997; Greenspan & Wieder, 1998; MacDonald, 1989; Prizant, Schuler, Wetherby, & Rydell, 1997; Schuler, Prizant, & Wetherby, 1997; Wetherby, Schuler, & Prizant, 1997). Contemporary behavioral approaches fall between these two ends of the continuum, incorporating aspects of each (Warren, 1993).

An Historical Perspective

For many years, approaches to enhancing language and communication abilities for young children with ASD have varied greatly in content (goals) and in teaching strategies. In the 1960s and 1970s, traditional behavioral approaches primarily based on a discrete trial teaching format conducted outside everyday social contexts (e.g., Lovaas, 1977) received much attention mostly because such approaches were the first to objectively demonstrate that children with ASD were capable of acquiring a variety of skills through systematic teaching efforts. The same teaching procedures were used for skills as varied as receptive and expressive speech (Lovaas, 1977) and sequences of motor behaviors such as those involved in self-help skills (Lovaas, 1981). These teaching procedures were primarily characterized by a one-to-one massed trial drill format to train early "readiness" skills in eye contact, attention, and sitting, followed by more advanced skills in matching, verbal imitation, receptive and expressive language, play, and so forth. The justification for a highly repetitive one-to-one approach was the belief that children with autism were not able to learn in more natural environments because of their extreme learning and attentional difficulties and the lack of practice opportunities and systematic reinforcement in more natural events (Lovaas, 1981).

In contrast to DT-TB approaches that were driven by operant behavior explanations of language development, cognitively based developmental psychologists, psycholinguists, and speech-language pathologists rebuked operant models as valid explanations of how typical children and children with disabilities could learn to communicate spontaneously or acquire a generative and creative language system (Warren, 1993). Questions were raised as to whether DT-TB approaches actually interfered with children's ability to engage in spontaneous and initiated communication, a process that appeared to be antithetical to what children were being taught in the discrete trial training regimen (Fay & Schuler, 1980; Prizant, 1982). One primary reason for this concern is that a competent communicator is one who is able to demonstrate a balance in sociocommunicative skills including initiating, maintaining, and responding to communicative partners. DT-TB approaches traditionally emphasized adult-directed methodologies that primarily placed children in a respondent role. Thus, the focus of training was on teaching children to become competent at responding, resulting in a lack of initiation and even passivity (Prizant, 1982).

Concerns about discrete trial approaches to "training" communication and language also were fueled by the revolution in developmental pragmatics (i.e., the study of language and communication development in social contexts). In the late 1970s and in the 1980s, this movement dramatically shifted the study of language and communication development (Bates, 1976, 1979) and also had a significant impact on the applied fields of special education and speech-language pathology (Bricker, 1993; McLean & Snyder-McLean, 1978). The study of pragmatics engendered a number of principles that guided clinical and educational practice with children with ASD and other severe communication disabilities and appeared to be antithetical to DT-TB approaches in theory and practice. First, the social context of naturally occurring interactions, including routines and events that occurred in everyday life with family members and peers, was considered to be of primary importance for communication and language development. Second, the child was viewed as an active learner and social participant rather than as a learner primarily under the control of the teacher utilizing a specific reinforcement schedule and a variety of instructional variables. Third, the role of the caregiver was seen as going well beyond presenting discriminative stimuli, prompting and shaping targeted responses, and responding to the child's behavior with consequent events (e.g., reinforcement, punishment), elements considered to be the primary components of teaching interactions in DT-TB accounts of language and communication development.

Research in developmental pragmatics documented that caregivers of children with and without disabilities facilitate communication and language development in many ways, including the following: creating motivating contexts, routines, and activities for communication; following the child's lead and attentional focus in activities; interpreting children's unconventional, preintentional, and early intentional behavior as meaningful; adjusting communicative style to best match a child's developmental capacities; modeling, supporting, and scaffolding for the child; and supporting emotional regulation and expression in communicative interactions (Bruner, 1981; MacDonald, 1989; Mahoney & Powell, 1988; McLean, 1990; McLean & Snyder-McLean, 1978; Prizant & Meyer, 1993; Prizant & Wetherby, 1990a).

Fourth, in practice, the developmental pragmatics movement emphasized the importance of deriving individualized goals and strategies in communication based on each child's current communication abilities as well as learning strengths and needs (Prizant & Wetherby, 1989, 1990b; Wetherby & Prizant, 1992). This was in contrast to programs using the same sequence of goals and teaching curriculum, as was common in some DT-TB approaches, especially in early stages of training (Bricker, 1993). Finally, the pragmatics movement has emphasized the need to focus on meaningful preverbal and verbal language and functional communication abilities at the outset rather than to build repertoires of speech sounds, words, and sentences largely devoid of conceptual understanding and social impact. Based on the research literature in developmental pragmatics for typically developing children and children with ASD (Bates, 1979; Wetherby, 1986; Wetherby & Prutting, 1984), the practice of understanding and documenting children's communicative intentions became central in research and in practical application in working with nonverbal as well as verbal individuals with ASD (Durand, 1990; Prizant & Duchan, 1981; Prizant & Wetherby, 1987; Wetherby, 1986), a notion inconsistent with the traditional behavioral doctrine of dealing primarily with observable behavior.

Citing the lack of generalization and communicative spontaneity in children who had nonetheless mastered speech goals in discrete trial training, practitioners with expertise in communication and language disorders in ASDs began to seriously question the efficacy of DT-TB procedures in enhancing true spontaneous communication and language abilities (Fay & Schuler, 1980; Prizant, 1982). Even Lovaas, who has been credited with introducing discrete trial approaches for children with ASD, stated that "the training regime . . . its use of 'unnatural' reinforcers, and the like may have been responsible for producing the very situation-specific, restricted verbal output which we observed in many of our children" (1977, p. 170). On the basis of this finding, he spoke of the need for spontaneity training, a concept that stands as an oxymoron in the eyes of specialists in communication development and disorders. That is, the concept of *training* implies establishing teacher or instructional control, a basic tenet of traditional behavioral approaches, whereas initiation and spontaneity in communication is viewed as affect driven based on internal motivation and internal locus of control by developmental researchers and clinicians (Greenspan, 1992; Prizant & Wetherby, 1990a).

In a retrospective critique of the use of DT-TB approaches (Lovaas, 1977) in language intervention for children with ASD, Koegel noted that "not only did language fail to be exhibited or generalize to other environments, but most behaviors taught in this highly controlled environment also failed to generalize" (1995, p. 23). Although coming from a contemporary applied behavioral analysis (ABA) orientation, Koegel stated the need to abandon discrete trial approaches in favor of more naturalistic approaches to language intervention on the contention that "early attempts to teach language, that emphasized repetitive practice, carefully controlled instructions, consistent and artificial reinforcers, highly structured and simple training environments, and so forth, might have actually retarded the efforts to achieve generalized intervention effects" (p. 23). It is interesting to note that these claims are remarkably consistent with earlier critiques of Fay and Schuler (1980), Prizant (1982), and Wetherby (1986), all of whom come from a DSP orientation.

The pragmatics revolution provided new methodologies and taxonomies for studying and documenting communication and language development in natural social contexts (Lund & Duchan, 1983). Advances in behavioral technology also led to functional assessment becoming recommended practice for understanding the variables that influence, or the motivations of, problem behaviors (see Carr et al., 1994; Donnellan, Mirenda, Mesaros, & Fassbender, 1984; Horner et al., 1990; and Meyer & Evans, 1986, 1993). This confluence of factors led to the emergence of contemporary behavioral approaches that drew from two primary sources: 1) the incorporation of behavioral research methodology and techniques to assess the functions of behavior and promote adaptive behavior (e.g., teaching positive, functionally equivalent alternative behaviors) (Carr & Durand, 1986; Dunlap, Vaughn, & O'Neill, 1998; Hart, 1985; Koegel & Johnson, 1989; Schreibman & Pierce, 1993) and 2) the infusion of knowledge derived from developmental pragmatics to promote the use of more natural and balanced social transactions in which learning opportunities are initiated by the child, with caregivers responding in a supportive and growth-inducing manner based on each child's motivations, attentional focus, and developmental strengths and needs. For example, Koegel and colleagues (Koegel & Koegel, 1995; Koegel, O'Dell, & Koegel, 1987) and Schreibman and Pierce (1993), who come from a contemporary ABA orientation, developed a more child-centered approach that drew heavily from social-pragmatic principles, which they referred to as the *natural language paradigm.*

These contemporary behavioral researchers helped to move behavioral approaches away from a primary reliance on discrete trial approaches and simple operant accounts of learning on which discrete trial approaches are grounded, and they embraced the use of ecobehavioral and functional assessment in broadening the appreciation of contextual and individual determinants and influences in learning (Strain et al., 1992). Thus, more natural routines with adults and peers and child-centered motivating activities including routines and events that recurred in everyday life with family members and peers became the primary intervention contexts (Koegel & Johnson, 1989; Schreibman & Pierce, 1993). This shift, along with the increasing influence of attempts to understand the communicative functions of challenging behavior using taxonomies from the pragmatic literature (Donnellan et al., 1984; Durand, 1990; Reichle & Wacker, 1993), further merged the perspectives of contemporary ABA approaches and DSP approaches.

Discrete Trial Training or Traditional Behavioral Approach

The discrete trial training approach has been defined as a strategy to teach new skills to children and has been called one of "several methods that increase the likelihood that a child will give the desired response so that it can be reinforced" (Anderson, Taras, & Cannon, 1996, p. 187). A *trial* is considered to be a "single teaching unit" (Lovaas, 1981) that begins with the presentation of a stimulus (teacher's instruction), the child's response, the consequence, and a pause (between-trial interval) before presentation of the next stimulus by the teacher (Anderson et al., 1996). Teacher instructions are given just once, and the child's response, which must then be evaluated as correct, incorrect, or no response, is followed by a consequence, based on correctness of the child's response relative to a predetermined criterion. Correct responses are reinforced with praise or primary reinforcers (e.g., food); incorrect responses are consequated with verbal feedback such as "no" or "wrong," followed by physical guidance of the child to a correct response (referred to as a *correction trial*) (Anderson et al., 1996). The purpose is to delineate each teaching episode clearly; this trial also provides an opportunity for the teacher to record data on each response. Schreibman, Kaneko, and Koegel offered this description of DT-TB approaches:

> In discrete trial training, the therapist chooses the stimuli to be used in training and the nature of the interaction, only correct responses are reinforced, indirect reinforcers (e.g., tokens, food) are typically used, several consecutive trials on a new task are presented, and the therapist initiates trials. (1991, p. 480)

Proponents of DT-TB indicate that it is but one strategy for teaching new skills (Johnson, 1994; Anderson et al., 1996). The most frequently cited and recommended volumes published by proponents of DT-TB (Lovaas, 1981; Maurice, Green, & Luce, 1996), however, focus on discrete trial programs as the initial and predominant strategy for teaching children with ASD. The primary elements descriptive of DT-TB include the following:

1. The teaching structure is highly prescribed, including choice of the stimuli presented, the responses targeted, and the consequences provided. Physical arrangements such as seating are often predetermined and should be adhered to faithfully.
2. There is a focus on teaching discrete and objectively defined behaviors. Traditionally, there has been a focus on speech as a primary communicative mode, beginning with vocal imitation and followed by word imitation.
3. The learning context involves a 1:1 child–teacher ratio, with the adult determining the activity and focus of attention and following a prescribed, sequenced curriculum.
4. Predetermined criteria are provided for correctness of response. Each response is evaluated as correct or incorrect, with predetermined consequences following the response. "Off-task" responses, even if communicative or relevant to some aspect of the training context, are ignored, or the child's behavior is redirected.
5. Initial focus is on adult control and child compliance. In a section of *Teaching Developmentally Disabled Children: The "Me" Book* entitled "Adult Is Boss," Lovaas (1981) outlined his rationale for initially providing "structured and authoritative" environments followed by lessening adult control.

6. Curricula used in discrete trial programs may not be informed by literature on sequences or processes on child language and communication development, unless the curricula chosen are developmentally based.
7. There is minimal use of contextual supports, such as accompanying use of gestures by the clinician/educator (unless specified in a hierarchy of prompts), activity boards, or picture schedules. Teaching is largely organized and directed through oral language.

The Middle Ground (Contemporary Applied Behavioral Analysis Approaches)

In response to the persistent problem of a lack of generalization of trained skills "noted time and time again" in the behavioral literature (Schreibman & Pierce, 1993, p. 184), behaviorally oriented researchers introduced teaching strategies in the 1980s that diverged significantly from earlier DT-TB approaches. Among the best known of such strategies discussed in the contemporary ABA literature are incidental language teaching (Hart, 1985), natural language paradigm (NLP) including pivotal response training (Koegel & Johnson, 1989; Schreibman & Pierce, 1993), and enhanced milieu approaches (Kaiser, Yoder, & Keetz, 1992). These approaches were developed as methods of achieving a more naturalistic approach to enhancing language and communication development for children with ASD and other childhood communication disabilities. These approaches were based, in part, on principles and interactive processes drawn from developmental literature on caregiver–child interaction (Snow & Ferguson, 1977) and developmental pragmatics (Bates, 1979; Bates, O'Connell, & Shore, 1987), as well as ABA.

There are a number of striking and significant distinctions between these more contemporary ABA approaches and traditional DT-TB approaches. First, "control" of the teaching interaction is either shared (Schreibman & Pierce, 1993), or shifted from "trainers" to children. Teachers are encouraged to follow the child's lead to encourage initiation and spontaneity in communication. Second, child-preferred and child-selected activities provide the primary contexts and topics for communicative exchange (Schreibman & Pierce, 1993). The trainer provides choice-making opportunities rather than select and impose teaching tasks. Third, because a child's attentional focus and preferences are followed, interactions are more natural and loosely structured rather than unfolding according to a prescribed training protocol followed in a contrived one-to-one teaching setting.

A fourth major distinction involves the specifics of how adults interact with children. As noted, in incidental teaching, NLP, or milieu teaching, it is most preferable for communicative exchanges to be initiated by the child with the adult being highly responsive to children's spontaneous communication (whether verbal, vocal, or gestural). For example, in NLP, any goal-directed attempts at communication are reinforced (i.e., accepted); thus, there is no requirement that the child produce a predetermined, targeted behavior to receive reinforcement. Similar to DSP approaches (described in the next section), the focus and ultimate goal of contemporary ABA approaches are to facilitate spontaneous communication and interaction. Incidental teaching, NLP, and milieu strategies have been found to enhance generalization in teaching language and communicative skills to children with disabilities, including ASD (see Hart, 1985; Kaiser & Hester, 1994; and Schreibman & Pierce, 1993, for reviews).

Underpinnings of a Developmental Social-Pragmatic Model

DSP approaches emphasize from the outset the importance of focusing on initiation and spontaneity in communication, following the child's attentional focus and motivations (to the extent possible), building on a child's current communicative repertoire (even if a child uses unconventional means to communicate), and using more natural activities and events as contexts that support the development of children's sociocommunicative abilities. The elements and justification for DSP approaches are as follows.

Use of Interactive-Facilitative Strategies

Interactive-facilitative strategies are ways in which communicative partners spontaneously interact with and respond to young children that are supportive of their sociocommunicative growth. The importance of this dimension of intervention is underscored by a number of facts. First, opportunities for communicative growth occur naturally throughout the day; therefore, a primary reliance on scheduled "lessons" or "programs" does not take advantage of multiple opportunities for communication enhancement. Second, research has demonstrated that caregivers' style of interaction and responsivity in interactions have an important influence on language and communication development (Hart & Risley, 1995). Third, research on the transactional nature of communication development indicates that with caregivers' appropriate modifications of interactive style, children develop a sense of efficacy and competence in communication (Mahoney & Powell, 1988). This growing sense of efficacy results in greater active participation and increased motivation in social exchange, which, in turn, reinforces caregivers' sense of efficacy and competence (Dunst, Lowe, & Bartholomew, 1990).

Thus, the role of the communicative partner is to build on children's initiations and provide models and responses that convey to children that their responses are meaningful and accepted. The goal is to have children construct a self-generated (self-constructed) knowledge base of communicative routines, means, and functions, and eventually for them to communicate flexibly and spontaneously across people and contexts. The purpose for interacting and communicating is motivated by the children's interests and goals and is largely under internal control rather than under external (or stimulus/instructional) control.

Interactive-facilitative strategies encompass aspects of verbal as well as nonverbal behavior. Based on ongoing assessment, decisions are made by educators, clinicians and caregivers as to the modifications in language and interactive styles that will best support an individual child's sociocommunicative development and enable a child to communicate intentions as independently as possible. The following non–mutually exclusive dimensions of interactive-facilitative strategies are drawn, in part, from Duchan (1986, 1989), MacDonald (1989), MacDonald and Gillette (1988), and McCormick (1990).

Degree of Acceptance of Children's Communicative Bids Duchan (1989) noted that communicative partners provide differential feedback to young children, which may include acceptance of communicative attempts, rejection, conditional acceptance, and unqualified acceptance. In general, conditional and unqualified acceptance have been found to be more facilitative of communicative success and growth in children. Conditional acceptance includes corrections that accept and acknowledge a child's attempt and provide positive corrective feedback. Conditional acceptance may also include corrections with explanations. In both cases, although corrective feedback is given, the child's meaning and intent is acknowledged, and further information is provided in a nonjudgmental and positive manner. Unqualified or unconditional acceptance includes positive feedback including attention, verbal and nonverbal expressions of acceptance (e.g., head nods, "yeah," "uh-huh," exact imitations), and expressions of positive affect. Unconditional acceptance is characteristic of very early caregiver–child interactions and helps young children to learn about the reciprocal nature of communicative exchange.

Degree of Directiveness Marfo (1990) discussed degree of directiveness or facilitativeness of partner style. A highly directive style, which is characteristic of traditional behavioral approaches, is typified by adult-selected topics and activities, frequent use of imperatives (commands) and test questions (i.e., questions to which the answers are known that are asked to test a child's knowledge), and intrusiveness on the child's behavior through a reliance on physical prompting for appropriate responses (Clark & Seifer, 1985). A directive style has been found to result in fewer child initiations, less elaborate responses, a limited range of communicative functions expressed, and even conversational reticence or passivity (Duchan, 1989). In specific regard to children with ASD, Rydell and Mirenda (1994) found a high association between the degree of adult directiveness and unconventional verbal behavior in children with ASD. They also found that although higher frequencies of verbalizations were found after adult-directed utterances, these verbalizations were mostly echolalic, serving a turn-taking function, with reduced comprehension.

A facilitative style, which is currently advocated by the DSP and some contemporary behavioral literature, is characterized by following the child's attentional focus, offering choices and alternatives within activities, responding to and acknowledging children's intent, modeling a variety of communicative functions including commenting on a child's activities, and expanding and elaborating on the topic of a child's verbal and nonverbal communication. The benefits of a more facilitative style include 1) providing a child with a sense of social control and communicative power, which has been found to result in increased initiations and more elaborate communicative attempts (Mirenda & Donnellan, 1986; Peck, 1985); 2) following a child's attentional focus and motivations, which reduces problems of compliance and may result in increased learning due to motivation and affective involvement; and 3) providing elaborated information and feedback appropriate to a child's level, which supports a child's communicative and language development through modeling of vocabulary and more varied language forms and functions. Mirenda and Donnellan (1986) found that compared with a "directive" style, the use of a "facilitative" style resulted in higher rates of student-initiated interactions, question asking, and conversational initiation in students with ASD. Rydell and Mirenda (1994) found that higher frequencies of generative utterances, initiations, and increased comprehension followed adult-facilitative utterances. Facilitative strategies have also been found to increase communicative initiation and social-affective signaling of children with ASD with limited or no language abilities (Dawson & Adams, 1984; Peck, 1985; Tiegerman & Primavera, 1984).

Appropriateness of style along the continuum from facilitativeness to directiveness is a child-specific issue and can only be determined by observing the effect of partner style on interactions. Relative to a child's typical abilities, a good stylistic match should result in 1) increased self-regulation of attention (i.e., ability to maintain a mutual focus of attention with minimal prompting), 2) active involvement in selecting and participating in activities, 3) frequent verbal and nonverbal communicative initiations, 4) more elaborate communicative initiations, and 5) positive affective involvement with the partner. A style may be thought to be more facilitative when these characteristics can be observed in children's behavior. For example, for a highly active and distractible child, a style that promotes a mutual attentional focus and more active involvement must be viewed as facilitative for that child even though it may have some directive qualities (e.g., physical prompting, limit setting). This same style, however, may have detrimental effects for a child with a lower activity level and greater attentional regulation. As Marfo (1990) has noted, the function of adult directiveness in supporting interactions is of overriding concern, not the presence or absence of features thought to be directive. In DSP approaches, however, educators and clinicians attempt to incorporate facilitative features in their interactions and gradually modify style along the facilitativeness–directiveness continuum until an optimal match is found.

Adjusting Language and Social Input The timing and complexity of language and social input to a young child may have a dramatic impact on the child's ability to sustain attention to others, to take turns in interactions, and to comprehend others' intentions expressed through language and gestures. Features of language input that support children's communicative growth have been documented in literature on mother–child interaction (Snow & Ferguson, 1977). The specific adjustments that have been shown to facilitate and support interactions and communicative growth include the following: 1) simplified vocabulary and reduced sentence length; 2) exaggerated intonation, slower rate, and clear segmentation of speech; and 3) contingent responding and scaffolding.

A Focus on Communicative Events and Functions

Communication enhancement efforts following a DSP approach are concerned with all dimensions of communication—that is, with enhancing communicative means or behaviors and providing a better understanding of the function of communicative behavior and of the dyadic and reciprocal nature of communicative events. This is seen as essential because individuals of all ability levels with ASD are so challenged in their understanding of communicative events in social contexts. Communicative events are defined by two or more participants' engaging in social interactions cooperatively to accomplish particular goals (e.g., sharing information, solving a problem, playing a game). The structure of such events involves reciprocal exchanges in which all participants understand that they each have a role and a responsibility to fulfill in the exchange toward a shared goal. In other words, intervention must support children in "making sense" of communicative transactions (Duchan, 1986). "Activity-based interventions" and "joint action routines" provide the contexts for learning how to communicate meaningfully (Bricker, 1998; Snyder-McLean, Solomonson, McLean, & Sack, 1984; Wetherby et al., 1997). Efforts to enhance communication development are thus not so much a matter of specifying desirable response topographies but of providing motivating contexts, including opportunities and needs to communicate (McLean & Snyder-McLean, 1978).

We believe that three significant principles, drawn from the literature on communication development, are crucial to understanding and enhancing communication abilities of children with ASD on the basis of DSP principles (Prizant & Wetherby, 1989). First, communication development involves continuity from prelinguistic to linguistic communication. That is, the development of preverbal communication is a necessary precursor to the development of the intentional use of language to communicate. Words are "mapped" onto prelinguistic communication skills; thus, for children with ASD who are not speaking, an emphasis should be placed on developing functional social and preverbal communication skills. Second, being a competent communicator is the outcome of a developmental interaction of cognitive, socioemotional, linguistic, and motor capacities. An individual's developmental profile across these domains should provide the basis for decision making for communication enhancement. Third, in a DSP approach, all behavior should be viewed in reference to the child's relative level of functioning across developmental domains. Many of the challenging behaviors developed by children with ASD can be understood as attempts to communicate when such behavior is interpreted relative to developmental discrepancies and as coping strategies in the face of significant linguistic and sociocommunicative limitations (Prizant & Wetherby, 1987).

Learning Is Transactional and Affectively Based

The DSP approach is transactional in nature, meaning that it addresses the interdependent and reciprocal influences among the child with ASD, the social environment, and the interaction between the individual and the environment over time (Sameroff & Fiese, 1990). Within this model, it is believed that if newly acquired skills are to be integrated within one's current behavioral repertoire and cognitive understanding, then teaching should extend current knowledge and incorporate self-generated behaviors. The focus is on helping children communicate about things they know or emotions they feel. Similarly, language is learned as a tool to help organize experiences and plan and regulate behavior, allowing for the integration of experiences across environments and times of occurrence. Language experience is thus used to mediate thinking and problem solving and serves to support emotional regulation (Prizant & Meyer, 1993; Wertsch, 1985).

DSP approaches use rich, affectively charged social interactions as the contexts of language learning and communicative exchange (Greenspan, 1992; Greenspan & Wieder, 1997b, 1998; MacDonald, 1989; Prizant & Wetherby, 1990a; Wieder, 1997). The natural reactions of others in reciprocal interactions refine and reinforce communicative behaviors in terms of both function and structure. Through social interaction, individuals experience and come to understand the impact of their communicative attempts on their environment (Snow, Midkiff-Borunda, Small, & Proctor, 1984). Through affective exchange and attunement, children learn to build trusting relationships with others, which provides the foundation for social, cognitive, and communicative growth (Greenspan, 1997). This underscores the need for consistent and clear responses in interactions with children with ASD, allowing them to form hypotheses about the behaviors and intentions of others, and to develop an understanding of the reciprocal nature of social interaction (Prizant et al., 1997; Quill, 1995).

In summary, DSP approaches are defined by the following characteristics:

1. The focus is on enhancing spontaneous social communication within a more flexible structure and more varied and motivating activities.
2. There is an emphasis on building multimodal communicative repertoires (e.g., speech, gestures, augmentative and alternative communication [AAC]) to enable children to have a range of strategies to express intentions.

3. To the extent possible, interactions are characterized by shared control, turn taking, and reciprocity.
4. Learning contexts involve meaningful activities or events, chosen for interest and motivation.
5. The relevance of a child's response is considered in reference to the ongoing context and activities, including acknowledgment of unconventional means or behaviors as legitimate attempts to communicate.
6. Use of a variety of social groupings is desirable because children's life experiences will involve increasingly complex social experiences.
7. Information about the sequences and processes of child development is used to frame the sequence of goals and to measure progress in a broader developmental context.
8. Contextual (visual, gestural) supports are seen as essential to help children "make sense" of activities and interactions rather than to "strip down" learning contexts.
9. There is a focus on helping children acquire socially acceptable means for social control (e.g., means to protest, means to make choices) to preclude behavioral difficulties.
10. Emotional expression and affect sharing are seen as central to the interactive and learning process.

It is important to note that for different approaches within the DSP end of the continuum, different goals may be emphasized despite clear similarities in philosophy and practice. For example, Greenspan and Wieder (1997b, 1998) stated their primary goals in terms of helping children master increasingly complex levels of socioemotional growth, which they saw as the foundation and impetus for communicative and language development (see Chapter 12). In contrast, Prizant and colleagues (Prizant et al., 1997; Schuler et al., 1997; Wetherby et al., 1997) focused on more specific sociocommunicative goals in enhancing children's abilities to express communicative intentions and emotions in increasingly more conventional and sophisticated ways, resulting in a growing sense of social competence and increased capacities in emotional regulation.

Distinctions Between Contemporary ABA and DSP Approaches

Given the shared characteristics of contemporary ABA approaches and DSP approaches, one may ask how these approaches differ. In our opinion, there are a number of important distinctions. First, some contemporary behavioral approaches do not draw as much from research on sequences of language development in typically developing children and children with ASD. Second, in DSP approaches, there is less of an emphasis on eliciting and measuring discrete behavioral responses as the primary measures of success and more of an emphasis on children's successful participation in extended interactive sequences and episodes. Third, in contemporary ABA approaches, more intensive on-line data collection based on frequency counts of isolated behaviors (e.g., words, vocalizations) is advocated in measuring behavioral change, consistent with the behavioral tradition. In contrast, in DSP approaches, there is greater emphasis on multimodal communication and more natural teaching; thus, multiple goals are often targeted within a particular activity (e.g., communication, social-affective signaling, *and* play goals), and multilevel analysis of functional communicative acts involving verbal, vocal, and nonverbal components often is performed (see, e.g., Prizant & Duchan, 1981; Prizant & Rydell, 1984; Wetherby, Prizant, & Hutchinson, 1998). Such analyses may be more informative of developmental progress and more reflective of true communicative behavior in daily activities; however, they clearly are more challenging to perform than discrete counts of specific behaviors. Because of these challenges, in DSP approaches, on-line data collection tends to be less intensive, with the goal of allowing educators and clinicians to be freed up to participate more fully in and support a child's success in social interaction. Often, videotaping is the method of choice in data collection, with the use of time-sampling procedures to measure change over time. Other methods for measuring developmental progress and shifts, such as collection and analysis of language and communication samples and enlisting significant others (e.g., family members) as informants about progress, may also be used in lieu of frequency counts of behavior.

Fourth, DSP approaches are driven by an understanding of the interdependency of different aspects of development, such as relationships between communication and socioemotional development (Greenspan & Wieder, 1998; Prizant & Wetherby, 1990a) and between language and play development (Westby, 1988). Thus, in addition to developmental progress being measured based on acquisition of new communicative skills (e.g., words, gestures), it is also conceptualized in reference to development shifts and progression through developmental stages, informing future goal setting. Fifth, DSP interventions place greater emphasis on enhancing communication abilities within meaningful events and routines, with clear beginnings, a sequence of logical steps, and a sense of completion, to enhance a child's cognitive grasp of the structure of events that occur in everyday life (Duchan, 1995; Quill, 1995).

Finally, with few exceptions (e.g., Schreibman et al., 1991), DSP approaches give more emphasis than most contemporary ABA approaches to addressing communication development within the context of developing relationships and socioemotional growth. Such goals include understanding and expressing emotions and mastering increasingly complex stages of emotional and social-cognitive development (Greenspan & Wieder, 1998; MacDonald, 1989; Prizant & Wetherby, 1990b). Prizant and Wetherby (1990a, 1990b) and Wetherby and Prizant (1992) argued for the central role of children's ability to share emotions with others and expression of positive affect in underscoring the interrelationships between communication and socioemotional development, and in clinicians' and educators' targeting goals and measuring outcomes in children with communication and socioemotional difficulties. In contrast, the role of affect and emotional expression in motivation and learning is minimized in the contemporary behavioral as well as the traditional behavioral literature (Prizant & Wetherby, 1998).

SCERTS MODEL FOR ENHANCING COMMUNICATION AND SOCIOEMOTIONAL ABILITIES

The latest incarnation of our model for enhancing communication and socioemotional abilities for young children with ASD focuses on **s**ocial-**c**ommunication, **e**motional **r**egulation, and **t**ransactional **s**upport as the primary dimensions for intervention planning. We refer to this model as the *SCERTS model of intervention.* We believe that this model addresses in a comprehensive manner the core, underlying deficits affecting children with ASD and that it reflects recommended practices (Dawson & Osterling, 1997) as well as the greatest challenges faced by families and all communicative partners.

Treatment philosophy and practice in the SCERTS model are based on a highly individualized approach, requiring that intervention programs, goals, and objectives be designed for the specific developmental challenges experienced by a child. The need for such an approach is based on the fact that although children with ASD and related disabilities share similar developmental challenges in the areas of communication, social relatedness, and sensory processing, there is great heterogeneity within this population of children (see Chapter 12). Similarly, families raising children with ASD vary greatly in the skills, resources, and support that are available to them in supporting their children's development. Therefore, the SCERTS model draws from a variety of empirically supported treatment methodologies to best meet the needs of each individual child and family. This is in contrast to approaches that are constrained in philosophy, methodology, and practice and therefore cannot meet the varied needs of children with ASD and their families. To circumvent problems of generalization, which is one of the great treatment challenges acknowledged in research literature on ASDs, treatment involves both clinical and school-based as well as home-based strategies, including family support, training, and education. These components—an individualized approach focusing on communication, social relatedness and sensory processing, and family-centered practices and support—reflect acknowledged "best practices" in the contemporary literature on ASDs (Dawson & Osterling, 1997; Wetherby & Prizant, 1999).

More specifically, the SCERTS model directly addresses what are considered to be the core deficits observed in children with ASD (Dawson & Osterling, 1997). Communication and language deficits are addressed through social-pragmatic language therapy, which emphasizes the functional use of preverbal and verbal communication skills in natural and semistructured interactions (Prizant & Wetherby, 1998). The effectiveness of this approach is supported by research on children with ASD and other developmental disabilities (McLean & Cripe, 1997), including validated and effective strategies to support the use of nonspeech communication systems such as picture symbols (see Chapter 14). As noted previously, social-pragmatic approaches are now practiced in both contemporary ABA programs as well as developmentally based programs (Prizant & Wetherby, 1998).

Deficits in social relatedness and social-emotional reciprocity are addressed through strategies developed as part of Greenspan's (Greenspan, 1992; Greenspan & Wieder, 1998) Developmental, Individual-Difference, Relationship-Based (DIR) model, more commonly known as the *floor time approach* (see Chapter 12). The effectiveness of this approach has been supported by follow-up research on 200 children with ASD, the largest outcome research sample to date (Greenspan & Wieder, 1997a).

Sensory processing deficits are addressed through sensory integration therapy and environmental adaptations and supports. These approaches involve techniques to support children's processing of sensory input to maintain optimal states of attention, arousal, and emotional regulation. Many children with ASD also have motor planning issues affecting daily living skills, which are also addressed. The effectiveness of sensory integration therapy for children with ASD is also supported by research (Fallon, Mauer, & Neukirch, 1994; see also Chapter 8).

It is essential to emphasize that within the SCERTS model, the whole is greater than the sum of the parts. The developmental challenges experienced by children with ASD do not occur in an isolated manner and cannot be treated as such. For example, activities for daily living such as dressing involve social interaction, communication, and sensory processing, as well as motor abilities. Furthermore, treatment approaches draw on children's developmental strengths and natural motivations to address areas of weakness. Thus, to the extent possible, intervention occurs within the natural routines across home, school, and community environments to support the development of critical skills. Finally, because the SCERTS model recognizes that the family context is the most important context for a child's development (Prizant & Meyer, 1993; see also Chapters 13 and 15), there is an emphasis on supporting and educating family members, including parents, brothers, and sisters, to best enhance the development of the child with ASD. This family-centered practice is recognized as another core characteristic of effective programs for children with ASD (Dawson & Osterling, 1997). Critical components of each domain of the model are delineated in the following sections from an assessment and intervention perspective.

Social-Communication

A number of basic tenets underlie the social-communication component of the SCERTS model.

Communicative Intent as the Underlying Construct

The most functional and relevant communicative abilities that children will acquire emerge from self-generated and self-motivated goals. Such goals have been referred to as *communicative intents* or *communicative intentions* in the developmental literature (Bates, Benigni, Bretherton, Camaioni, & Volterra, 1979). When a child is able to direct behavior to others such that desired goals are achieved, it may be said that communicative attempts have functioned as intended. The term *communicative functions of behavior* is used to refer to this concept in both the developmental and contemporary ABA literature (Donnellan et al., 1984; Durand, 1990; Prizant & Wetherby, 1987). Thus, assessment of the intentions expressed by young children and of the communicative functions served by communicative acts is essential in assessment of young children's abilities, for these provide the foundation for developing a more sophisticated and elaborated communicative repertoire (Prizant & Bailey, 1992; Wetherby & Prizant, 1989).

Range of Functions

The purposes of a child's behavior may vary in the communicative intentions expressed or functions achieved, ranging from relatively nonsocial purposes (i.e., behavior regulation, or communicating to regulate others' behavior to meet immediate needs) to very social purposes (i.e., joint attention, or communicating to share observations and experiences). Prior to the emergence of words, typically developing children use intentional communicative signals for three major functions: behavior regulation, social interaction, and joint attention. These three general functional categories represent a continuum of sociability or social motivation in communication. Wetherby (1986) first suggested that the easiest and first-emerging communicative intention for children with ASD is behavior regulation and that the most difficult is joint attention, presumably because of the differing social underpinnings of these abilities. Research has demonstrated repeatedly that young children with ASD are most challenged in generating goals and expressing intentions that are more social in nature, such as communicating for joint or shared attention (see Wetherby et al., 1998, for a review). This profile of communicative functions has important implications for early identification of ASDs (see Chapter 2), as well as for focusing communication enhancement efforts on expanding communicative functions. A priority of intervention is to expand communicative acts to more social purposes, which contributes to more functional, relationship-based communication. In doing so, it is essential that activities are selected and environments are engineered to create multiple opportunities for communicating for a variety of purposes (see Wetherby et al., 1997, for further discussion).

Developmental Sequences in Communication

Another significant aspect of enhancing communicative competence is application of a comprehensive understanding of developmental sequences. Earlier, misguided attempts at speech training (e.g., Lovaas, 1977) for many children who were clearly not yet "ready" to acquire this highly complex and symbolic form of communication were made because of a lack of knowledge of the very fundamentals of the evolution of communicative and linguistic competence as documented in the developmental literature. Application of knowledge from the developmental literature has had a tremendous impact on current practices of assessing and enhancing language and communication abilities for children with ASD.

Continuum of Presymbolic to Symbolic Communication It is now widely accepted that children with ASD vary greatly in their capacities to acquire and use symbolic systems of communication such as language-based systems including oral language and sign language. Because of developmental literature and intervention research since the 1980s, however, nonspeaking, presymbolic children with ASD are now able to benefit from instructional strategies that focus on the acquisition of nonsymbolic (e.g., natural gestures, nonspeech vocalizations) as well as quasi-symbolic (e.g., photographs, picture symbols) means to communicate intentions (see Chapter 14 for a review of the AAC literature).

Continuum of Echolalia to Creative Language A developmental perspective in understanding echolalia and other forms of unconventional verbal behavior (Prizant & Rydell, 1993) has had a significant impact on both assessment and intervention efforts. Prizant (1983) described the transition from echolalic speech as following a predictable progression. For many children with ASD, early speech typically is predominantly echolalic and serves limited communicative functions. With social-cognitive and linguistic growth, echolalic speech is used for a greater variety of communicative functions, and more creative patterns of language begin to emerge. With the development of a more rule-governed and generative linguistic system, echolalic speech decreases and speech repetition becomes more flexible and less rigidly produced.

For children more able to move on to primarily creative and spontaneous language, echolalia may not completely disappear but may be observed primarily during states of confusion and fatigue or during highly adult-directed interactions, when it serves the function of conversational turn taking (i.e., participation in the reciprocity of communicative exchange) (Rydell & Mirenda, 1994). For other children, patterns of echolalia and other forms of unconventional verbal behavior may not demonstrate progressive change. Therefore, intervention strategies must be based on systematic analyses of echolalia and other forms of unconventional verbal behavior, taking individual differences and situational factors into account. In general, however, echolalia usually represents a transitional phenomenon and is a positive prognostic indicator for further communicative growth and change (McEachin, Smith, & Lovaas, 1993; Prizant, 1983).

Continuum of Communicative Means: Unconventional to Conventional Conventionality in communicative signaling refers to the degree to which the meaning of signals is shared or understood by a social community. In communication development, all young children demonstrate a progression from less conventional forms to forms with greater conventionality at both prelinguistic and linguistic levels. Children with ASD acquire unconventional behavior to express communicative intentions in the absence of more conventional means (Prizant & Wetherby, 1987). Even speech production (e.g., delayed echolalia, metaphorical language) may be unconventional in both form and function (Prizant & Rydell, 1993). Thus, it is essential that assessment efforts document unconventional communicative means and that intervention efforts focus on helping individuals acquire more conventional and socially acceptable forms to communicate rather than simply ignore unconventional means as inconsequential or, even worse, include attempts to eradicate such behavior.

In summary, the SCERTS model emphasizes that communication enhancement efforts must address the following core issues: expressing communicative intent; expanding the range of communicative functions; targeting presymbolic, quasi-symbolic, or symbolic communicative means depending on a child's abilities; supporting a child's transition from echolalic speech to creative language; and continually supporting the acquisition of more conventional means to communicate at both nonverbal and verbal levels. Intervention efforts, however, cannot address these goals in isolation. It is essential that children be "available" attentionally and emotionally in the context of supportive relationships and transactions to benefit optimally from efforts to enhance communicative competence, which is addressed by the last two dimensions of the SCERTS model.

Emotional Regulation

Emotional regulation is a core developmental process underlying attention, engagement, and the establishment of secure relationships. Emotional regulatory capacity has been defined as "an individual's ability to develop and use various means to control or modulate his or her level of emotional arousal" (Prizant & Meyer, 1993, p. 57). Such capacities allow a child to stay calm and focused, to problem-solve, to maintain social engagement, to communicate effectively, and to benefit from the rich learning opportunities in everyday experiences. Strategies for emotional regulation vary from sensorimotor and presymbolic means to higher-level conceptual and linguistic means. Sensorimotor and presymbolic means may include repetitive movement (e.g., rocking, spinning), tactile and oral self-stimulation (e.g., massage, deep pressure, sucking), or blocking out and shutting oneself down from sensory input (e.g., gaze aversion, placing hands over the ears or eyes, physical withdrawal from overstimulating circumstances). Higher-level means of emotional regulation may include talking about potentially dysregulating events, such as changes in routine or schedule, and/or engaging in role-playing to prepare for and become desensitized to stressful events (e.g., visits to the dentist).

Researchers have identified two types of capacities, self-regulatory and mutual/interactive regulatory capacities, that are believed to be essential for maintaining emotional regulation, especially during confusing, highly arousing, and stressful circumstances (Tronick, 1989). Self-regulatory capacities involve the use of sensorimotor or higher-level symbolic means that can be applied independently to regulate emotional arousal. Many so-called stereotypic behaviors of children with ASD such as rocking and repetitive hand movements may serve a self-regulatory function (see Chapter 7 for further discussion). Higher-level means may include self-directed language or delayed echolalia for self-calming (e.g., a child sitting in the back of a car repeating, "Don't worry, the dentist is not going to hurt you," on the way to the dentist).

Mutual or interactive regulatory capacities involve helping children to develop the ability to solicit and secure the assistance of others in regulating emotional arousal. With less competent communicators, the more competent partners must be sensitive and responsive to the often unconventional, subtle, and idiosyncratic behaviors that indicate a need to support a child's regulation of emotional arousal. For example, when one child is distressed as indicated by vocalization, bodily tension, or agitated movement, a partner may respond by speaking in a slow, calm voice, and by hugging or giving a child some deep pressure on the shoulders or arms. For another child, playing soothing music and/or moving a child to a calming space may be a more effective strategy. Higher-level strategies that children may acquire or may be taught include requesting assistance from others to preclude frustration during difficult tasks, expressing emotions in an effort to seek support or comfort from others, or requesting information about uncertain or anxiety producing events. Preparing individuals for unpredictable changes in routine, a common dysregulating event for children with ASD, may be accomplished through pictures and through language and thus may serve a mutual regulatory function.

In the SCERTS model, both self- and mutual emotional regulation are addressed in assessment and intervention. In assessment, the goal is to determine the types of strategies a child already demonstrates for mutual or self-regulation. Potential strategies that may be helpful for an individual child based on his or her sensory integration needs and communicative profiles are identified and targeted as intervention goals. It is also important to assess the availability of activities and contexts to support emotion regulation. For example, the use of soothing activities such as listening to music or looking at favorite books, the application of a "sensory diet" throughout the day (see Chapter 7), and having a quiet relaxing space may help a child to maintain emotional regulation throughout the day.

Transactional Support

We have proposed that the "transactional model" of development, which shares many principles with social-pragmatic approaches to enhancing communication, is the most relevant model in designing effective interventions for young children with ASD (Prizant & Wetherby, 1989). This model stipulates that developmental outcomes are "the result of interplay between child and context over time, in which the state of one impacts on the next state of the other in a continuous dynamic process" (Sameroff, 1987, p. 274). Thus, in a transactional model of intervention, the active role of the child in learning is acknowledged, and partners respond actively and flexibly to a child's communicative attempts and reactions in social exchange. The transactional model also emphasizes that developmental facilitators include all of the people, including parents, other caregivers, siblings, and peers, who interact and engage with children with ASD on a regular basis. The concept of transactional support implies that clinicians and educators must expand their role from focusing primarily on enhancing children's abilities to supporting others in growth-inducing interactions and activities designed to enhance children's developmental capacities. Furthermore, environmental adaptations and modifications, such as the use of visual supports, enable children to benefit from learning strengths when faced with the challenges of communication and social interaction.

Transactional Support to Families

The most critical sociocommunicative experiences for most children occur in their interactions with family members, both when they are learning the basic elements of communicative exchange and when they expand their communicative mastery. Daily routines and family events provide the experiential opportunities in which children learn and practice communicative abilities (Manolson, 1992). In supporting families, clinicians and educators must be cognizant of the whole range of possible reactions that family members may experience when raising a child with ASD. Parents and caregivers should be asked to discuss their child's strengths and difficulties and to articulate the primary concerns and expectations regarding their child's development. When appropriate, caregivers may be encouraged to share their sense of competence as well as limitations in fostering communicative and socioemotional development. Successful and unsuccessful strategies that family members may have employed to promote social and communicative interactions must also be explored. Information about a child's and family's strengths and needs and family priorities, as gathered in assessment, form the basis from which specific intervention goals are derived. Caregivers are supported in reference to communicative and interactive styles that are most appropriate in enhancing their child's development. Issues discussed previously such as degree of directiveness and developmentally appropriate language and communicative modeling in everyday routines are important considerations in ongoing support of caregivers.

When working with families, it also is essential that clinicians and educators understand various family structures and functions and how these can be influenced by economic, ethnic, and cultural factors. For example, because of cultural and pragmatic factors, biological parents may not necessarily be the primary caregivers in some families; thus, other family members such as grandparents or older siblings may play a more active role in intervention. When practitioners design intervention strategies to be used by family members and integrated into daily family routines, it is critical that recommendations be compatible with the family's belief systems and sociocultural characteristics (Lynch & Hanson, 1998).

Helping parents to develop appropriate expectations and realistic goals in communication is another important dimension of transactional support. This involves helping parents to learn to recognize and celebrate even the smallest meaningful gains in sociocommunicative and socioemotional development. Meaningful progress may involve less dramatic changes (e.g., increase in the variety of communicative intentions expressed, increase in the rate of communicative acts, progress in emotional regulation) that may not be as apparent as more striking developmental gains (e.g., acquisition of first words).

Transactional Support to Peers and Siblings

Inclusive programming is now recognized as an integral component of programming for many children with ASD. A variety of models are now available to support the development of relationships, play, and reciprocal communication among children with ASD and their peers. Some examples include Integrated Play Groups (Wolfberg, 1995; Wolfberg & Schuler, 1993), Circle of Friends (McTarnaghan, 1998), and Peer Mediated Intervention (PMI; Strain & Kohler, 1998). These models serve to promote peer-related competencies, which include the ability to initiate and maintain conventional social-communication interactions with peers across people, environments, and circumstances. In this chapter, we use the acronym PMI as a generic term to refer to these approaches.

A systematic approach to PMI becomes increasingly important for a child with ASD as practitioners have come to understand 1) how children with ASD learn best; 2) how their learning style differs from that of typical peers, which may be both challenging and beneficial (e.g., strengths in visuospatial processing); and 3) what difficulties children with ASD experience in social, communication, and play development. In addition, the field has become more aware that the development and use of conventional sociocommunicative skills with peers often requires systematic support and opportunities for successful interaction.

A transactional approach to PMI offers children with ASD opportunities to learn with and from peers and to develop enduring relationships. Approaches vary in the degree of structure and adult guidance provided to children who are learning and applying social, communication, and play skills in predictable and scaffolded activities. Of primary importance is teaching children with ASD *how* and *when* to use their communication and interaction skills by reading and understanding social cues and conventions, as well as by following the rules of the social, communication, and play schemes inherent in play interactions. These approaches suggest that by engineering the environment to increase the child's familiarity and expectancy of interactional routines, practitioners increase the likelihood of the child's applying interactional skills in a more conventional and goal-directed manner with peers. Conversely, if the environment is unfamiliar and a high degree of novelty is present, then there is a greater likelihood that interactional breakdowns with peers will occur and that opportunities for success in initiating and maintaining communicative and play interactions will be reduced.

Principles of Peer Mediated Intervention

PMI draws from and, therefore, fits well with developmental and transactional philosophy and practice on supporting language and communication development. The following principles, some of which were highlighted previously, are reviewed with specific regard to the role of peers in enhancing abilities.

Use of Naturalistic Interactions and Settings The ultimate goal in PMI is for a child to learn and practice emerging social skills in naturalistic interactions across people, settings, and circumstances. Learning involves a child's understanding and following natural cues, conventions, and rules of interactions with peers in a variety of contexts. The focus becomes contingent interaction, reciprocal exchange, and interpersonal anticipatory behaviors between a child and his or her peers.

Engineering Environments Naturally occurring activities and play routines can be engineered to provide consistent, predictable, and familiar environments in which a child can develop sociocommunicative abilities. Thus, the requisite abilities for successful interaction can be more consistently learned, understood, and applied by a child with ASD when interactions and expectancies are very clear and the child's sociocommunicative attempts are followed by consistent peer responses.

Control for Novelty For children with ASD, interactional breakdowns and challenging behaviors most often occur in unpredictable, novel circumstances. Novelty and unexpected interactional and environmental variables often lead to dysregulation, disorganization, confusion, agitation, and heightened anxiety (Klinger & Dawson, 1992), precluding attention and responsiveness to the environment and to partners. Novelty can be presented unknowingly in many environments, such as in busy, highly stimulating classrooms; large-group activities; or other similar environments where unpredictable events may occur. PMI, by its very nature, increases novelty when a child is being presented with unfamiliar social, communication, and play schemes in less structured settings. Systematic control of novel elements becomes an important consideration with PMI, especially in the initial stages of program development. The importance of controlling novel events, however, will vary depending on a child's developmental capacities because coping with increased novelty and unpredictability is an important goal as children develop.

Shared Control/Reciprocity Natural interactions among friends and peers are largely based on reciprocal sociocommunicative exchange and sharing of control. Typical peer interaction does not allow for one partner to dominate or control the other partner; rather, partners engage in a process of initiating and maintaining sociocommunicative acts as well as contingently responding to social overtures of others. When an interaction is dominated by one partner, the other partner often loses interest or interactional breakdowns occur. Ideally, a child with ASD should have some familiarity with the sociocommunicative requirements and play schemes prior to being placed in typical peer interactions to increase his or her understanding of how and when to engage in sociocommunicative initiations with peers. In addition, when a child is allowed opportunities to both take the lead in play interactions as well as follow the peer's lead, shared control is fostered with the peer and the child is not automatically relegated to a respondent role within the interaction.

Unconventional Verbal and Social-Play Behaviors PMI recognizes that children with ASD may initially engage in purposeful and intentional sociocommunicative acts even though these acts may appear unconventional. Children with ASD should not be precluded from participating in functional peer-mediated interactions due to atypical communicative patterns (e.g., echolalia, incessant questioning). Rather, peers should be supported in recognizing and understanding the purpose and intent of these unconventional behaviors. Interventions are designed to systematically increase multiple means of exchange in sociocommunicative interactions (verbal and nonverbal) while replacing less conventional with more conventional means of interaction.

Enhancing Motivation to Communicate in Everyday Interactions Naturally occurring daily routines and joint action routines (Snyder-McLean et al., 1984) selected for their potential in supporting mutually enjoyable interactions among children with ASD and peers are used as foundations for PMI. These routines incorporate 1) an obvious theme or purpose, 2) a joint focus for the interaction, 3) exchangeable roles, 4) a clear sequence and structure, 5) multiple repetitions of turns, and 6) opportunities for controlled variation of structure and expectation (Prizant et al., 1997; Snyder-McLean et al., 1984).

Highly predictable joint action routines that are meaningful, purposeful, and intrinsically motivating for the child with ASD are well suited to maintaining extended interactions with peers.

Expression of Communicative Intent PMI targets natural opportunities within joint action routines for the child to understand and use a variety of sociocommunicative acts for 1) behavioral regulation (e.g., requesting objects or action, protesting), 2) social interaction (e.g., requesting social games or routines, maintaining routines, greeting, calling to others), and 3) joint attention (e.g., commenting, providing information). Multiple opportunities are also presented for a child to increase his or her persistence in maintaining routines or for repairing interactional breakdowns with peers using conventional means of communication. A transactional approach to PMI de-emphasizes teaching syntactically and semantically correct sentence forms in favor of promoting the child's understanding of how and when to participate in reciprocal social exchange.

Adult Participant's Role The adult's role is one of 1) creating naturalistic and motivating sociocommunicative opportunities; 2) modeling appropriate means of communication based on the child's developmental level and intervention goals; 3) prompting to enable the child to achieve sociocommunicative success; 4) repairing breakdowns, if necessary; and 5) offering repeated opportunities for predictable interactions as more conventional means of communication are learned. The initial role of the adult participant is one of helping the child to become familiar with the social, communication, and play expectancies in a highly predictable environment. The adult engineers a learning environment that controls for novelty, and he or she initially serves as a primary communicative partner while a child's interactional skills are first being taught. The role of the adult fades as a primary interactant as peers are systematically supported in replacing the adult in these familiar routines.

DIRECTIONS FOR FUTURE RESEARCH

Except for research addressing the relationships between challenging behavior and communication (see Chapter 13), intervention research on communication of children with ASD has focused primarily on acquisition of specific communicative means and on strategies to teach those communicative means in contexts ranging from highly structured to more naturalistic. The challenge for the next generation of research is to examine the complex relationships among the acquisition of communicative abilities, socioemotional factors (e.g., emotional regulation), and types of transactional supports that allow for better sociocommunicative outcomes for children with ASD. In other words, we believe the critical question regarding treatment outcomes is "Which combinations of treatment elements are most effective in developing individualized approaches for individual children and families?" (Prizant & Wetherby, 1998, p. 347). We plan to address these issues in research on the SCERTS model as it is being applied in center- and home-based environments.

Furthermore, in measuring efficacy of intervention, researchers need to go beyond traditional measures of communicative and language skills such as improvement on standardized tests and include broader characteristics, such as degree of success in communicative exchange, related dimensions of emotional expression and regulation, sociocommunicative motivation, social competence, peer relationships, and the child's competence in natural environments (Prizant & Wetherby, 1998). Intervention research on children with ASD has been negligent in documenting a range of meaningful outcome measures. Therefore, extreme caution should be taken in drawing conclusions about the efficacy of a particular intervention approach. Future research should strive to document meaningful changes that reflect the core domains associated with ASDs as well as measures of family functioning.

CONCLUSIONS

From a developmental, transactional perspective, enhancing the development of sociocommunicative and language abilities for children with ASD is far more complex and challenging than teaching a sequence of speech or nonverbal behaviors. The ultimate goal is for a child with ASD to participate as a partner in sociocommunicative exchange with peers and family members and to experience interactions as successful and emotionally fulfilling. The development of trusting and secure relationships is both a foundation for and a product of success in social communication with others.

In this chapter, we have provided an historical perspective on approaches to enhancing language and communicative abilities and what we believe to be a contemporary, comprehensive model for enhancing sociocommunicative and related abilities. Facilitating true progress in these abilities will only occur through a more comprehensive understanding of the interdependent aspects of a child's development, within the context of his or her family and broader social network.

REFERENCES

Anderson, S., Taras, M., & Cannon, B. (1996). Teaching new skills to young children with autism. In C. Maurice, G. Green, & S. Luce (Eds.), *Behavioral interventions for young children with autism* (pp. 181–194). Austin, TX: PRO-ED.

Bates, E. (1976). *Language and context: The acquisition of pragmatics.* San Diego: Academic Press.

Bates, E. (1979). *The emergence of symbols: Cognition and communication in infancy.* San Diego: Academic Press.

Bates, E., Benigni, L., Bretherton, I., Camaioni, L., & Volterra, V. (1979). *The emergence of symbols: Cognition and communication in infancy.* San Diego: Academic Press.

Bates, E., O'Connell, B., & Shore, C. (1987). Language and communication in infancy. In J. Osofsky (Ed.), *Handbook of infant development* (pp. 149–203). New York: John Wiley & Sons.

Bricker, D. (1993). Then, now, and the path between: A brief history of language intervention. In S.F. Warren & J. Reichle (Series Eds.) & A.P. Kaiser & D.B. Gray (Vol. Eds.), *Communication and language intervention series: Vol. 2. Enhancing children's communication: Research foundations for intervention* (pp. 11–31). Baltimore: Paul H. Brookes Publishing Co.

Bricker, D. (with Pretti-Frontczak, K., & McComas, N.). (1998). *An activity-based approach to early intervention* (2nd ed.). Baltimore: Paul H. Brookes Publishing Co.

Bruner, J. (1981). The social context of language acquisition. *Language and Communication, 1,* 155–178.

Carr, E., & Durand, V.M. (1986). The social-communicative basis of severe behavior problems in children. In S. Reis & R. Bootzin (Eds.), *Theoretical issues in behavior therapy* (pp. 219–254). San Diego: Academic Press.

Carr, E.G., Levin, L., McConnachie, G., Carlson, J.I., Kemp, D.C., & Smith, C.E. (1994). *Communication-based intervention for problem behavior: A user's guide for producing positive change.* Baltimore: Paul H. Brookes Publishing Co.

Clark, G., & Seifer, R. (1985). Assessment of parents' interactions with their developmentally delayed infants. *Infant Mental Health Journal, 6,* 214–225.

Dawson, G., & Adams, A. (1984). Imitation and social responsiveness in autistic children. *Journal of Abnormal Child Psychology, 12,* 209–226.

Dawson, G., & Osterling, J. (1997). Early intervention in autism. In M.J. Guralnick (Ed.), *The effectiveness of early intervention* (pp. 307–326). Baltimore: Paul H. Brookes Publishing Co.

Donnellan, A., Mirenda, P., Mesaros, R., & Fassbender, L. (1984). Analyzing the communicative functions of aberrant behavior. *Journal of The Association for Persons with Severe Handicaps, 9,* 201–212.

Duchan, J.F. (1986). Language intervention through sensemaking and fine-tuning. In R. Schiefelbusch (Ed.), *Communicative competence: Assessment and language intervention.* Baltimore: University Park Press.

Duchan, J. (1989). Evaluating adults' talk to children: Assessing adult attunement. *Seminars in Speech and Language, 10,* 17–27.

Duchan, J. (1995). *Supporting language learning in everyday life.* San Diego: Singular Publishing Group.

Dunlap, G., Vaughn, B.J., & O'Neill, R. (1998). Comprehensive behavioral support: Application and intervention. In S.F. Warren & J. Reichle (Series Eds.) & A.M. Wetherby, S.F. Warren, & J. Reichle (Vol. Eds.), *Communication and language intervention series: Vol. 7. Transitions in prelinguistic communication* (pp. 343–364). Baltimore: Paul H. Brookes Publishing Co.

Dunst, C., Lowe, E., & Bartholomew, P. (1990). Contingent social responsiveness, family ecology, and infant communicative competence. *National Student Speech-Language-Hearing Association, 17,* 39–49.

Durand, V.M. (1990). *Severe behavior problems: A functional communication training approach.* New York: Guilford Press.

Fallon, M., Mauer, D., & Neukirch, M. (1994). The effectiveness of sensory integration activities on language processing in preschoolers who are sensory and language impaired. *Infant–Toddler Intervention,* 4, 235–243.

Fay, W.H., & Schuler, A.L. (Vol. Eds.). (1980). *Emerging language in autistic children.* In R.L. Schiefelbusch (Series Ed.), *Language intervention series* (Vol. 5). Baltimore: University Park Press.

Greenspan, S. (1992). *Infancy and early childhood: The practice of clinical assessment and intervention with emotional and developmental challenges.* Madison, CT: International Universities Press.

Greenspan, S. (1997). *The growth of the mind and the endangered origins of intelligence.* Reading, MA: Addison Wesley Longman.

Greenspan, S.I., & Wieder, S. (1997a). Developmental patterns and outcomes in infants and children with disorders in relating and communicating: A chart review of 200 cases of children with autistic spectrum diagnoses. *Journal of Developmental and Learning Disorders, 1,* 87–141.

Greenspan, S.I., & Wieder, S. (1997b). An integrated developmental approach to interventions for young children with severe difficulties in relating and communicating. *ZERO TO THREE Bulletin,* 5–17.

Greenspan, S.I., & Wieder, S. (1998). *The child with special needs: Encouraging intellectual and emotional growth.* Reading, MA: Addison Wesley Longman.

Hart, B. (1985). Naturalistic language training techniques. In S. Warren & A.K. Rogers-Warren (Eds.), *Teaching functional language: Generalization and maintenance of language skills* (pp. 63–88). Baltimore: University Park Press.

Hart, B., & Risley, T.R. (1995). *Meaningful differences in the everyday experience of young American children.* Baltimore: Paul H. Brookes Publishing Co.

Horner, R., Dunlap, G., Koegel, R., Carr, E., Sailor, W., Anderson, J., Albin, R., & O'Neill, R. (1990). Toward a technology of "nonaversive" behavioral support. *Journal of The Association for Persons with Severe Handicaps, 15,* 125–147.

Johnson, C. (1994, November–December). Interview with Dr. Ivar Lovaas. *Advocate: Newsletter of the Autism Society of America.*

Kaiser, A., & Hester, P. (1994). Generalized effects of enhanced milieu teaching. *Journal of Speech and Hearing Research, 37,* 63–92

Kaiser, A.P., Yoder, P.J., & Keetz, A. (1992). Evaluating milieu teaching. In S.F. Warren & J. Reichle (Series & Vol. Eds.), *Communication and language intervention series: Vol. 1. Causes and effects in communication and language intervention* (pp. 9–47). Baltimore: Paul H. Brookes Publishing Co.

Klinger, L.G., & Dawson, G. (1992). Facilitating early social and communicative development in children with autism. In S. Warren & J. Reichle (Series & Vol. Eds.), *Communication and language intervention series: Vol. 1. Causes and effects in communication and language intervention* (pp. 157–186). Baltimore: Paul H. Brookes Publishing Co.

Koegel, L.K. (1995). Communication and language intervention. In R.L. Koegel & L.K. Koegel (Eds.), *Teaching children with autism: Strategies for initiating positive interactions and improving learning opportunities* (pp. 17–32). Baltimore: Paul H. Brookes Publishing Co.

Koegel, R., & Johnson, J. (1989). Motivating language use in autistic children. In G. Dawson (Ed.), *Autism: New perspectives on diagnosis, nature and treatment* (pp. 310–325). New York: Guilford Press.

Koegel, R.L., & Koegel, L.K. (Eds.). (1995). *Teaching children with autism: Strategies for initiating positive interactions and improving learning opportunities.* Baltimore: Paul H. Brookes Publishing Co.

Koegel, R., O'Dell, M.C., & Koegel, L.K. (1987). A natural language paradigm for teaching nonverbal autistic children. *Journal of Autism and Developmental Disorders, 17,* 187–199.

Lovaas, O.I. (1977). *The autistic child: Language development through behavior modification.* New York: Irvington Press.

Lovaas, O.I. (1981). *Teaching developmentally disabled children: The "me" book.* Baltimore: University Park Press.

Lund, N., & Duchan, J. (1983). *Assessing children's language in naturalistic contexts.* Upper Saddle River, NJ: Prentice-Hall.

Lynch, E.W., & Hanson, M.J. (1998). *Developing cultural competence: A guide for working with children and their families* (2nd ed.). Baltimore: Paul H. Brookes Publishing Co.

MacDonald, J. (1989). *Becoming partners with children.* San Antonio, TX: Special Press.

MacDonald, J., & Gillette, Y. (1988). Communicating partners: A conversational model for building parent–child relationships with handicapped children. In K. Marfo (Ed.), *Parent–child interaction and developmental disabilities.* New York: Praeger.

Mahoney, G., & Powell, A. (1988). Modifying parent–child interaction: Enhancing the development of handicapped children. *Journal of Special Education, 22,* 82–96.

Manolson, A. (1992). *It takes two to talk* (2nd ed.). Toronto: Hanen Early Language Resource Centre.

Marfo, K. (1990). Maternal directiveness in interactions with mentally handicapped children: An analytical commentary. *Journal of Child Psychology and Psychiatry and Allied Disciplines, 31,* 531–549.

Maurice, C., Green, G., & Luce, S. (1996). *Behavioral intervention for young children with autism.* Austin, TX: PRO-ED.

McCormick, L. (1990). Intervention processes and procedures. In L. McCormick & R. Schiefelbusch (Eds.), *Early language intervention* (pp. 215–260). Columbus, OH: Merrill.

McEachin, J.J., Smith, T., & Lovaas, O.I. (1993). Long-term outcome for children with autism who received early intensive behavioral treatment. *American Journal on Mental Retardation, 97,* 359–372.

McLean, L. (1990). Communication development in the first two years of life: A transactional process. *ZERO TO THREE Bulletin, 11*(1), 13–19.

McLean, L.K., & Cripe, J.W. (1997). The effectiveness of early intervention for children with communication disorders. In M. Guralnick (Ed.), *The effectiveness of early intervention* (pp. 349–428). Baltimore: Paul H. Brookes Publishing Co.

McLean, J., & Snyder-McLean, L. (1978). *A transactional approach to early language training: Derivation of a model system.* Columbus, OH: Charles Merrill.

McTarnaghan, J. (1998). *Circle of friends.* Unpublished training manuscript, Community Autism Resources, Fall River, MA.

Meyer, L.H., & Evans, I.M. (1986). Modification of excess behavior: An adaptive and functional approach for educational and community contexts. In R.H. Horner, L.H. Meyer, & H.D.B. Fredericks (Eds.), *Education of learners with severe handicaps: Exemplary service strategies* (pp. 315–350). Baltimore: Paul H. Brookes Publishing Co.

Meyer, L.H., & Evans, I.M. (1993). Meaningful outcomes in behavioral intervention: Evaluating positive approaches to the remediation of challenging behaviors. In S.F. Warren & J. Reichle (Series Eds.) & J. Reichle & D.P. Wacker (Vol. Eds.), *Communication and language intervention series: Vol. 3. Communicative alternatives to challenging behavior: Integrating functional assessment and intervention strategies* (pp. 407–428). Baltimore: Paul H. Brookes Publishing Co.

Mirenda, P., & Donnellan, A. (1986). Effects of adult interactional style on conversational behavior of students with severe communication problems. *Language, Speech, and Hearing Services in Schools, 17,* 126–141.

Peck, C. (1985). Increasing opportunities for social control by children with autism and severe handicaps: Effects on student behavior and perceived classroom climate. *Journal of The Association for Persons with Severe Handicaps, 4,* 183–193.

Prizant, B. (1982). Speech-language pathologists and autistic children: What is our role? *Asha, 24,* 463–468, 531–537.

Prizant, B. (1983). Language acquisition and communicative behavior in autism: Toward an understanding of the ''whole'' of it. *Journal of Speech and Hearing Disorders, 48,* 296–307.

Prizant, B., & Bailey, D. (1992). Facilitating the acquisition and use of communication skills. In D. Bailey & M. Wolery (Eds.), *Teaching infants and preschoolers with disabilities* (pp. 299–361). Columbus, OH: Merrill.

Prizant, B.M., & Duchan, J.F. (1981). The functions of immediate echolalia in autistic children. *Journal of Speech and Hearing Disorders, 46,* 241–249.

Prizant, B.M., & Meyer, E.C. (1993). Socioemotional aspects of communication disorders in young children and their families. *American Journal of Speech-Language Pathology, 2,* 56–71.

Prizant, B.M., & Rydell, P.J. (1984). An analysis of the functions of delayed echolalia in autistic children. *Journal of Speech and Hearing Research, 27,* 183–192.

Prizant, B.M., & Rydell, P. (1993). Assessment and intervention strategies for unconventional verbal behavior. In S.F. Warren & J. Reichle (Series Eds.) & J. Reichle & D.P. Wacker (Vol. Eds.), *Communication and language intervention series: Vol. 3. Communicative approaches to challenging behavior* (pp. 263–297). Baltimore: Paul H. Brookes Publishing Co.

Prizant, B.M., Schuler, A.L., Wetherby, A.M., & Rydell, P. (1997). Enhancing language and communication: Language approaches. In D. Cohen & F. Volkmar (Eds.), *Handbook of autism and pervasive developmental disorders* (2nd ed., pp. 572–605). New York: John Wiley & Sons.

Prizant, B.M., & Wetherby, A.M. (1987). Communicative intent: A framework for understanding social-communicative behavior in autism. *Journal of the American Academy of Child and Adolescent Psychiatry, 26,* 472–479.

Prizant, B., & Wetherby, A. (1989). Enhancing language and communication in autism: From theory to practice. In G. Dawson (Ed.), *Autism: Nature, diagnosis, and treatment* (pp. 282–309). New York: Guilford Press.

Prizant, B.M., & Wetherby, A.M. (1990a). Incorporating a socioemotional perspective in early communication assessment. *ZERO TO THREE Bulletin, 11,* 1–12.

Prizant, B., & Wetherby, A. (1990b). Toward an integrated view of early language and communication development and socioemotional development. *Topics in Language Disorders, 10,* 1–16.

Prizant, B.M., & Wetherby, A.M. (1998). Understanding the continuum of discrete-trial traditional behavioral to social-pragmatic, developmental approaches in communication enhancement for young children with autism/PDD. *Seminars in Speech and Language, 19,* 329–353.

Quill, K.A. (Ed.). (1995). *Teaching children with autism: Methods to enhance communication and socialization.* Albany, NY: Delmar.

Reichle, J., & Wacker, D.P. (Vol. Eds.). (1993). *Communicative alternatives to challenging behavior: Integrating functional assessment and intervention strategies.* In S.F. Warren & J. Reichle (Series Eds.), *Communication and language intervention series: Vol. 3.* Baltimore: Paul H. Brookes Publishing Co.

Rydell, P.J., & Mirenda, P. (1994). Effects of high and low constraint utterances on the production of immediate and delayed echolalia in young children with autism. *Journal of Autism and Developmental Disorders, 24.*

Sameroff, A. (1987). The social context of development. In N. Eisenburg (Ed.), *Contemporary topics in development* (pp. 273–291). New York: John Wiley & Sons.

Sameroff, A., & Fiese, B. (1990). Transactional regulation and early intervention. In S. Meisels & J. Shonkoff (Eds.), *Handbook of early childhood intervention* (pp. 119–149). Cambridge, England: Cambridge University Press.

Schreibman, L., Kaneko, W., & Koegel, R. (1991). Positive affect of parents of autistic children: A comparison across two teaching techniques. *Behavior Therapy, 22,* 479–490.

Schreibman, L., & Pierce, K. (1993). Achieving greater generalization of treatment effects in children with autism: Pivotal response training and self-management. *The Clinical Psychologist, 46,* 184–191.

Schuler, A.L., Prizant, B.M., & Wetherby, A.M. (1997). Enhancing language and communication: Prelinguistic approaches. In D. Cohen & F. Volkmar (Eds.), *Handbook of autism and pervasive developmental disorders* (2nd ed., pp. 539–571). New York: John Wiley & Sons.

Snow, C., & Ferguson, C. (1977). *Talking to children: Language input and acquisition.* Cambridge: Cambridge University Press.

Snow, C., Midkiff-Borunda, S., Small, A., & Proctor, A. (1984). Therapy as social interaction: Analyzing the context for language remediation. *Topics in Language Disorders, 3,* 72–85.

Snyder-McLean, L., Solomonson, B., McLean, J., & Sack, S. (1984). Structuring joint action routines: A strategy for facilitating communication and language development in the classroom. *Seminars in Speech and Language, 5,* 213–228.

Strain, P., & Kohler, F. (1998). Peer mediated social intervention for children with autism. *Seminars in Speech and Language, 19,* 391–405.

Strain, P., McConnell, S., Carta, J., Fowler, S., Neisworth, J., & Wolery, M. (1992). Behaviorism in early intervention. *Topics in Early Childhood Special Education, 12,* 121–141.

Tiegerman, E., & Primavera, L. (1984). Object manipulation: An interactional strategy with autistic children. *Journal of Autism and Developmental Disorders, 11,* 427–439.

Tronick, E. (1989). Emotions and emotional communication in infancy. *American Psychologist, 44,* 112–149.

Warren, S. (1993). Early communication and language intervention: Challenges for the 1990s and beyond. In S.F. Warren & J. Reichle (Series Eds.) & A.P. Kaiser & D.B. Gray (Vol. Eds.), *Communication and language intervention series: Vol. 2. Enhancing children's communication: Research foundations for intervention* (pp. 375–395). Baltimore: Paul H. Brookes Publishing Co.

Wertsch, J. (Ed.). (1985). *Culture, communication and cognition: Vygotskian perspectives.* New York: Cambridge University Press.

Westby, C. (1988). Children's play: Reflections of social competence. *Seminars in Speech and Language, 9,* 1–13.

Wetherby, A.M. (1986). The ontogeny of communicative functions in autism. *Journal of Autism and Developmental Disorders, 16,* 295–316.

Wetherby, A., & Prizant, B. (1989). The expression of communicative intent: Assessment guidelines. *Seminars in Speech and Language, 10,* 77–91.

Wetherby, A.M., & Prizant, B.M. (1992). Profiling young children's communicative competence. In S.F. Warren & J. Reichle (Eds.), *Causes and effects in language disorders and intervention* (pp. 217–251). Baltimore: Paul H. Brookes Publishing Co.

Wetherby, A., & Prizant, B. (1999). Enhancing language and communication development in autism: Assessment and intervention guidelines. In D. Zager (Ed.), *Autism:*

Identification, education, and treatment (pp. 141–174). Mahwah, NJ: Lawrence Erlbaum Associates.

Wetherby, A.M., Prizant, B.M., & Hutchinson, T.A. (1998). Communicative, social/affective, and symbolic profiles of young children with autism and pervasive developmental disorders. *American Journal of Speech-Language Pathology, 7,* 79–91.

Wetherby, A.M., Schuler, A.L., & Prizant, B.M. (1997). Enhancing language and communication: Theoretical foundations. In D. Cohen & F. Volkmar (Eds.), Handbook of autism and pervasive developmental disorders (2nd ed., pp. 513–538). New York: John Wiley & Sons.

Wetherby, A.M., & Prutting, C.A. (1984). Profiles of communicative and cognitive-social abilities in autistic children. *Journal of Speech and Hearing Research, 27,* 364–377.

Wieder, S. (1997). Creating connections: Intervention guidelines for increasing interaction with children with Multisystem Developmental Disorder (MSDD). *ZERO TO THREE Bulletin,* 19–27.

Wolfberg, P. (1995). Enhancing children's play. In K.A. Quill (Ed.), *Teaching children with autism: Strategies to enhance communication and socialization* (pp. 193–218). Albany, NY: Delmar.

Wolfberg, P.J., & Schuler, A.L. (1993). Integrated play groups: A model for promoting the social and cognitive dimensions of play in children with autism. *Journal of Autism and Developmental Disorders, 23,* 467–489.

10

More Able Children with Autism Spectrum Disorders

Sociocommunicative Challenges and Guidelines for Enhancing Abilities

Diane Twachtman-Cullen

> One dark evening a young man happened on an inebriated man frantically searching the ground under a streetlight.
>
> "May I help you?" the young man asked.
> "I lost my keys back there in the alley," the inebriated man replied.
> "If you lost them in the alley, then why are you looking for them over here?"
> "'Cause there isn't any light over there in the alley!"

> An American man walked into a bank in Italy. When the receptionist looked up at him, he smiled and said, "Parla italiano?" The woman standing next to him whispered, "She's not Italian, she's English speaking." The American promptly corrected his utterance. "Parla inglese?"

INTRODUCTION: THE PLIGHT OF MORE ABLE CHILDREN

The absurdity reflected in these two passages illustrates two corresponding issues that plague more able children with autism spectrum disorders (ASDs; e.g., autistic disorder, Asperger syndrome, and pervasive developmental disorder). For example, the subtle nature of their language and sociocommunicative challenges often goes undetected, particularly when masked by language form and content that appear typical or even high level. Even when language and sociocommunicative difficulties are confirmed, their underlying complexities and the cognitive substrates that govern them often escape attention. In education and intervention, this can result in problems being viewed as superficial and isolated, although in reality they are complex and multifaceted. Blinded by the impressive strengths of more able children, practitioners often either cast their scientific beam of light in the wrong place or focus it too narrowly to address adequately the complex challenges of these children.

Parents of more able children speak poignantly of people's tendency to be blinded by the strengths of their children. One mother of an 8-year-old boy with Asperger syndrome described her son's plight in the following manner: "The good news is he's high functioning, and the bad news is he's high functioning!" The flip language of today's culture belies the poignancy of the paradoxical message: The very strengths observed in more able children may mask their deficits in social understanding and expression and in language comprehension and use. In the absence of such knowledge, areas of true deficit often are given superficial, behaviorally based explanations that do not acknowledge the child's neurological compromises, characterizing them instead as issues of willful noncompliance.

Another mother spoke eloquently of the uneven pattern of skill development that further obfuscates the underlying issues in more able children:

> My 9-year-old high-performing autistic son is in his public school's gifted and talented program. He learned to read at 3 years and 5 months of age and read 26 phonics readers within the next month. On the other hand [he] has no imagination, and takes everything he hears literally. He is rigid and impulsive. He has frequent tantrums. He plays with his saliva a lot. He has no friends, due to his lack of social skills.

Such widely disparate skills obscure rather than facilitate understanding. To further complicate matters, many of the assessment tools that practitioners customarily employ provide a false sense of security because many of the most popular instruments tap into the relatively preserved, discrete skills in more able children, leaving skill areas that are more subtle and complex unnoticed. Thus, unmindful of the specific nature of the weaknesses of more able children, adults inadvertently "allow" these children either to "fall through the cracks" regarding intervention or to find themselves in the absurd position of the American in Italy—that is, sometimes they make illogical adjustments!

This chapter is concerned with redirecting the focus of attention in addressing the needs of more able children with ASD so that practitioners are able to make the adjustments and accommodations that not only are appropriate to the children's intervention needs but also lead to increased academic success. The premise of this chapter is that to meet the sociocommunicative needs of more able children with autism, it is necessary for practitioners to widen their focus of attention, that is, to be guided by an expanded research base that, in addition to language, takes into account information processing as well as the interrelated cognitive and social-cognitive constructs that are an integral part of sociocommunicative functioning.

The first section of this chapter addresses the crucial role of research in understanding the challenges of more able children. The importance of adopting a multidimensional research perspective is stressed. This approach takes into account language comprehension, higher-level pragmatics, information processing, and the related cognitive and social-cognitive constructs of theory of mind (ToM) and executive function (EF). The initial focus on typical development sets the stage for the discussion of ways in which the sociocommunicative deficits in autism and related disorders reflect compromises in these areas. The final sections of the chapter address general guidelines for enhancing abilities in more able children, as well as implications for both clinical and educational practice and future research.

THE COMPLEXITY OF SOCIOCOMMUNICATIVE BEHAVIOR: LESSONS FROM THE WORLD OF TYPICAL DEVELOPMENT

Oliver Sacks described language as "the symbolic currency, to exchange meaning" (1989, p. 39). This depiction of language has many advantages over more technical definitions. For example, it underscores the dynamic nature of language use. Although language may be used for more solitary purposes (e.g., rehearsal, self-monitoring), it is also true that the *highest* and *best* use of language is for the exchange of meaning (i.e., communication). Well-respected conceptualizations of language (Bates, 1976, 1979; Bloom & Lahey, 1978; Bruner, 1990; McLean & Snyder-McLean, 1978; Muma, 1978) also highlight several important features of language use: Language is purposeful; it is a vehicle by which to convey communicative intent; its use involves reciprocity; language is representational (i.e., symbolic); and most important, language is an ideal medium by which meaning may be exchanged among individuals. In Sacks' definition of language, as well as in those of early child language theorists, one sees the essence of the relationship between language and communication. A closer look at the individual elements that make the exchange of meaning possible reveals the complexities and interrelationships involved in the process of communication.

The Establishment of Meaning: The Scaffold for Language Acquisition

A baby's first word is one of the most cherished and heralded events of childhood, preserved in his or her baby book and ensconced in parents' memories. In contrast, the events leading up to that most memorable event—the process of meaning making that sets the stage for production—are largely ignored (Adamson, 1996; Sevcik & Romski, 1997; Twachtman-Cullen, 1997a). Traditionally, research efforts have focused on expression rather than on comprehension (Hirsh-Pasek & Golinkoff, 1991; Huttenlocher, 1974).

It is interesting to note that some of the most remarkable insights into the crucial role of comprehension in language acquisition come from the study of nonhuman primates, specifically bonobo apes, also known as pygmy chimpanzees (*Pan paniscus*) (Savage-Rumbaugh, 1991; Savage-Rumbaugh & Lewin, 1994; Sevcik & Savage-Rumbaugh, 1994). Perhaps most remarkable of all is that the essentiality of comprehension to the overall process of language acquisition in primates was discovered quite by accident!

Savage-Rumbaugh and Lewin (1994) chronicled the story of Kanzi, a bonobo ape raised in captivity, close to his adoptive mother Matata. The latter had been the focus of systematic, discrete trial-based language training designed to teach her a small number of symbols with which to communicate. After 2 years of what was termed "meager success," Matata was dropped from language training and replaced by 2½-year-old Kanzi. According to Savage-Rumbaugh and Lewin (1994), Kanzi *spontaneously* began to use the keyboard that was placed in front of him on more than 120 occasions on the very first day of training. Savage-Rumbaugh described the events as follows:

> I was hesitant to believe what I was seeing. Not only was Kanzi using the keyboard as a means of communicating, but he also knew what the symbols meant—in spite of the fact that his mother had never learned them. For example, one of the first things he did that morning was to activate "apple," then "chase." He then picked up an apple, looked at me, and ran away with a play grin on his face. Several times he hit food keys, and when I took him to the refrigerator, he selected those foods he'd indicated on the keyboard. Kanzi was using specific lexigrams to request and name items, *and* to announce his intention—all important symbol skills that we had not recognized Kanzi possessed. (Savage-Rumbaugh & Lewin, 1994, p. 135)

Although the exact nature of Matata's minimal progress in symbol use may never be fully understood, one difference between Kanzi and his mother was consummately apparent. There was a significant discrepancy between the two bonobo apes in their level of *comprehension* of the symbols on the keyboard; that is, not only did Kanzi demonstrate an impressively higher level of comprehension than did Matata, but even more significant, his comprehension was born *not* of systematic training but of natural language learning in the social environment. This led Savage-Rumbaugh and Lewin to conclude that "Kanzi's language acquisition seemed to announce dramatically that language acquisition was first and foremost a feat of understanding" (1994, p. 136).

Savage-Rumbaugh's work with Kanzi revolutionized thinking not only about the conduct of primate research in general (i.e., naturalistic learning versus systematic, discrete trial-based training) but also about the powerful relationship between the natural environmental context and comprehension. The importance of this research to the understanding of both typical and atypical language development, particularly with respect to the crucial, albeit intangible role of comprehension, cannot be overstated.

Research related to early brain development also highlights the importance of experiential, naturalistic learning to the child's understanding of his or her world. It is important to note that although one had to rely on conventional wisdom alone in the past, there is now compelling evidence of heightened metabolic activity in infants, in those parts of the brain responsible for the regulation of emotions, interactions, and sequencing *at the time that the infants are involved* in activities related to reciprocal interactions, choice making, and search behavior (Bell & Fox, 1994). Likewise, Chugani, Phelps, and Mazziotta (1994) have provided additional evidence of the intimate relationship between experience and neural connectivity at a time when infants are forming the crucial apperceptions that set the stage for meaningful expression.

Pragmatics: The "Driver" of Discourse

Bates (1976) revolutionized the language-learning literature through her introduction of the concept of *pragmatics,* delineating three specific aspects of pragmatic language use. The first, and perhaps best understood, is the use of speech acts to express intentionality in order to accomplish a given purpose (i.e., function). According to Dore the speech act is central to conversational discourse for "it is the unit most capable of conveying propositional, intentional, and interactional meanings simultaneously" (1986, p. 11). Lower-level functions include such tasks as making simple requests and engaging in protest behavior, whereas higher order functions include such complex behaviors as negotiating and expressing opinions.

In addition to knowledge regarding specific communicative functions, Bates (1976) stated that competent language use also requires that communicators make judgments about what their listeners already know and what information their listeners need to be given to comprehend the intentions of the speaker. These judgments are known as *presuppositions,* and typical language users employ them so effortlessly that they are essentially automatic. For example, one would not enter a room and say, "Can you imagine that!?" without first grounding the listener with respect to the information needed to make sense of the utterance (e.g., "He just asked me to increase my work hours from 35 to 40 hours per week without compensation. Can you imagine that!?"). It should be obvious that presuppositional judgments require social understanding and perspective-taking ability. Such knowledge enables individuals to regulate speech style and content to suit listener and situational needs. Thus, one would speak differently to a child than to an adult acquaintance and differently still to an authority figure.

The third area of pragmatic knowledge originally delineated by Bates (1976) involves the ability to apply the rules of discourse in order to engage in cooperative conversational exchanges. Grice's (1975) conversational maxims with respect to *quantity, quality, relevance,* and *clarity* addressed this area of pragmatics by providing a rule system for cooperative dialogic exchanges. Table 1 in Twachtman (1996) provided descriptions of Grice's maxims, as well as examples of ways in which these conversational rules may be violated.

Clearly, the ability to engage in cohesive conversational discourse is a complex process requiring many different types of knowledge and competencies. Labov and Franshel captured the essence of the intrinsic blending of linguistic features and sociocultural understandings and reciprocations that are deeply embedded within conversational discourse: "Conversation is not a chain of utterances, but rather a matrix of utterances and actions bound together by a web of understandings and reactions" (1977, p. 30). The conventions of discourse related to topicality, nonverbal cues, and the use of strategies to repair communicative breakdown further enhance the "matrix of utterances" into a richly textured tapestry for the exchange of meaning.

Two additional constructs essential to this exchange of meaning are ToM and EF. Both require a representational view of the world. In the former case, mental representations afford an a priori understanding of human behavior, whereas in the latter case, they afford a "blueprint" for future execution.

The Role of Theory of Mind

Frith defined ToM as "the ability to predict relationships between external states of affairs and internal states of mind" (1989, p. 157). For example, if a child screams at the sight of a dog, we infer that he or she is afraid. Likewise, if the child's face "lights up" at the sight of a parent, we infer that he or she is happy to see the parent. The ability to infer states of mind based on external behavior and circumstance has also been referred to as the act of *mentalizing* (Baron-Cohen, 1995; Frith, 1989), an activity that Frith linked to the brain's internal drive for meaning and coherence.

It is interesting to note that it was not until relatively recently that the concept of ToM was applied to young children (Perner, 1991; Wellman, 1990). Whereas earlier it was felt that children were largely unaware of the existence of states of mind until 6 or 7 years of age, now there is consensus that children as young as 3 or 4 years of age have some level of awareness of such mental states (Wellman, 1993). The importance of a developing ToM cannot be overstated because, according to Tager-Flusberg, it enables the child to "interpret human behavior within a causal-explanatory framework, [and affords] understanding that the mind does not simply copy reality but provides a representation of the world" (1997, p. 135). It should be obvious that a representational view of the world is necessary to the establishment of meaning and to effective communication, overall.

ToM is also important to an understanding of language acquisition and use. According to Tager-Flusberg (1993, 1997) there is a close correlation between the development of language and ToM, such that they are integrated with each other and progress according to similar timetables. Indeed, one of the crowning achievements of early language development—joint attention (specifically triadic attention)—is intimately related to ToM, for it involves the child's ability to both use and respond to visual signals and conventional gestures for the purpose of sharing attention regarding an object or event with another person. This form of nonverbal behavior represents a significant advance in the child's social-cognitive/sociocommunicative development. Not only is it viewed as an early indicator that another person has a different point of view (mental state) than the child's own (Bretherton, McNew, & Beeghly-Smith, 1981; Sigman, 1989; Twachtman-Cullen, 1997b), but it also marks the onset of intentional communication (Tager-Flusberg, 1997) and undergirds the development of representational thought (Bates, Benigni, Bretherton, Camaioni, & Volterra, 1979; see Chapters 4 and 5 for further discussion of ToM).

The Role of Executive Function

As of 2000, although there is no universally accepted definition of EF, threads of commonality exist among different conceptualizations of this complex neuropsychological construct. The most basic area of agreement is that EF activities are carried out primarily by the frontal lobes of the brain, though the importance of interconnectedness and communication with other brain areas is acknowledged. As such, EF is considered a domain-general, as opposed to a domain-specific, construct (Denckla, 1996). Denckla concentrated on the cognitive aspects of EF, defining the latter as "control processes [that] involve inhibition and delay of responding" (p. 265) with respect to the organization of behavior. This view of EF underscores its metacognitive and organizational components.

Pennington, Bennetto, McAleer, and Roberts (1996) approached the subject of EF from a neuropsychological perspective, emphasizing, like Denckla (1996), inhibition of irrelevant or inappropriate actions, as well as planning, future orientation, and mental representation of those plans (i.e., keeping one's plans in mind or "on-line" for later execution). The latter activity is known as *working memory* and is considered central to the concept of EF. In addition, there is widespread agreement that EF serves an overseeing function regarding behavioral self-regulation, the sequencing of behavioral actions, and the ability to be flexible in response to changing circumstances (Eslinger, 1996).

Although EF is interrelated with other constructs such as memory and attention, EF clearly transcends the more fundamental psychological processes in its gatekeeping role as the "manager" of the complex skills that subserve adaptive behavior. According to Eslinger many scientists view EFs as the "crowning achievement of human development" (1996, p. 368). EFs are remarkable for their richly textured, complex roles in diverse areas of human functioning. Thus, EF ability not only is important in problem-solving and other acts of cognition and metacognition but also is thought to play an important role in socioemotional behavior, information processing, and in overall adaptive functioning. (See Chapters 4 and 5 for further discussion of EF.)

The Management of Information: A Multilayered Process

Information processing may be construed as the domain in which comprehension, pragmatic knowledge, ToM, and EF intersect. Twachtman-Cullen and Twachtman-Reilly defined information processing as "the act of receiving, interpreting, assimilating, organizing, controlling, storing, monitoring, retrieving, formulating, and expressing knowledge" (1998, p. 31). Thus, the information-processing system is at once complex and multidimensional, involving a number of brain systems and functions as well as cognitive decision making that is largely automatic and therefore below the level of consciousness. All of the parameters (comprehension, pragmatic ability, ToM, and EF) discussed previously are intertwined within the information-processing system.

The most basic level of information processing is that of sensation because information to be processed must first enter the brain through the sensory system. Because the amount of information coming in through each of the senses is ongoing in individuals with intact sensory systems, there must be mechanisms for filtering the raw sensory data and for coordinating sensation across modalities (e.g., coordinating what is heard with what is seen). Attentional deployment decisions may be thought of as the brain's filtering system; that is, the brain must deploy attention selectively to attend to those critical environmental features necessary for the establishment of meaning, a process that requires considerable understanding and judgment. Attentional deployment also plays an important role in sensory modulation (i.e., the regulation of incoming information) and is intimately related to perception (i.e., awareness). To attach meaning to what is perceived, there must be mechanisms for interpreting the information selected for processing. Interpretation involves relating incoming (i.e., new) information and experiences with old information and experiences. At a certain point in time, the brain's storage system takes over so that information may be retained for later use. This storage, too, involves unconscious cognitive decision making with respect to whether the information is more appropriately stored in short- or long-term memory. It should be obvious that this decision must flow from an implicit understanding of the uses to which the information is to be put. Finally, information processing also involves the ongoing use of organizing and monitoring strategies for the control, efficient handling, retrieval, and use of information. Remarkably, this entire process is largely unconscious and automatic and, for the most part, takes place in milliseconds (see Chapter 7 for further discussion).

Over the years, several different information-processing theories have been postulated. These include "bottom-up," data-driven models as well as "top-down," conceptually driven models. Although there is overlap between them, each one emphasizes different ways of manipulating information. Although an in-depth consideration of these models is beyond the scope of this chapter, it is important to note that competent and efficient information processing would seem to involve a blend of both data- and conceptually driven approaches, as well as a level of processing sufficiently deep to be effective.

In summary, the process of human communication is both multidimensional and intricate, for it requires the interweaving of many complex cognitive and social-cognitive understandings and skills. Stated succinctly, the management of information for the exchange of meaning as opposed to the mere exchange of words requires *communicative competence* on the part of both interactants (i.e., the message sender and receiver). As such, the use of language for communication is a consummately transactional act, encompassing three interdependent areas of competence: linguistic, interpersonal, and cultural competence. Clearly, communicative competence requires knowledge of the complex interrelationships among linguistic rules, structures, and vocabulary, as well as an in-depth understanding of both interpersonal social behaviors and the larger cultural context in which these are embedded (Rice, 1986; see Chapter 3 for further discussion of cultural learning).

SOCIOCOMMUNICATIVE INTERDEPENDENCE: A GAME OF DOMINOES

Because the many facets of social communication are interdependent, problems in one area or another in turn affect functioning in each other area, in much the same way that cascading dominoes affect each of the following dominoes in succession.

The Process of Meaning-Making

There is an oxymoronic quality to our understanding of the term *comprehension* because the construct is as multidimensional and far-reaching as it is taken for granted and ignored. This is particularly apparent when considered with respect to more able children with ASD, for their superficial verbal skills often mask their cavernous weaknesses in comprehension. For example, memorized chunks of echolalic utterances have lulled many a caregiver into assuming comprehension of the linguistic elements where none exists. This assumption of receptive language competence commonly results in the practice of attempting to build expressive language skills on a foundation too weak to support understanding and sense making.

Twachtman-Cullen characterized comprehension as "the power that fuels expression" (1997a, p. 9)—a view that elevates comprehension to a central (and in my view, *proper*) place in the acquisition of language. Similarly, Savage-Rumbaugh & Lewin defined comprehension as "the essence of language" (1994, p. 174), stating that it "drives language acquisition" (p. 168). These characterizations support the view that comprehension is both basic to and intertwined with expression. In other words, meaningful expression (i.e., the exchange of meaning)—not the mere recitation of memorized strings of words—

is dependent on comprehension and sense making. Indeed, notwithstanding the multipurpose usefulness of echolalia to children with ASD, at least some of the functions served by both immediate and delayed echolalia have proved to be reliable indicators of comprehension difficulty (Prizant & Duchan, 1981; Prizant & Rydell, 1984). Likewise, according to the results of a study by Roberts (1989), children with autism who had more advanced receptive language ability exhibited fewer echolalic utterances.

Twachtman-Cullen (1997b; 1998) argued for a more expanded view of comprehension in more able children and linked their problems in understanding and sense making to their well-known expressive language anomalies, particularly literalness and the use of metaphorical language. For example, a 10-year-old girl with Asperger syndrome appeared horrified when her teacher said, "Eyes on the board." The child's literal interpretation demonstrated her failure to comprehend her teacher's communicative, albeit figurative, intent (i.e., to obtain the girl's attention). Even the most able children with ASD have difficulty with sarcasm and double entendre, for both require understanding of paralinguistic features such as facial expression and tone of voice, as well as an appreciation for culturally based idiosyncratic expressions, in order to derive meaning. Because these nonverbal, intangible aspects of communicative behavior require complex social understanding and are mediated by subtle social cues, children with ASD fail to recognize their message value. This is particularly devastating when the entire meaning of the message is carried by such features. Consider the sarcastically conveyed utterance, "Just what I need—another tie!" A literal interpretation clearly misses the communicative intent of the utterance.

Metaphorical language use, long recognized as an idiosyncratic form of expression, is intimately related to comprehension as well. At its most basic level, metaphorical communication represents the child's lack of knowledge regarding the importance of shared social understanding (Twachtman-Cullen, 1998). At a deeper level, it may also represent the child's lack of understanding of that aspect of ToM known as *perspective taking.* Thus, when a child gets upset because a caregiver does not understand what he or she means by a metaphorical utterance such as "The king's quest is over, so now he shall rest" (used to ask for a break), that child is demonstrating a lack of understanding regarding the important role of shared knowledge in communication as well as a lack of appreciation for the different mindset and knowledge needs of the interactant. Without this information, the child is unable to repair his or her message so that it makes sense to the listener. Indeed, he or she would not even be aware of the necessity for conversational repair.

Similar to a snowball rolling down a hill, comprehension difficulty becomes cumulative. Thus, not only does it affect language expression and information processing, it also has a significant impact on academic skills as well because all of these processes are interdependent. Support for this contention may be found in the neuropsychological and language literature in ASD. Minshew, Goldstein, Muenz, and Payton reported that "language tests revealed that the autistic subjects had a rather profound impairment in complex linguistic processes involving language comprehension" (1992, p. 757). Minshew, Goldstein, Taylor, and Siegel documented "deficits in comprehension of complex linguistic constructions, semantic-pragmatic language, verbal reasoning and abstraction, all of which likely contribute to the overall difficulty with comprehension of oral and written information" (1994, p. 267). This same trend is seen in reading. Performance related to word recognition and the decoding of words was at a higher level than that of reading comprehension (Frith & Snowling, 1983; Minshew et al., 1994; Whitehouse & Harris, 1984).

Comprehension issues may well be the unsung linchpin around which the many symptoms of autism and their effects on academic performance turn. Several studies have revealed that individuals with high-functioning autism, in contrast to their strengths in *procedural* knowledge (i.e., knowledge for *doing* things), demonstrate weaknesses in *declarative* knowledge (i.e., knowledge *about* things) (Goldstein, Minshew, & Siegel, 1994; Minshew, Goldstein, & Siegel, 1995; Minshew et al., 1994). Thus, their oft-seen skills in procedural tasks such as rote memorization, word recognition, spelling, and reading decoding stand in sharp contrast to their significant difficulties in concept formation, language and reading comprehension, complex information processing, problem solving, inferential reasoning, and the analysis and synthesis of information (Goldstein et al., 1994; Minshew et al., 1995; Minshew et al., 1994). Not only do all of these skills involve declarative knowledge, at the heart of which is comprehension, but they also further illustrate the interdependence among constructs.

Theory of Mind Impairment

Baron-Cohen (1995) coined the term *mindblindness* to characterize the difficulty that people with autism have with reading the mental states (i.e., thoughts, feelings, and beliefs) of others, a process that Baron-Cohen refers to as *mindreading*. The latter is considered an essential function of the cognitive construct *ToM*.

When compared with typical peers, children with autism demonstrate important differences regarding aspects of language acquisition reflective of ToM difficulty. These differences are particularly apparent with respect to pragmatics, given the linkages between the latter and ToM. For example, the pragmatic functions of requesting and commenting develop concurrently in typical children (Bates, Camaioni, & Volterra, 1975), whereas in children with autism, the more social function of commenting develops *after* the instrumental function of requesting (Wetherby, 1986; Wetherby & Prutting, 1984). Tager-Flusberg provided a direct link to ToM stating that "it is primarily the comment functions that exploit the ability to attribute intentions to others" (1997, p. 139).

The discrepancy between instrumental and social functions is also apparent in prelinguistic communicative behaviors, the precursors to representational thinking (Bates, 1979; Bates et al., 1979; Curcio, 1978; Mundy, Sigman, Ungerer, & Sherman, 1986; Wetherby, 1986; Wetherby & Prutting, 1984). In fact Curcio's (1978) seminal observation regarding the paucity of joint attention gestures in children with autism brought to light the strikingly different pattern of prelinguistic development in these children. More recently, a study by Baron-Cohen (1989) found that when children with autism did use pointing gestures, they used them as *protoimperatives* (i.e., to request), as opposed to as *protodeclaratives* (i.e., to comment). These discrepancies, at the very least, reflect a lack of sophistication in representational ability in children with autism (Baron-Cohen, 1989), even at higher levels of functioning.

Additional areas of deficit in autism reflective of ToM impairment include impoverishment in the use of denial negation, in the use of *wh-* questions, and, conversationally, in the provision of new information based on an understanding of listener needs (Tager-Flusberg, 1997). All of these uses of language require an appreciation for mental states in others that ToM deficits impede, if not preclude. Moreover, because ToM knowledge is fundamental to perspective taking, socioemotional behaviors related to empathy, sharing, comforting, and the like are also necessarily compromised. Clearly, these areas of impairment extend beyond proficiency in phonology, morphology, syntax, and lexicality (i.e., discrete linguistic elements) into the richly textured area of communicative competence (i.e., sociality and pragmatics). In fact, the pattern of skill development usually seen in more able children with ASD reveals both their strengths in linguistic skills and their concomitant deficits in communicative competence at the level of discourse. Tager-Flusberg provided the following summary:

> Even when children with autism have acquired both lexical and syntactic forms, they remain at very primitive levels of communicative competence, hampered by their inability to add new information and extend a conversational topic over several communicative turns. . . .These conversational impairments stem from a lack of awareness that people communicate not only to achieve goals but also to exchange information, and indeed, that people may have access to different information. (1997, p. 140)

ToM deficits have also been linked to higher-order language impairments in more able children. These include problems in reading comprehension and in the interpretation and analysis of both oral and written information (Minshew et al., 1995). Narrative discourse is particularly problematic, given that it involves the blending of cognitive, linguistic, and social knowledge. The ability to engage in narrative discourse activities will be negatively affected by such ToM deficits as the tendency to "see things in black and white," difficulty in understanding the intentions and viewpoints of others, problems with inferential reasoning, and the literal interpretation of behavior. It should be obvious that all of these deficits are also rooted in different facets of comprehension difficulty. It follows then that ToM impairment significantly weakens the reserve of background mental state knowledge needed for sense making and the meaningful exchange of information overall.

It is important to note that despite the significant weaknesses in ToM that occur in autism, there are at least some individuals at the very highest levels of functioning who are able to mentalize to some degree (Happé, 1993). Even so, Gillberg and Ehlers (1998) struck a cautionary note regarding formal testing by noting that adequate performance on formal tests of ToM does not necessarily translate to skilled mentalizing in functional situations.

Executive Function Impairment

EF ability has received a great deal of attention in the literature related to attention-deficit/hyperactivity disorder (ADHD). Research into EF with respect to autism is a relatively recent phenomenon (Prior & Hoffman, 1990; Rumsey, 1985). Notwithstanding, more than 80% of studies performed before 1998 have documented EF deficits in individuals with ASD (Ozonoff, 1998). Furthermore, research findings indicate that EF deficits appear to be common across the entire autism spectrum (Ozonoff, 1998) and across a wide chronological and mental age range (Ozonoff, 1995). The latter finding caused Ozonoff (1995) to speculate that EF impairment may be a central deficit of autism. EF impairment includes problems in the following areas: mental planning, the ability to maintain set (i.e., a readiness stance), impulse control, flexibility in both thought and action, and the ability to keep plans and goals in mind or "on line" (i.e., in working memory). Impairment in these areas often translates to the following behavioral manifestations: distractibility; impulsivity (resulting from difficulty in delaying gratification and inhibiting inappropriate responses); rigidity and inflexibility; repetitive, stereotypic behavior; transition difficulty; and problems in self-regulation and self-monitoring. The latter two also contribute to difficulty that children with ASD have in *applying* information that is already within their repertoires (Ozonoff, 1998). It is important to note that although many of the foregoing behavioral symptoms are common to ASDs and ADHD, virtually no research has compared the attentional problems in the two disorders. Despite the areas of overlap vis-à-vis executive dysfunction that autism shares with ADHD, it has been suggested that frontal lobe executive dysfunction alone is probably not sufficient to cause all of the symptomatology associated with autism (Ozonoff, 1995; Prior & Hoffman, 1990); hence, this may explain the substantial differences that also exist between ADHD and autism.

EF deficits have a negative impact on problem solving ability in several ways. Distractibility makes it difficult for the child to maintain the necessary state of readiness to work on the problem. Once engaged, children with EF deficits also experience difficulty shifting from the use of ineffective problem solving strategies to other, more effective ones. Problems here reflect both perseveration and cognitive inflexibility—two well-known features of autistic symptomatology.

In addition to the previously noted aspects of EF difficulty, Ozonoff (1998) suggested that *stimulus overselectivity* (i.e., the tendency to focus on a small, often irrelevant subset of cues) may also reflect such impairment. The child who turns over a small toy car and spins only one wheel typifies stimulus overselectivity. It should be obvious that such a narrow focus of attention would severely restrict concept development. Similarly, EF deficits likely contribute to the tendency for individuals with ASD to "miss the forest for the trees" (Frith, 1989). For example, a child with Asperger syndrome described a picture of people being taken from a flooded house by rowboat as follows: "I see a house. I see water. There are people in a boat." Clearly, the child saw the "trees" (i.e., the details in the picture), while at the same time, he missed the "forest" (i.e., the flood, which was the picture's intent). Unfortunately, meaning and sense making can only be derived by organizing discrete parts into a cohesive whole—a process made all the more difficult by EF deficit.

It would be nearly impossible to overstate the centrality of EF ability to overall functioning. Because of the expansive nature of the processes affected by EF impairment and the multifold ramifications for overall adaptive behavior, EF difficulty has links to several areas of functioning, including those related to language understanding and use, ToM, and information processing. As such, EF is considered to be the "executive overseer" of behavior.

Despite individual differences in the ways in which discrete aspects of EF impairment may affect individuals with ASD, commonality is nevertheless seen in two more general, though interrelated areas: automaticity and control. Lacking the automaticity that properly working EF ability lends to the brain–behavior system, children with ASD either lack the organizational strategies needed to effectively and efficiently deal with the information that impinges on them (Ameli, Courchesne, Lincoln, Kaufman, & Grillon, 1988; Minshew & Goldstein, 1993) or fail to apply them in a time-efficient or appropriate manner. This leads to manifold difficulty not only with the recall of complex information but also with information processing in general. Thus, the myriad mental decisions and control processes governing adaptive behavior, which for most of us are executed effortlessly and automatically, take on effortful and cumbersome qualities for children with autism, creating an additional "drag" on an already compromised system. The cumulative effects of these difficulties are widespread. Consequently, they have a negative impact on the individual skills that scaffold overall adaptive function, while at the same time they cause processing delays that further disrupt information exchange. Furthermore, given the importance of attention, working memory, planning, and organizational ability to the development of critical thinking skills and overall learning, these difficulties also wreak havoc with respect to academic performance. Worse yet, the symptoms of EF impairment (e.g., distractibility, inflexibility) are often misinterpreted as acts of *willful noncompliance* rather than as the sequelae of significant neurological deficit (Ozonoff, 1998). These misattributions can set the stage for additional failure by adversely affecting the child's self-esteem and closing off avenues of needed personal and academic support.

Pragmatic Underpinnings

Of all of the features of possible language deficit in autism (e.g., semantic, syntactic, phonological), the one that is pathognomonic of the syndrome itself is that of pragmatic impairment. Notwithstanding, given the subtlety of such impairment in more able children, deficits in language use are often missed, unless one adopts a discourse perspective. Indeed, the exchange of meaning, with its various links to all of the constructs discussed previously, takes on the aura of an art form at the level of discourse. In addition to deficits with obvious connections to ToM difficulty, three additional areas of weakness with more subtle ToM linkages loom large for more able children with ASD.

The first of these concerns presuppositional judgments regarding listener needs. Specifically, adjustments in speech style vis-à-vis situational needs require complex social and cultural understanding. This is a well-known area of difficulty in autism. Likewise, judgments regarding the type and amount of information needed by the listener are rooted in the knowledge that other people have different minds and, hence, different requirements for information. Children with autism demonstrate their lack of presuppositional knowledge when they fail to ground the listener in the subject matter prior to delivering the essential point. For example, Twachtman (1995) cited a child, Ryan, who in noticing an irritation on his leg began to chant, "South America, South America," as his way of commenting on how the shape of the mark on his leg was remarkably similar to the map of South America. Typical children would not "cut to the chase" as Ryan did. They would implicitly know that more grounding was required (e.g., that they would need to say, "That spot on my leg looks just like the map of South America").

Application of the four maxims of conversational discourse (Grice, 1975) is the second area fraught with difficulty for more able children with ASD because knowledge of discourse rules requires social and presuppositional judgment, sensitivity to listener needs, and an appreciation for context—all of which are areas of grave difficulty for children with autism. Children who violate the rules of topicality by engaging in lengthy monologues or who tangentially shift the conversation to their own areas of interest (even in the face of social distress signals from the listener) violate the respective maxims of *quantity* and *relevance.* Furthermore, it should be obvious that many of the conversational violations that occur in autism reflect the lack of appreciation of lis-

Table 10.1. The four maxims of conversational interaction

Maxim 1: Quantity Be informative without being verbose. Speaking "nonstop" without regard to "social distress" signals is an example of difficulty with quantity.

Maxim 2: Quality Be truthful. Confabulation (i.e., filling in knowledge gaps with false information that the speaker believes to be true) is an example of difficulty with quality.

Maxim 3: Relevance Contribute only information that is pertinent to the topic and situation. Tangential comments constitute difficulty with the rule of relevance.

Maxim 4: Clarity The information conveyed should be clear and understandable to the listener. Initiating a conversation in the middle of a thought without providing background information is an example of a problem with the rule of clarity.

From Twachtman, D.D. (1996, Summer). There's a lot more to communication than talking! *The Morning News,* 3–5; based on Grice (1975); reprinted by permission.

tener needs and as such are rooted in poor presuppositional judgment. Other examples are given in Table 10.1.

The third area of pragmatic deficit concerns socioemotional expression. Problems here stand in stark contrast to competence in the recitation of factual information, at least from the point of view of ease of information access. Compare the following two language samples generated during approximately the same period of time by the same fourth-grade boy, Brian. Directed to write an *essay* on what he wanted in a wife, based on the book *Sarah, Plain and Tall* (MacLachlan, 1985), Brian did communicate a wealth of factual information about the qualities he desires in a wife; however, he did so via a "chain of utterances" rather than the "matrix of utterances" required of cohesive discourse (Labov & Franshel, 1977) and essay writing:

> My future wife should be a good bowler.
> A person who constantly goes to Boston.
> Likes hot dogs.
> Doesn't mind that I'm allergic to milk.
> Is sincere!
> Likes puzzles.
> Can read road maps.
> Likes computers and golfing.

Notwithstanding that Brian was able to express a good deal of concrete information vis-à-vis what he wants in a wife, he was at a loss to express his feelings with respect to the book *The Witch of Blackbird Pond* (Speare, 1958):

Q: How did you feel when Kit first met the Wood family?
A: I felt that this was a shocking surprise that Kit would live such a different lifestyle than what she was used to.
Q: How did you feel when Matthew ordered his family to give the fancy clothing back to Kit?
A: I felt that Matt should've changed his mind.
Q: How did you feel when Kit saved Hannah from the angry mob?
A: Dramatic, too dramatic, trying to kill Hannah, a poor old defenseless woman.

In none of these cases was this child able to express socioemotional information. Instead, he clung to more concrete descriptions of events. This is not to say that children with ASD do not have feelings but rather that the expression of them—with their abstract, socioemotional, and mentalistic underpinnings—is very difficult. To wit, consider the same child's expression of deep emotion in answer to the question, "How did you feel when the mob burned Hannah's house?": "Sad as a tiger dying." These examples lead one to speculate that socioemotional information may be somewhat easier to express when feelings are unequivocal and explicit, as opposed to subtle and amorphous, and/or when they can be tied to a circumstance or event that has meaning for the child. Finally, even when more able children are able to express socioemotional information, they often do so in an awkward and circuitous manner. Brian's expression of gratitude to his grandmother showed poignantly his deep feelings, yet at the same time it revealed his difficulty in expressing them: *All my honesty is in the Heart of my soul released on this sheet.*

Information Processing: The Final Domino

Nowhere is the whole greater than the sum of its individual parts than in the multifaceted, highly complex realm of information processing. The ability to process information requires competency in all of the areas already discussed: *comprehension,* in its most expansive form; *EF,* in its many managerial and control operations; *ToM,* in its richly textured mentalizing functions; and *social-pragmatics,* in all its interpersonal and culturally based receptive and expressive subtleties. But these alone, as encompassing as they are, do not add up to the *whole* of information processing. Issues related to depth, manner, and speed of processing, as well as those related to the many intangibles, such as cohesion, vigilance, and metacognitive/metalinguistic awareness, reach beyond the sum of the individual parts to make possible the exchange of information in a communicatively competent manner. In this way, information processing may be construed as the final common pathway at which all of the competencies needed for the successful handling of information for the exchange of meaning come together. Thus, as research has shown, even the most able children with ASD experience difficulty with information processing (Goldstein et al., 1994; Minshew et al., 1995; Minshew et al., 1994). A closer look at the ways in which information processing may be compromised not only serves to illustrate the intricacies in the system but also reveals the interconnectedness of the processes discussed previously.

Information processing requires a complex matrix of understandings from single words, sentences, and discourse to nonverbal elements such as body language, tone of voice, and facial expressions. It also requires sensitivity to context. Compromises in comprehension and knowledge of pragmatics make the processing of information unwieldy. Even when more able children with ASD can comprehend some of the more obvious, straightforward elements of language use, they nonetheless experience significant difficulty with the comprehension of subtle, nonverbal cues; figurative language; and contextual information. These difficulties, of course, adversely affect comprehension, processing time, and verbal expression. Moreover, a superficially impressive lexicon does not ensure that the child has a grasp on multiple meanings of words, knowledge of culturally based colloquialisms, or a cohesive sense of how one sentence relates to another. All of these understandings, however, are basic not only to comprehending incoming information but also to knowing how to handle and deploy it in the service of language expression. Clearly, if children with ASD do not know what something means or fail to appreciate its socioemotional significance, then it will be impossible for them to manage it effectively, that is, relate it to existing information; assimilate it into their fund of knowledge; transfer it to the appropriate storage area of the brain (i.e., short- or long-term memory); or retrieve it in an efficient or contextually appropriate manner.

ToM deficits also have an impact on information processing by interfering with the "causal–explanatory framework" (Tager-Flusberg, 1997), which is integral to the interpretation of human behavior and abstract, inferential reasoning. Weaknesses here compromise metalinguistic and metacognitive awareness, both of which are foundational to the type of high-level pragmatic knowledge that undergirds figurative language and humor. Consequently, it is not surprising that children with such deficits have a concrete, literal interpretation of behavior and events rather than one that is based on abstract, inferential information.

Correspondingly, Eslinger (1996) suggested that compromises in EF—particularly working memory—also relegate the individual to greater literalness. He described "utilization behavior," observed in patients with frontal lobe injury, as the routinized, concrete response to the literal aspects of environmental circumstances. This behavior contrasts sharply with the purposeful, goal-directed behavior in typical people that results from their using the information that working memory keeps "on line" to guide responses that are adaptive to specific situations. The parallels between utilization behavior and procedural knowledge and between purposeful behavior and declarative knowledge are striking.

Other aspects of EF impairment place additional demands on the already overburdened information-processing system by compromising access to the necessary cognitive resources, attentional "filters," and organizational controls that oversee and regulate adaptive behavior. Without these automatic controls the manipulation of incoming and outgoing information becomes a conscious, effortful, and time-consuming process that depletes the child's energy and resources and undoubtedly interferes with the vigilance and depth of processing required to effectively and efficiently manage information. Given the interdependence of all of the constructs discussed in this chapter, each of the compromises in the system, in domino-like fashion, creates additional problems for the other parts of the system. The end result is the well-documented difficulties that children with autism have with complex or late information processing (Minshew, 1996; National Institutes of Health, 1995) and the problems in academic performance that these difficulties create.

CLINICAL AND EDUCATIONAL IMPLICATIONS

Indeed, this discussion has come full circle, back to the "good news—bad news" plight of more able children with ASD. Specifically, all too often these children are denied services by speech-language pathologists, based on standardized scores that highlight their superficial strengths in the form and structure of language, while at the same time, their deficits in more subtle aspects of communication go undetected. Unfortunately, standardized tests, by their very nature, are inadequate to judge the subtle, complex, cross-domain deficits that characterize the pattern of language-learning difficulty that is seen in more able children with ASD. Furthermore, the isolated and artificial test conditions associated with standardized instruments can actually create an artifactual elevation in the scores of these children, because the simplicity and low-level stimulation of the test environment may well be more hospitable to their language-processing constraints than the high-load, high-stress, "real world" environment. Clearly then, it is imperative that clinicians adopt an integrative stance that looks beyond discrete skills, standardized instruments, and global test scores, into the multifaceted area of language use in context (i.e., discourse), to determine sociocommunicative strengths and weaknesses, as well as into the ramifications of deficits in ToM, EF, and overall information processing.

The four maxims of conversational interaction may be used as a guideline for informally assessing the difficulty that more able children have in applying the rules of interactive discourse in their everyday lives, as well as the extent to which they are able to make use of presuppositional information to guide their interactions. By obtaining language samples under varying contextual conditions, speech-language pathologists can gain excellent, albeit informal, information regarding not only the child's implicit understanding of his or her listener's needs (i.e., presuppositional knowledge) but also the extent to which the child is able to flexibly and competently apply the various conversational rules during the cognitively demanding moment. Trouble spots can be addressed within the context of conversational role plays wherein children can practice applying learned strategies by which to monitor their discourse behavior.

The related discourse problem of difficulty with narration has implications for both speech-language pathologists and educators, given its significant negative impact on the development of critical thinking skills and concept formation. Like its conversational counterpart, narration, too, requires an integrative approach that focuses on the interplay of cognitive and social-cognitive skills that fuel it. This is particularly important because children with ASD evidence difficulty in *all three* of the areas of narrative disability described by Westby (1984). This is in contrast to students with specific language-learning disabilities, who typically evidence difficulty in one area or another. Specifically, inefficient or delayed processing in children with ASD is often marked by word retrieval difficulty that does not necessarily reveal itself in confrontation naming tests. In addition, these children also evidence problems with the EF tasks of organizing and planning oral narratives and with the deeper, more conceptually based representations of schema (i.e., world) knowledge necessary for a cohesive understanding of events. Without the latter, events are experienced as separate occurrences, devoid of the linkages that support meaning and scaffold the production of oral and written narratives.

Situational vignettes provide an excellent vehicle to assess and later address the subtle and overlapping difficulties that more able children have with the comprehension of complex linguistic information; inferential, abstract reasoning; presuppositional judgments; higher-order pragmatic ability; and the social-cognitive constructs of EF and ToM. The information in this chapter will enable clinicians to design intervention protocols based on the unique pattern of deficits and strengths demonstrated by these children. Situational vignettes embedded in role-play activities are particularly germane to the needs of more able children and offer a distinct advantage over more didactic approaches. Specifically, because of the dynamic, interactive nature of role plays, they afford opportunities for children with ASD to apply and hence fortify newly acquired skills in a context that is relevant and meaningful. Role plays also mirror the pattern of skill acquisition in typical development. Conversely, didactic approaches in which the child is required to respond to information presented in a teacher–pupil instructional format are not only static and contrived but also are devoid of opportunities for the child to *demonstrate* his or her understanding through the application of learned strategies. Furthermore, given the difficulty that children with ASD have in *applying* information that they may actually be able to verbalize, mere recitation of information in a formal instructional situation in no way ensures the understanding and internalization necessary for later application.

Clearly, the knowledge gained from clinical observation and both formal and informal assessment will be of immeasurable importance to educators in helping them to understand their students' needs as well as in providing them with a framework for making the adjustments, adaptations, and modifications required to accommodate these children in their classrooms. To this end, it is crucial for teachers and clinicians to understand that behavior that *appears* willful and volitional or appears to be the result of laziness and disorganization is more likely a reflection of the child's response to his or her neurological impairments (e.g., deficits in EF, ToM, or pragmatics). Furthermore, it also is essential for teachers and clinicians to understand the ways in which comprehension difficulty, EF deficits, and ToM impairment can affect not only the child's interpretation of a story character's intentions and motivations but also his or her ability to comprehend, infer, abstract, apply, and process information in general. Such knowledge can alert the teacher to the necessity of providing direct teaching and environmental supports to scaffold learning. Moreover, if educators understand that despite strengths in procedural knowledge, more able children with ASD nonetheless demonstrate significant weaknesses in the more conceptually based declarative knowledge, educators will be less likely to be blinded by the strengths of these children and more likely to intensify early efforts to address the foundational skills that support the development of critical thinking skills and concept formation.

Finally, if there is a "bottom line" to serving the more able child with ASD, it is perhaps best encapsulated by the reversal of the popular adage: "What you don't know (about the strengths, weaknesses, and needs of these children) *will* bother you!" Worse yet, what is not known will compromise the social and academic success of these children, given that such success is dependent on direct and informed teaching in an educational milieu cognizant of and responsive to their unique and complex needs.

DIRECTIONS FOR FUTURE RESEARCH

It is important that research efforts reflect the paradigm shift in autism from the earlier domain-specific view to the domain-general conceptualization because the deficits that more able children manifest are both subtle and reflective of difficulty at the level of more diffuse neural systems. This requires that researchers adopt a discourse perspective and an expanded research focus that shifts attention from discrete language elements per se to those complex language processes and social-cognitive constructs that are involved in information exchange. Moreover, given that language is the conduit through which all other learning flows, it is essential that researchers also investigate the effects that deficits in comprehension, pragmatic ability, and ToM have on the development of critical thinking, problem solving, and similar conceptually based academic skills. In addition, if practitioners are to meet the needs of more able individuals with ASD, then there must be better ways of assessing the specific nature of their sociocommunicative challenges than those that are currently available. Specifically, many of the language assessment tools lack sensitivity to the subtle problems that these children manifest and/or tap into relatively preserved discrete skills. In either case, test scores are artifactually enhanced, even as deficit areas go unnoticed. A discourse perspective also will be of immense value, particularly with respect to obtaining a holistic view of the more able child's multifaceted sociocommunicative needs. Finally, the subtle and complex nature of the sociocommunicative impairment in more able children requires not only increased sensitivity to different research perspectives but also an expanded and deeper knowledge base that takes into account the interplay among the cognitive and social-cognitive constructs that are an integral part of the sociocommunicative process. Only then will a richly textured view of the many facets of this complex disorder emerge to guide intervention efforts.

CONCLUSIONS

This chapter has considered the sociocommunicative challenges and needs of more able children with ASD. It has done so from the perspective of an expanded research base that takes into account the interrelationships among language understanding and use, and the social-cognitive constructs that undergird information processing and communication. Sociocommunicative behavior is a highly complex, interdependent process that reflects competencies derived from several different, interrelated cognitive substrates. As such, to derive an understanding of the problems that more able children have with language understanding and use, it is vitally important to look beyond their discrete language skills. Thus, it is necessary to examine the ways in which deficits in comprehension, pragmatic knowledge, ToM, and EF adversely affect the processing of information in an efficient or effective manner. The importance of a discourse perspective is stressed as the vehicle by which to judge communicative competence. Implications for future research call for continued expansion into related cognitive and social-cognitive areas, and for the development of assessment tools that pinpoint rather than obfuscate the subtle deficits that more able children possess. Finally, clinicians and educators are cautioned to look beyond the superficial strengths of these children, to be creative in their efforts to discover ways to address their weaknesses, and to be willing to make the adjustments and provide the supports that enable children with ASD to be more successful in sociocommunicative and academic endeavors.

REFERENCES

Adamson, L.B. (1996). *Communication development during infancy.* Boulder, CO: Westview.

Ameli, R., Courchesne, E., Lincoln, A., Kaufman, A.S., & Grillon, C. (1988). Visual memory processes in high-functioning individuals with autism. *Journal of Autism and Developmental Disorders, 18,* 601–615.

Baron-Cohen, S. (1989). Perceptual role taking and protodeclarative pointing in autism. *British Journal of Developmental Psychology, 7,* 113–127.

Baron-Cohen, S. (1995). *Mindblindness: An essay on autism and theory of mind.* Cambridge, MA: MIT Press.

Bates, E. (1976). *Language and context: The acquisition of pragmatics.* San Diego: Academic Press.

Bates, E. (1979). *The emergence of symbols: Cognition and communication in infancy.* San Diego: Academic Press.

Bates, E., Benigni, L., Bretherton, I., Camaioni, L., & Volterra, V. (1979). *The emergence of symbols: Cognition and communication in infancy.* San Diego: Academic Press.

Bates, E., Camaioni, L., & Volterra, V. (1975). The acquisition of performatives prior to speech. *Merrill-Palmer Quarterly, 21,* 205–226.

Bell, M.A., & Fox, N.A. (1994). Brain development over the first year of life: Relations between EEG frequency and coherence and cognition and affective behaviors. In G. Dawson & K. Fischer (Eds.), *Human behavior and the developing brain* (pp. 314–345). New York: Guilford Press.

Bloom, L., & Lahey, M. (1978). *Language development and language disorders.* New York: John Wiley & Sons.

Bretherton, I., McNew, S., & Beeghly-Smith, M. (1981). Early person knowledge as expressed in verbal and gestural communication: When do infants acquire a theory of mind? In M. Lamb & L. Sherrod (Eds.), *Infant social cognition* (pp. 333–373). Mahwah, NJ: Lawrence Erlbaum Associates.

Bruner, J. (1990). *Acts of meaning.* Cambridge, MA: Harvard University Press.

Chugani, H.T., Phelps, M.E., & Mazziotta, J.C. (1994). Positron emission tomography study of human brain functional development. *Annals of Neurology, 22,* 487–497.

Curcio, F. (1978). Sensorimotor functioning and communication in mute autistic children. *Journal of Autism and Childhood Schizophrenia, 8,* 281–287.

Denckla, M.B. (1996). A theory and model of executive function: A neuropsychological perspective. In G.R. Lyon & N.A. Krasnegor (Eds.), *Attention, memory, and executive function* (pp. 263–278). Baltimore: Paul H. Brookes Publishing Co.

Dore, J. (1986). The development of conversational competence. In R.L. Schiefelbusch (Ed.), *Language competence: Assessment and intervention* (pp. 3–60). San Diego: College-Hill.

Eslinger, P.J. (1996). Conceptualizing, describing, and measuring components of executive function: A summary. In G.R. Lyon & N.A. Krasnegor (Eds.), *Attention, memory, and executive function* (pp. 367–395). Baltimore: Paul H. Brookes Publishing Co.

Frith, U. (1989). *Autism: Explaining the enigma.* Cambridge, MA: Blackwell.

Frith, U., & Snowling, M. (1983). Reading for meaning and reading for sound in autistic and dyslexic children. *British Journal of Developmental Psychology, 1,* 329–342.

Gillberg, C., & Ehlers, S. (1998). High-functioning people with autism and Asperger syndrome: A literature review. In E. Schopler, G.B. Mesibov, & L.J. Kunce (Eds.), *Asperger syndrome or high-functioning autism?* (pp. 79–106). New York: Plenum.

Goldstein, G., Minshew, N.J., & Siegel, D.J. (1994). Age differences in academic achievement in high-functioning autistic individuals. *Journal of Clinical and Experimental Neuropsychology, 16,* 671–680.

Grice, H. (1975). Logic and conversation. In D. Davidson & G. Harmon (Eds.), *The logic of grammar.* Encino, CA: Dickinson.

Happé, F. (1993). Communicative competence and theory of mind in autism: A test of relevance theory. *Cognition, 48,* 101–119.

Hirsh-Pasek, K., & Golinkoff, R. (1991). Language comprehension: A new look at some old themes. In N. Krasnegor, D. Rumbaugh, R. Schiefelbusch, & M. Studdert-Kennedy (Eds.), *Biological and behavioral determinants of language development* (pp. 301–320). Mahwah, NJ: Lawrence Erlbaum Associates.

Huttenlocher, J. (1974). The origins of language comprehension. In R.L. Solso (Ed.), *Theories of cognitive psychology* (pp. 331–368). Mahwah, NJ: Lawrence Erlbaum Associates.

Labov, W., & Franshel, D. (1977). *Therapeutic discourse.* San Diego: Academic Press.

MacLachlan, P. (1985). *Sarah, plain and tall.* New York: HarperCollins.

McLean, J., & Snyder-McLean, L. (1978). *A transactional approach to early language training.* Columbus, OH: Merrill.

Minshew, N. (1996). Autism. In B.O. Berg (Ed.), *Principles of child neurology* (pp. 1713–1729). New York: McGraw-Hill.

Minshew, N.J., & Goldstein, G. (1993). Is autism an amnesic disorder?: Evidence from the California Verbal Learning Test. *Neuropsychology, 7,* 209–216.

Minshew, N.J., Goldstein, G., Muenz, L.R., & Payton, J.B. (1992). Neuropsychological functioning in nonmentally retarded autistic individuals. *Journal of Clinical and Experimental Neuropsychology, 14,* 749–761.

Minshew, N.J., Goldstein, G., & Siegel, D.J. (1995). Speech and language in high-functioning autistic individuals. *Neuropsychology, 9,* 255–261.

Minshew, N.J., Goldstein, G., Taylor, H.G., & Siegel, D.J. (1994). Academic achievement in high functioning autistic individuals. *Journal of Clinical and Experimental Neuropsychology, 16,* 261–270.

Muma, J. (1978). *Language handbook.* Upper Saddle River, NJ: Prentice-Hall.

Mundy, P., Sigman, M., Ungerer, J., & Sherman, T. (1986). Defining the social deficits in autism: The contribution of nonverbal communication measures. *Journal of Child Psychology and Psychiatry and Allied Disciplines, 27,* 657–669.

National Institutes of Health. (July 1995). *Preliminary report of the autism working group* (pp. 1–30). Bethesda, MD: NIH Inter-Institute Autism Coordinating Committee.

Ozonoff, S. (1995). Executive functions in autism. In E. Schopler & G.B. Mesibov (Eds.), *Learning and cognition in autism* (pp. 199–215). New York: Plenum.

Ozonoff, S. (1998). Assessment and remediation of executive dysfunction in autism and Asperger syndrome. In E. Schopler, G.B. Mesibov, & L.J. Kunce (Eds.), *Asperger syndrome or high-functioning autism?* (pp. 263–290). New York: Plenum.

Pennington, B.F., Bennetto, L., McAleer, O., & Roberts, R.J., Jr. (1996). Executive functions and working memory: Theoretical and measurement issues. In G.R. Lyon & N.A. Krasnegor (Eds.), *Attention, memory, and executive function* (pp. 327–348). Baltimore: Paul H. Brookes Publishing Co.

Perner, J. (1991). *Understanding the representational mind.* Cambridge, MA: MIT Press.

Prior, M., & Hoffman, W. (1990). Neuropsychological testing of autistic children through an exploration with frontal lobe tests. *Journal of Autism and Developmental Disorders, 20,* 581–590.

Prizant, B.M., & Duchan, J.F. (1981). The functions of immediate echolalia in autistic children. *Journal of Speech and Hearing Disorders, 46,* 241–249.

Prizant, B.M., & Rydell, P.J. (1984). An analysis of the functions of delayed echolalia in autistic children. *Journal of Speech and Hearing Research, 27,* 183–192.

Rice, M.L. (1986). Mismatched premises of the communicative competence model and language intervention. In R.L. Schiefelbusch (Ed.), *Language competence: Assessment and intervention* (pp. 261–280). San Diego: College-Hill.

Roberts, J.M.A. (1989). Echolalia and comprehension in autistic children. *Journal of Autism and Developmental Disorders, 19,* 271–281.

Rumsey, J.M. (1985). Conceptual problem-solving in highly verbal, nonretarded autistic men. *Journal of Autism and Developmental Disorders, 15,* 23–36.

Sacks, O. (1989). *Seeing voices: A journey into the world of the deaf.* Berkeley: University of California.

Savage-Rumbaugh, E.S. (1991). Language learning in the bonobo: How and why they learn. In N. Krasnegor, D.M. Rumbaugh, R.L. Schiefelbusch, & M. Studdert-Kennedy (Eds.), *Biological and behavioral determinants of language development* (pp. 209–233). Mahwah, NJ: Lawrence Erlbaum Associates.

Savage-Rumbaugh, S., & Lewin, R. (1994). *Kanzi: The ape at the brink of the human mind.* New York: John Wiley & Sons.
Sevcik, R.A., & Romski, M.A. (1997). Comprehension and language acquisition: Evidence from youth with severe cognitive disabilities. In L.B. Adamson & M.A. Romski (Eds.), *Communication and language acquisition: Discoveries from atypical development* (pp. 187–202). Baltimore: Paul H. Brookes Publishing Co.
Sevcik, R.A., & Savage-Rumbaugh, E.S. (1994). Language comprehension and use by great apes. *Language and Communication, 14,* 37–58.
Sigman, M. (1989). *Bridges between psychology and medical research* [Audiocassette]. Silver Spring, MD: Autism Society of America.
Speare, E.G. (1958). *The witch of Blackbird Pond.* Boston: Houghton Mifflin.
Tager-Flusberg, H. (1993). What language reveals about the understanding of minds in children with autism. In S. Baron-Cohen, H. Tager-Flusberg, & D.J. Cohen (Eds.), *Understanding other minds: Perspectives from autism* (pp. 138–157). New York: Oxford University Press.
Tager-Flusberg, H. (1997). Language acquisition and theory of mind: Contributions from the study of autism. In L.B. Adamson & M.A. Romski (Eds.), *Communication and language acquisition: Discoveries from atypical development* (pp. 135–160). Baltimore: Paul H. Brookes Publishing Co.
Twachtman, D.D. (1995). Methods to enhance communication in verbal children. In K.A. Quill, (Ed.), *Teaching children with autism: Strategies to enhance communication and socialization* (pp. 133–162). New York: Delmar Publishers Inc.
Twachtman, D.D. (1996, Summer). There's a lot more to communication than talking! *The Morning News,* 3–5.
Twachtman-Cullen, D. (1997a, Spring). Comprehension: The power that fuels expression. *The Morning News,* 9–11.
Twachtman-Cullen, D. (1997b). *A passion to believe: Autism and the facilitated communication phenomenon.* Boulder, CO: Westview.
Twachtman-Cullen, D. (1998). Language and communication in high-functioning autism and Asperger syndrome. In E. Schopler, G.B. Mesibov, & L.J. Kunce (Eds.), *Asperger syndrome or high-functioning autism?* (pp. 199–225). New York: Plenum.
Twachtman-Cullen, D., & Twachtman-Reilly, J. (1998). *Meeting the needs of more able children with autism spectrum disorders: Translating what we know into what we need to do.* Unpublished manuscript.
Wellman, H.M. (1990). *The child's theory of mind.* Cambridge, MA: MIT Press.
Wellman, H.M. (1993). Early understanding of mind: The normal case. In S. Baron-Cohen, H. Tager-Flusberg, & D.J. Cohen (Eds.), *Understanding other minds: Perspectives from autism* (pp. 10–39). New York: Oxford University Press.
Westby, C.E. (1984). Development of narrative language abilities. In G.P. Wallach & K.G. Butler (Eds.), *Language learning disabilities in school-age children* (pp. 103–127). Baltimore: Lippincott Williams & Wilkins.
Wetherby, A.M. (1986). Ontogeny of communicative functions in autism. *Journal of Autism and Developmental Disorders, 16,* 295–316.
Wetherby, A.M., & Prutting, C.A. (1984). Profiles of communicative and cognitive-social abilities in autistic children. *Journal of Speech and Hearing Research, 27,* 364–377.
Whitehouse, D., & Harris, J.C. (1984). Hyperlexia in infantile autism. *Journal of Autism and Developmental Disorders, 14,* 281–289.

11

Promoting Peer Play and Socialization

The Art of Scaffolding

Adriana L. Schuler and Pamela J. Wolfberg

> In play a child always behaves beyond his average age, above his daily behavior; in play it is as though he were a head taller than himself. As in the focus of a magnifying glass, play contains all developmental tendencies in a condensed form and is itself a major source of development. (Vygotsky, 1978, p. 102)

With impairments in reciprocal social interaction, communication, and imagination as the defining features of autism spectrum disorders (ASDs), it is no surprise that the development of symbolic play and peer interaction has presented such a challenge to interventionists. Although it is not unusual for individuals with autism to accumulate an often astounding verbal repertoire, they seldom use their verbal skills to relate to their peers and/or to engage in pretend play. Gains typically documented pertain to speech production and use of tangible language functions, such as concrete requests and protest (for reviews see Howlin, 1981, 1986; Schuler, Gonsier-Gerdin, & Wolfberg, 1990), as opposed to functions that are more social in nature, such as commenting, describing, or sharing (Curcio, 1978; Fay & Schuler, 1980; Mundy, Sigman, Ungerer, & Sherman, 1986; Wetherby & Prutting, 1984; see also Chapter 6). Motivations to communicate seem to revolve around properties of the physical world (for a more in-depth discussion, see Papy, Papy, & Schuler, 1995; Schuler, 1995) rather than around the expression of socioemotional concerns or more playful social intentions. Socially referenced, spontaneous, and meaningful use of speech often remains merely an elusive objective rather than a reality of intervention.

This chapter argues that the teaching of both the social and the dynamic dimensions of play presents a major challenge to practitioners and that peer play is of critical importance if one wants to expand and diversify the communicative repertoires of children with ASD. Following a discussion of the paucity of play in children with autism and the pitfalls of overly directive approaches, it is argued that practitioners need to become more cognizant of the culture of play and that more socially referenced forms of learning need to be imposed on more mechanistic and adult-controlled modes of learning, which are so prevalent. The need for scaffolding and the power of more flexible child-centered structures are discussed along with the type of skills that are critical to effective scaffolding. Subsequently, an overview of the integrated play group model is presented along with a case vignette that illustrates how facilitators provide the guidance and support that allow children with ASD to use objects in more conventional and collaborative ways and to expand and diversify their communicative repertoires. Directions for future research also are discussed.

PROMOTING PLAY: PROMISES AND CHALLENGES

The challenges encountered in promoting communication that is both meaningful and functional are even further exacerbated when teaching play skills. That highly structured educational approaches have been reported to be most effective in teaching children with autism presents a special set of challenges to anyone trying to promote peer play and socialization. Although speech and language skills are generally the primary target of intervention efforts, play skills may be equally if not more important, particularly when the social dimensions of communication are taken into consideration. Engagement in peer play may well be the ultimate antidote against the behavioral rigidity that epitomizes ASDs because the negotiation of themes and variations constitutes the essence of play. Defined by joint action and attention, play provides a prime context for the coordination of joint action and social referencing. In their negotiation of access to toys and play structures, partners in play flexibly shift gaze between themselves and their physical environment. In doing so, they learn to interact with and relate to people and objects at the same time.

Without specific support or guidance, children with autism gravitate to repetitive play activity ranging from manipulating objects and enacting elaborate routines to pursuing obsessive and narrowly focused interests. They are less likely to exhibit functionally appropriate play and rarely produce pretend play (Harris, 1993; Jarrold, Boucher, & Smith, 1993, Wing & Gould, 1979). Similarly, they have problems entering and sustaining social play activities with peers. In free play situations, they typically either avoid and resist social overtures, passively enter play with little or no self-initiation, or approach peers in an obscure and one-sided fashion (Lord, 1984; Wing & Attwood, 1987; Wolfberg, 1999).

That the essence of the autistic spectrum may be best captured by a restricted range of interests and a seemingly obsessive insistence on sameness may speak to the detrimental impact of social isolation. When children with autism seem to engage in pretend play, a closer examination of the behaviors involved may reveal them to be highly repetitive. In sharp contrast to the rich, thematic variations evident in the play of typically developing children, the play of children with autism seems almost obsessive in its literal repetition of identical acts. Analogous with the literal quality and the apparently meaningless repetition of speech in echolalia, the play of children with autism might be described more aptly as "echo*play*lia."

Nevertheless, one might argue that both echolalia and "echoplaylia" are not far removed from the delayed imitation processes that are so characteristic of typical development (for a more in-depth discussion, see Schuler, 1979). After all, typically developing children start out with highly restricted play repertoires. These are gradually broadened through participation in ongoing verbal and nonverbal negotiations, which constitute the core of peer play. The unprecedented expansion and diversification of the behavior repertoire of typically developing children engaged in peer play may speak to the value of these experiences. The capacity to understand and relate to the social world and, ultimately, to participate in the culture of childhood hinges on play skills. It is therefore critical that children with autism are supported in peer play and related socialization processes.

Despite its therapeutic potential, play—particularly peer play—has not received much attention in the education of or intervention for children with autism. Yet, a number of studies have shown autistic children to be capable of engaging in more complex and diverse forms of play when supported by an adult (Boucher & Lewis, 1990; Greenspan & Wieder, 1997; Lewis & Boucher, 1988; Mundy, Sigman, Ungerer, & Sherman, 1986, 1987; Riquet, Taylor, Benaroya, & Klein, 1981; Sigman & Ungerer, 1984; Van Berckelaer-Onnes, 1994), and more experienced peers (Goldstein & Cisar, 1992; Kohler, Strain, Hoyson, & Jamison, 1997; Lord, 1984; Lord & Hopkins, 1986; McHale, 1983; Roeyers, 1996; Strain & Kohler, 1995; Wolfberg, 1999; Wolfberg & Schuler, 1993).

Although these findings speak to the need for interventions that capitalize on the potential for peer play and socialization, very few comprehensive interventions have been reported. Interventions that do target play generally focus on specific skills that serve either as a context or as a presumed developmental prerequisite. The limited success in teaching play has unfortunate repercussions in terms of the quality of life of many children with autism. Without the interpersonal skills and flexible modes of representation that manifest themselves in the context of play, it is difficult for individuals with autism to develop friendships or nurture social relations. Without the benefits of participation in play culture many people with autism remain isolated. Their attempts to socialize are often poorly timed and mistaken as a sign of deviance and limited social interest.

From a transactional perspective the neglect of peer play comes at a high price. We believe that the pervasive dynamics of social exclusion impose a secondary level of disability over a more basic deficit in the processing of social information. Because the ever-decreasing opportunities to socialize serve to amplify the skill deficits already encountered, social exclusion, if unmitigated, leads to ever-increasing social deficits. Yet, our own experiences with our "integrated play groups" (Wolfberg, 1995b; Wolfberg & Schuler, 1993) have convinced us that many children with autism are much more capable of play than is typically assumed. We believe that the lack of access to and support for peer play is primarily responsible for the skill deficits encountered. Despite its secondary nature, the effects of exclusion may be more pervasive and disabling than are more primary, biologically based impairments in the processing of social information.

For children with autism to fully participate in a range of peer play experiences in inclusive environments, interactions with more competent peers need to be supported. Although interventions may integrate children with autism and peers without disabilities in the context of play activity, they tend to focus on specific interaction skills rather than on play as an area of competence (see, e.g., Odom & Brown, 1993; Odom & Strain, 1984; Roeyers, 1996). Moreover, the few interventions that do focus on play tend to operate without a cohesive conceptual framework. For instance, interventions tend to be highly structured and focus on adult-directed rather than child-initiated activity or lack structure altogether, led by the assumption that play is what children do when left to their own devices. Such interventions may not tap into the full potential of children with ASD. What is needed is a better understanding of how play naturally evolves and influences social and symbolic development, along with an appreciation of the obstacles encountered by children with ASD.

ROLE AND CULTURE OF PLAY

An appreciation of the role of play in peer culture and child development should be the centerpiece of any efforts to enhance the socialization and play of children with autism. Research shows that play fulfills a number of interrelated functions for developing social, communicative, and linguistic competence (Bretherton, 1984; Bruner, 1986; Corsaro & Schwarz, 1991). Children's participation in mutually enjoyed activities offers a foundation on which to establish positive social relationships and friendships (Hartup & Sancilio, 1986; Parker & Gottman, 1989). Within the context of mutually constructed play activity, children gain skill and practice in the use of increasingly complex verbal and nonverbal sociocommunicative strategies. They learn to initiate, interpret, and respond to one another's social cues to successfully extend invitations and gain entry into peer group activities (Dodge, Schlundt, Schocken, & Delugach, 1983). To achieve interpersonal coordination in play, children learn how to negotiate and compromise while exploring social roles and issues of intimacy and trust (Dunn, 1991; Garvey, 1977; Howes, Unger, & Matheson, 1992; Parker & Gottman, 1989; Rubin, 1980).

Social pretend play is an especially important context for children to learn new vocabulary, complex language structures (Ervin-Tripp, 1991), and the rules of conversation (Garvey, 1977). By reconstructing symbolic play scripts abstracted from life experiences, children develop narrative competence and story comprehension (Pellegrini, 1985). They also learn to construct a shared understanding of literal and nonliteral meaning (Garvey, 1977; Howes et al., 1992), which underlies the capacity to develop a "theory of mind" (ToM; Baron-Cohen, Leslie, & Frith, 1985; Leslie, 1987).

Peers perform a distinct role in offering opportunities for socialization and play that cannot be duplicated by adults (Hartup, 1979, 1983). Within the first year of life, infants begin to take notice of and show an interest in other children by looking, smiling, vocalizing, gesturing, reaching out, and touching one another. They also show that they recognize familiar peers by reacting to them in idiosyncratic ways (Hay, 1985). Early social exchanges tend to be brief and fleeting with a playful orientation as youngsters offer and accept toys, mutually manipulate objects, and occasionally imitate one another (Vandell & Wilson, 1982). As children enter the preschool years, they show an increasing desire and ability to coordinate social activity while actively seeking out peers for the purpose of play and companionship through participation in their peer culture.

Peer culture reflects the unique social worlds that children construct out of their everyday experiences separate from adults (Corsaro, 1985, 1988, 1992; Denzin, 1977; Wolfberg & Schuler, 1999). A pivotal feature of peer culture is that children develop a sense of collective identity in which they recognize themselves as members of a group created exclusively by and for children. Although the adult world is often represented within the content of peer culture, children pursue social activity that is most meaningful to them on their own terms regardless of adult expectations. Because play is the leading social activity in the lives of children, it is the very essence of their culture.

The term *play culture* may more accurately describe that realm in which children live their social and imaginary lives (Selmer-Olsen, 1993; Wolfberg, 1999). The culture is based on children's active participation in the types of social activities that are valued by their peer group. In a sense, play culture is living folklore that manifests itself in the rituals, narratives, and creations children produce and pass on to one another. The skills, values, and knowledge acquired through peer play experiences are a part of the cultural tradition transmitted to each new generation of children.

Along the same vein, Vygotsky (1933/1966, 1978) attributes a most active role to play as a primary social activity for acquiring symbolic capacities, interpersonal skills, and social knowledge. According to Vygotsky, play's significance extends beyond merely reflecting development to leading development. Thus, play is seen as a driving force rather than a mirror of development. Through participation in play, children construct shared meanings and transform their understanding of the skills, values, and knowledge inherent to society and culture at large. Vygotsky viewed even independent play as social activity because children's themes, roles, and scripts are a reflection of these larger sociocultural worlds. Not only does such a view have powerful implications for our understanding of symptomatology in autism, but it also provides a powerful testimony to the importance of play interventions.

LIMITATIONS OF INTUITIVE AND DIRECTIVE APPROACHES

Even when the importance of play is acknowledged, the learning mechanisms involved remain largely elusive. When caregivers manage to facilitate desired social interactions, they seem to be guided largely by intuitions and hunches rather than any formalized body of knowledge. Similarly, we have observed many gifted teachers providing impromptu scaffolding of playful interactions. Nevertheless, the pitfalls of this type of intuitive guidance lie in the fact that it is difficult to teach others to do so and that there is little recourse when scaffolding efforts fail. Problem solving is difficult without a more formalized body of knowledge and related measurement schemes to evaluate and reflect on options and choices.

Not knowing how to take corrective action, one may well give up and end up justifying instructional failure by labeling the child as "disabled" and/or deviant. Moreover, a practitioner's lack of comfort with the violations of his or her expectations may spark a need for increased predictability and order. Guided by remedial logic, practitioners may be tempted to take back control in an attempt to correct the perceived deficits. At odds with a transactional spirit, intervention efforts now target the behaviors of the least capable interactant, at the risk of intensifying the child's disability, as discussed by Lyons (1991) and Stanovich and Stanovich (1996). At odds with a spirit of play, the remediation of deficits and the need to regain control become the focal points of directive intervention.

One of the major problems with highly directive interventions, such as those promoted by Ivar Lovaas and his colleagues (Lovaas, 1987; McEachin, Smith, & Lovaas, 1993), is that in pursuit of compliance and accuracy, the interventions often fail to acknowledge child initiations. The practitioner is likely to redirect or ignore when the child responds in ways that were not anticipated or scripted in advance. The limitations of highly directive teaching methods may be best illustrated by the fact that no documentation has ever been provided of the successful use of principles of direct instruction in teaching play. Although the topographies of the behaviors involved may indeed be taught successfully, these behaviors remain dependent on external cues and are not readily generalized to other settings or interactants. Given that one of the defining features of play is positive affect, it seems easier to fool one's audience through the rote reproduction of trained speech than through the repetition of trained play scripts. Unlike a child who reproduces memorized speech, a child engaged in rote play does not project a sense of competence.

That principles of compliance directly violate the very nature of play as self-imposed activity (Smith & Vollstedt, 1985) may account for our instructional failures. After all, play ceases to exist when adults call the shots. The practitioner's dilemma is one of balance. Although more directive adult-structured approaches may be overly controlling, more child-centered approaches that attempt to acknowledge the child's state of mind and try to follow its lead are often too subtle to draw in the child's attention. One of the challenges in the design of effective intervention thus lies in the creation of child-centered structures that are neither too loose nor too rigid.

Another limitation of highly directive approaches is that their reliance on externally adult-imposed structures places them at odds with the essence of inclusion and the least restrictive environment. As discussed previously, interventions that take place in segregated, artificial settings are unlikely to counteract the insidious dynamics of exclusion and isolation. For instance, when children with ASD are removed from their peer culture during the critical preschool years, even intensive one-to-one programming cannot keep pace with or prepare them to reenter the dynamics of socialization in the mainstream. Even when these children are successfully engaged in carefully programmed responses to series of "discrete" instructional cues, the isolation from their peer culture serves to aggravate their social deficits. How could one ever prepare children for more social forms of learning and interaction through the completion of thousands of one-to-one drills?

Whereas principles of direct teaching are useful in teaching concrete skills, which need to be mastered independently, they may not be compatible with the hierarchical and reciprocal nature of communication and symbolic representation (see Chapter 9). Commonly reported problems with the generalization of social skills may result from reliance on overly rigid intervention structures that violate the nature of symbolic interaction. As discussed so eloquently by Frank Smith (1983, 1988), the acquisition of modes of symbolic interaction should not be reduced to supposedly prerequisite component pieces or be divorced from the cultural contexts in which those modes of representation have evolved. Because play is so entrenched in the symbolic transmission of culture, practitioners need to search for more compatible instructional alternatives.

STRUCTURE AND MEDIATION OF SUPPORT: CULTURAL MODES OF LEARNING

Newer insights into scaffolding and the capacity to engage in culturally referenced forms of learning hold great promise in the design of interventions that promote social reciprocity and symbolic representation. Practitioners need to acknowledge the very special ability that humans have to transmit and acquire knowledge from others and to consider and learn from the perspectives and experiences of others (Bruner, 1975; Vygotsky, 1934/1962). Tomasello, Kruger, and Ratner (1993) described the ontogeny of such cultural forms of learning, which culminate in the mutual construction of new meanings or ideas and the acknowledgement of the perspectives of others (see Chapter 3). They claimed that cultural learning extends beyond earlier, more mechanistic conceptualizations of social learning, in which the child's attention is drawn to specific objects and/or locations in his or her environment that might have otherwise gone unnoticed. Because shared reflection is not included in these more mechanistic forms of social learning, they are essentially solitary. Although the adult may deliver reinforcement and carefully structure the learning environment, highly adult-controlled teaching formats, such as discrete trial techniques, do not allow for the reciprocity that characterizes more cultural forms of learning.

The paucity of pragmatic communication and mentalizing skills in people with autism may speak to the need to include more socially referenced forms of learning to counter the overly lean instructional menus that are typically encountered by people with autism. When children with autism only have exposure to operant and more mechanistic forms of social learning, this experience limits their ability to benefit from more inclusive socially and culturally referenced forms of learning. When practitioners do not provide access to more cultural modes of learning they may inadvertently keep these children locked into a mechanistic view of the world. The results of a study by Hadwin, Baron-Cohen, Howlin, and Hill (1997), documenting the impact of specific instruction geared to teach children with autism to understand the emotions and beliefs of others, may expose the limitations of such an adult-controlled format. That the specific gains achieved through a highly structured question-and-answer format and corrective feedback did not generalize to conversations with others invites the investigation of alternative approaches.

Notions of cultural learning are most pertinent to those types of tasks that require the ability to compare one's own perspective to those of others, and, ultimately, to the emergence of ToM. Such notions ought to guide a search for instructional alternatives because they provide an account of how one learns through and with another rather than merely from another. Moreover, because of its inherent reciprocity, the scaffolding of peer play deserves careful consideration in such an endeavor. With joint attention, turn taking, and reciprocal imitation as the essential features of play, play may serve as the prime vehicle for children to learn to appreciate the needs and perspectives of others. Given these natural opportunities for the simulation of others' mental states and the formation of ToM, scaffolded play holds much promise. That solitary object-based rather than more reciprocal modes of learning are more congruent with thought patterns characteristic of autism may explain why these modes continue to dominate intervention efforts. Initially, linear and discrete intervention structures may indeed provide the child with the order and predictability that allow him or her to make accurate predictions about the actions of others. Nevertheless, if social connections are to be made, more reciprocal and collaborative modes of learning need to be superimposed on the type of linear skill progressions that typically characterize initial intervention efforts.

What has become apparent is that effective interventions (see Dawson & Osterling, 1997, and Harris & Handleman, 1985) are highly structured, providing individuals with autism with more routines and predictability than they typically would face in everyday interactions. Enabled by their anticipation of the daily course of events, they become increasingly able to participate. Therefore, interventionists need to somehow reconcile principles of cultural learning, scaffolding, and guided participation, which have been so astutely described by Bruner (1986) and Rogoff (1990), with the need for structure, predictability, and order that seems so pervasive in autism. Although this may seem an awesome task, we have, nevertheless, had the privilege of observing expert practitioners in action. We have learned much from conducting structured group interviews with expert teachers (Schoenwald, 1997). The observations and interview data collected lead us to believe that the mediation of interpersonal structures presents the biggest challenge in promoting reciprocal interactions.

Although the mediation of temporal and spatial structures may indeed capture the history and essence of special education practices, the parameters of interpersonal structure remain uncharted. Few conscious efforts have been made to clarify the structure of interpersonal interactions to individuals with minimal social understanding. The dynamics of social interaction need to be made more transparent if individuals with autism are to participate successfully in social interaction. To allow for ever-increasing participation, it is important that the support structures provided are indeed sufficiently transparent, flexible, and transitional. Following Vygotskian (1978) principles of guided participation and support in the zone of proximal development, these temporary support structures are removed with the unfolding of newly gained confidence and competence. This implies that these adjustable structures are child or client centered rather than rigidly adult controlled, providing those involved the needed room to breathe and grow, defying the institutionalization of rigidity. We believe that the selection of optimal structures needs to be made on a case-by-case basis for the benefit of individual children and not merely for the convenience of therapists, teachers, established curricula, and/or school systems.

Expert practitioners make carefully informed decisions about the type, intensity, and configurations of support structures needed. Such skilled practitioners manage to mediate successful interactions by staging enticing contexts and by adapting their own styles of interaction to effectively match the learning styles and levels of development of individual children. To gain and direct the attention of their pupils, these practitioners may use simpler words, more contextual support, and exaggerated affect. They know how to build as well as intentionally dismantle individually tailored support structures, allowing children with autism to anticipate and, eventually, participate in interactions with adults as well as peers. We believe that the actions of such highly competent practitioners are fueled by advanced theories of mind, which allow them to appreciate the mental states and communicative needs of individuals who express themselves in erratic and unconventional ways.

The need for individually tailored support structures underscores the importance of professional expertise and reflective practice. We have observed experienced teachers who masterfully scaffold the joint attention and action of children with autism but who are unable to explain their course of action. For instance, they might have known how to entice a child with autism to tolerate sitting in a chair surrounded by a circle of peers despite the fact that the same child might initially have thrown him- or herself on the floor in a screaming fit of temper. Guided by their intuitions, these practitioners might, nevertheless, lack the language to reflect on and share their expertise. What seems essential to the advancement of professional practice and growth is the proliferation of a metacognition about special education and related instruction (For a more extensive discussion, see Castaneda, Schuler, & Watanabe, 1997, and Schuler, 1998). A more formalized body of knowledge that builds on and expands teachers' intuitive grasp of the mediation of interpersonal structure is essential if practitioners are to effectively scaffold the peer interactions and socialization of children with autism. As an illustration of such a "translation" and expansion of intuitive knowledge of peer interactions and play, we describe the use of facilitated peer mediation to promote both the social and cognitive as well as the affective dimensions of play.

CLINICAL AND EDUCATIONAL IMPLICATIONS

Consistent with a transactional orientation, intervention efforts should foster successful social transactions in supportive contexts as opposed to aiming for context-stripped remediation of deficits. To arrive at more reciprocal, culturally grounded modes of learning, instruction should be built around the interests and initiatives of the individuals involved, even when most or all of such initiatives take unconventional forms. Close observation and ongoing evaluations of current levels of understanding and competence are therefore critical. Such observations should be designed to determine the highest level of competence to be targeted given the optimal amount of social assistance, allowing for scaffolded performance within the zone of proximal development, as defined by Vygotsky (1934/1962). Effective practitioners know how to mediate optimal configurations of structure that allow for ongoing progression along a developmental trajectory.

Skilled practitioners know when to break down and/or remodel support structures, as well as build new ones that center around the interests and levels of understanding exhibited. Building on their own perspective-taking skills, they compensate for the fact that individuals with autism have such limitations with regard to the state of mind of their communication partners and often are bewildered by the unpredictability of their actions. In mediating proper support structures, practitioners draw from those very unique human qualities that seem so compromised in autism, that is, the abilities to transmit and acquire knowledge from others and to consider and learn from the perspectives and experiences of others (Bruner, 1975; Vygotsky, 1934/1962).

Effective practitioners are guided by unusually refined theories of mind, allowing them to understand the perspectives and intentions of their students and clients despite their unusual nature and the unconventional ways in which they are expressed. Consistent with a transactional dynamic, teachers and therapists need to excel in those domains in which individuals with autism are so challenged. To achieve this proficiency, clinicians, educators, and caregivers may need to examine their own level of discomfort when common behavior expectations and norms are violated. It is conceivable that excessive structure imposed by practitioners is more a reflection of their anxiety and uneasiness, motivated by their need to reestablish control (on their own terms). Although a directive and controlling stance might make him or her feel more at ease, it typically leads to power struggles and is not conducive to play and peer interaction. To provide individuals with ASD with a sense of control and structure, teachers and practitioners need to acknowledge these individuals' interests and preoccupations. Building on these individuals' current behavior repertoire, the practitioner needs to select motivating materials and activity contexts that support a sense of competence (see Chapters 9 and 12).

To effectively promote peer play and socialization, practitioners need to draw from a number of different sources of knowledge and insight to accommodate varying developmental levels, learning styles, and interests. In fact, when applied to play, the meaning of the word *teaching* in the Western world needs to be broadened to include all of the different configurations of support needed to promote a child's participation in peer-mediated activities that characterize the culture of play. That many different dimensions of support are necessary to enhance socialization and play makes it difficult to rely on any single instructional algorithm or formula. Effective practitioners cannot afford to be too single minded; they need to be flexible and adopt a holistic style. In fact, the type of multidimensional teaching and support needed might be better portrayed as an "art" rather than as a discrete set of skills. In summary, we believe that skilled practitioners possess the following qualities.

Observation Skills

To build child-centered structures, it is critical that practitioners sharpen their observation skills so that they become more cognizant of how unconventional forms of expression may indicate particular needs, emotional states, desires, preferences, and intentions. For this purpose, practitioners need to be well versed in informal, qualitative assessment techniques as well as more formalized methods (see Chapters 9 and 13).

Knowledge of Autism Spectrum Disorders

Astute assessment and evaluation skills hinge on familiarity with the communicative, social, linguistic, and affective features associated with ASDs. To recognize the idiosyncrasies in social development, practitioners need to be informed about the unique learning styles and developmental profiles and discontinuities that individuals with autism and related disorders may have.

Understanding and Appreciating Play

Practitioners need a thorough understanding and appreciation of the pervasive role of play in child development and the construction of peer culture. A thorough understanding of play will help practitioners in mediating play scenarios; building on the interests of individual children; and capitalizing on the opportunities afforded by settings, play materials, and configurations of peer support.

Providing a Secure Base for Play

By providing a predictable and accepting play environment, children are encouraged to take risks in exploring their physical as well as social environment. Practitioners need to create an environment that gives children a sense of belonging as well as a feeling of competence by acknowledging their initiations and interests. Ensuring that children are familiar with the facilitator and striving for consistent group membership are helpful assets.

Setting the Stage for Play

Practitioners need to be skilled in organizing play spaces with props and visual supports that create enticing play environments. In doing so, practitioners nonverbally communicate an invitation for children to engage in playful interactions. Play spaces that are carefully selected and laid out well, with well-positioned toys, are tremendous assets in promoting peer play.

Ritualizing and Dramatizing Play

The ability to ritualize and dramatize events and emotions, incorporating exaggerated affect, serves to engage children who might otherwise seem aloof and nonattentive (see Chapter 12). Skilled practitioners manage to build anticipation through the effective use of rituals. In addition, a general sense of theater will help practitioners to not only entice children but also to sustain their attention.

Narrating Scripts

To promote the growth of language as well as play skills, effective practitioners are able to create play scenarios and narrate scripts following children's lead and to apply principles of semantic contingency. By expanding on children's actions, verbalizations, and social interactions, practitioners promote higher levels of thematic cohesion as well as communicative and linguistic competence. Practitioners use language primarily to coach rather than to direct children's play and language use.

Scaffolding

The art in scaffolding play lies in the construction and intentional dismantling of flexible, transparent, and child-centered structures that provide children not only with an anticipatory set but also with enough room for initiation. The provision of predictable and secure support structures allows children to increasingly participate in the social world around them as they proceed within their zone of proximal development. For this purpose, rigid adult-imposed and a priori structures are counterproductive because they violate the nature of play.

Facilitating Peer Mediation and Social Understanding

To facilitate peer play and socialization, effective practitioners assist peers in understanding the communicative behaviors of their playmates with autism and in strategizing new ways to engage them. Furthermore, the mediation of joint attention, action, and affect helps children make sense of the social interactions and language that surrounds them.

Theory of Mind

To effectively scaffold and accommodate the limited perspective-taking skills of children with autism, practitioners need to draw from their own ToM to better appreciate their pupils' view of the world, state of mind, affective states, intentions, and desires. A better understanding of their children's perspectives helps practitioners in building the type of anticipatory structures that incorporate children's current perceptions and motivations.

Reflective Practice

Guided by astute perceptions and monitoring of child skill levels, sensitivities, preoccupations, and idiosyncrasies, skilled facilitators make continual adjustments to the physical environment, sociocultural ecology, developmental status, appropriate play activities, themes, and scripts, as well as instructional strategies, modalities, and interactional styles.

AN ILLUSTRATION OF A PEER PLAY INTERVENTION

The concept of *integrated play groups* grew in response to the need to develop a comprehensive play intervention for children with autism that includes all of the previously mentioned features (Wolfberg, 1995a, 1995b, 1999; Wolfberg & Schuler, 1993). This model specifically incorporates variables documented to affect play and social interaction in children with ASD. Integrated play groups offer children who are less skilled in play (novice players) ongoing opportunities to participate in play with typically developing peers as playmates (expert players). The focus is on guided participation in play, described as the process through which children develop while actively participating in culturally valued activity with the guidance, support, and challenge of companions who vary in skill and status (Rogoff, 1990; Vygotsky, 1978). Novices thus gain expertise while playing with other more competent players under the guidance of a skilled practitioner.

The Ecology of Play

Play groups typically include three to five familiar peers and/or siblings with a higher ratio of expert to novice players. The children's ages, developmental status, and gender may vary, offering different types of beneficial experiences. Play groups take place in natural, integrated environments such as in the home, inclusive classrooms, integrated school sites, after-school programs, recreation centers, and neighborhood parks. Play spaces are thoughtfully designed and include a wide range of constructive and sociodramatic play materials with high potential for interactive and imaginative play to accommodate children's diverse interests, learning styles, and developmental needs.

Because *schedule* and *routines* offer the most tangible support structures, our groups meet on a regular basis over an extended period of time, two times or more per week for approximately 30–60 minutes. Personalized visual schedules or calendars help players anticipate future play sessions. Opening and closing rituals at the beginning and end of each play session, such as discussing a brief plan or review of events and/or singing a simple song, are used to further instill a sense of order and anticipation.

Spatial order is inherent in the way play materials and place spaces are organized. The latter are purposely restricted in size with clearly defined boundaries. Play materials are explicitly organized so that they are accessible, visible, clearly labeled, and logically arranged around activities and themes. A wide range of exploratory, constructive, and sociodramatic play materials with high potential for interactive and imaginative play are included. Toys and props vary in degree of structure and complexity to accommodate children's diverse interests, learning styles, and developmental levels.

Assessing Play

Becoming an astute observer and interpreter of how children play independently, beside, and with other children is key to being an effective play group guide. In the case of children with autism, one must be especially sensitive to the subtle qualities rather than obvious deficits observed when they play alone and with peers. Systematic observations of social and symbolic dimensions of play, sociocommunicative abilities, and play preferences provide a basis for intervention and evaluation.

We developed a framework for identifying characteristics associated with the symbolic as opposed to social dimensions of play. Within the symbolic dimension of play—ranging from simple sensorimotor explorations of objects to more complex imaginative play schemes—distinctions are made between nondifferentiated object *manipulation,* and *functional* (conventional and emerging symbolic) and *symbolic/pretend* play that may be directed toward objects or that signifies specific events (adapted from McCune-Nicholich, 1981; Piaget, 1962; and Smilansky, 1968). Within the social dimension of play, in reference to the child's distance to and involvement with one or more children, distinctions are made between *isolation, orientation, proximity* (parallel), *common focus,* and *common goal* (adapted from Parten, 1932). This assessment scheme allows us to document progress from brief and fleeting encounters to coordinated and sustained interactions and from undifferentiated, repetitive activity to more discriminative and imaginative object play.

The ways in which children communicate in the context of peer play activities are also examined in detail. The *functions* of communication (e.g., requests for objects, peer interaction and affection, protests, declarations, comments) may be accomplished through a variety of verbal and nonverbal *means* (e.g., facial expressions; eye gaze; proximity; manipulating another's hand, face, or body; showing or giving objects; gaze shift; gestures; intonation; vocalization; nonfocused or focused echolalia; one-word or complex speech/sign) (Peck, Schuler, Tomlinson, Thiemer, & Haring, 1984; Schuler, Prizant, & Wetherby, 1997). Documenting the play preferences of both novice and expert players in play groups offers a means by which to identify and match children's play interests. Play preferences include a child's attraction to certain toys or props (e.g., round objects, toys that move, realistic replicas), interactions with toys or props (e.g., spins toys, lines up toys, uses objects conventionally), choice of play activities (e.g., roughhousing, quiet play, constructive play), choice of play themes (e.g., familiar routines, invented stories, fantasy play), and choice of playmates (e.g., no one in particular, one or more peers).

Promoting Play

Intervention (guided participation) involves structuring opportunities for novice and expert players to coordinate play while also challenging novice players to practice new and increasingly complex forms of play. This entails enticing expert and novice players to discover common ground on which they can collaborate in mutually enjoyed activities. The adult must naturally modify his or her own behavior in response to the movement and patterns of activity in play groups. He or she acts as an interpreter to help the expert and novice players figure out what is meant by the others' words and actions. To start a play event, the adult sometimes directs the play group as though it were a stage performance, arranging props and assigning roles to ensure that everyone has a satisfying part. At other times he or she stands on the periphery of the group, questioning, commenting, and offering suggestions that enable the children to organize and direct their own play activities. Ultimately, the adult shifts this responsibility to the expert players as they demonstrate competence in carrying out play events on their own. The methods used to guide participation in play are described as monitoring play initiations, scaffolding interactions, sociocommunicative guidance, and play guidance.

To guide children in their play endeavors, it is essential to become an astute observer of children's play as a means to *monitor play initiations.* As noted previously, one must be especially sensitive to the subtle qualities rather than obvious deficiencies observed. Child initiations in play, even in unusual forms, serve as indices of present and emerging capacities in social and symbolic forms of play. Recognizing and interpreting all play acts as purposeful and adaptive and as meaningful attempts to initiate play with others and/or to express oneself in play with materials, roles, and events, is essential for guiding decisions on how to intervene on behalf of novice players. Thus, play initiations become a catalyst for building and extending each novice player's existing play repertoire along social and symbolic dimensions. In addition, these initiations provide a point of departure from which novice and expert players can establish a mutual focus on play activities.

Scaffolding, by definition, is the provision of adjustable and temporary support structures. In play groups, the adult scaffolds interactions by adjusting the amount of external support provided in relation to the children's play needs. Initially, most children require a great deal of assistance while they acclimate to the experience of being in play groups. As the children grow increasingly comfortable and competent in their play, the adult gradually lessens this support and withdraws from the play group. Remaining readily available on the periphery of the group, the adult offers the children a secure base from which to explore and try out new activities. At the same time, the adult monitors play initiations and provides assistance whenever necessary.

Sociocommunicative guidance strategies enable novices and experts to establish a mutual focus in play by recognizing and responding to initiations. Directed to both experts and novices alike, these strategies foster attempts to extend invitations to peers to play, to persist in enlisting reluctant peers to play, to respond to peers' cues and initiations in play, to maintain or expand interactions with peers, and to enter or join peers in an established play event. By interpreting the subtle verbal and nonverbal cues of novice players as meaningful and purposeful acts, experts learn to respond to and nourish these play initiations. By the same token, interpreting by breaking down the complex social cues of expert players allows novices to better understand and fully participate in the play context.

Practitioners also employ *play guidance strategies* to engage and fully immerse novice players in activities with expert players slightly beyond their present capacities for spontaneous play as exhibited in unstructured play sessions. To be fully immersed in play allows children to participate in the whole play experience, even if participation is minimal. This is similar to notions of *partial participation* (Baumgart et al., 1982; Ferguson & Baumgart, 1991), *community of learners* (Brown & Campione, 1990), *learner as cultural member* (Heath, 1989), and *legitimate peripheral participation* (Lave & Wenger, 1991). Thus, novices may carry out play activities and roles that they may not as yet fully comprehend. For example, a child inclined to line up objects may incorporate this scheme into a larger play theme of pretending to go grocery shopping. With the assistance of more capable peers, the child may take on the role of a store clerk who is responsible for arranging the groceries on the shelf.

Vignette: Teresa

The following vignette focuses on Teresa, a 9-year-old girl with a diagnosis of autism (for a detailed account of Teresa, see Wolfberg, 1999). Teresa attended a special day class for children with moderate to severe disabilities in a public elementary school. Guided by her special education teacher, she participated in an integrated play group with one other classmate with special needs (Freddy) and three typically developing peers (Sook, Keila, and Ronny) from third- and fourth-grade general education classes. These groups met twice weekly for 30 minutes in Teresa's classroom. Teresa's familiarity and personal fascination with food preparation in her daily life provided a logical context for play with her peer group.

In the scenario in Table 11.1, Teresa initially showed an interest in playing with groceries and cooking in the play kitchen by engaging in functional or emerging pretend play sequences while her peers requested to play with Play-Doh. To establish a common focus on the play, the teacher suggested combining the two activities into a joint pretend play theme (baking). While verbally

Table 11.1. Scene from Teresa's integrated play group

Play scene		Interpretation of novice player's actions	Interpretation of teacher's actions
The children enter the play area. Teresa unloads a basket of groceries into the play refrigerator while Freddy bangs on a piece of plastic fruit, Sook fools around with a timer by the stove, and Keila and Ronny dump miniature cars onto the floor.		Teresa shows her interest in playing house by enacting a functional play sequence.	
Teacher:	Okay…now what did you guys decide on playing together?		The teacher verbally guides children to establish a common focus by posing leading questions about their play preferences.
Ronny:	I want to play ah…whatchamacallit, ah…you know, that sticky stuff?		
Teacher:	Play-Doh?		
Ronny:	Yeah, Play-Doh.		
Teacher:	Okay, is that something that everyone wants to play? Do Freddy, Teresa, and Sook want to play with it? Does Keila?		
Teresa:	[Facing Sook] Wanna play kitchen? Wanna play kitchen?	Teresa initiates social play by asking a peer to join her in a preferred activity. As the peer responds, Teresa vocalizes her play interest.	
Sook:	[Taps Teresa's arm] Teresa...		
Teresa:	Play kitchen, I'll play kitchen.		
Teacher:	Okay, Teresa said she wants to play with the kitchen. Teresa, everyone else seems to want to play with the Play-Doh. Would you like to set up the table and have the Play-Doh?		The teacher interprets initiations of novice and expert players and suggests a way to connect their play interests.
Teresa:	We eat, it time for dinner, time for dinner, dinnertime.	Teresa expands on idea of playing with Play-Doh in the kitchen by suggesting a pretend play theme.	
Teacher:	How about if we get the Play-Doh, we can pretend we're cooking?		The teacher reinforces Teresa's idea along with that of her peers.
Freddy:	Play-Doh. [Raises his hand]	Teresa and her peers affirm their shared interest and expand the theme by assigning and taking on roles in pretend play.	
Ronny:	Yeah.		
Teresa:	You cook, you cooking.		
Keila:	I'm the mother.		

Teacher: [To Sook and Ronny] Why don't you help move the table so people can sit down, and Freddy and I will get the Play-Doh.		The teacher directs and assists the children in organizing the play space and materials.
Teresa unloads the grocery basket as Sook and Ronny set up the table, Keila examines the small stove, and Freddy helps bring the Play-Doh and tools to the table.	Teresa incorporates preferred play materials into the evolving play context.	
Teacher: Here are some rolling pins....Let's see what else you need, cookie cutters....Teresa, do you want to help bake some things?		The teacher visually and verbally guides Teresa by offering materials and suggesting related pretend play theme.
Teresa: Bake a cake?	Teresa elaborates on the pretend play theme with a novel idea.	
Teacher: In the stove? Teresa: Yeah.		The teacher reinforces and extends Teresa's idea.
Teacher: [To Teresa] Why don't you sit down with Keila, and...[To Keila] Why don't you go over and ask [Teresa]? Keila: Teresa...do you want to go play with this?		The teacher guides children to establish a common focus.
Teresa: Yeah. [Without hesitation, walks over and takes a place at the table, and begins playing with the Play-Doh] Play with Play-Doh. Wabby, wabby, wabby Play-Doh. *Keila follows Teresa and sits beside her.*	Teresa responds to peer's invitation and begins exploring the play materials.	
Teresa: Hi Keila. Keila: Hi. Teresa: What is your name? Keila: Hi.	Teresa greets peer and uses delayed echolalia to engage her.	
Teresa: Hi. [To the teacher] I'll cook on stove, I'll cook it. Teresa cooking, Teresa cook.	Teresa greets teacher and comments on her play.	

(continued)

Table 11.1. (*continued*)

Play scene		Interpretation of novice player's actions	Interpretation of teacher's actions
Keila:	[To the teacher] You know what I'd do if I didn't have one of these things? [Referring to rolling pin] I'd go like this. [Flattens Play-Doh with hands]		
Teacher:	Why don't you show Teresa?		The teacher redirects peer to establish common focus with Teresa using the play materials.
Teresa:	[Watching Keila] Gotta cook, gotta bake Keila? Gotta cook.	Teresa comments on the activity to peer, expanding the pretend play theme.	
Keila:	[To Teresa] I'm making cookies.		
Teresa:	[Copies Keila flattening the Play-Doh, announcing excitedly] I'm making cookies too. We all making, we hope, we happy, we bake cookies. We put in oven, we put in oven right here. Okay Keila? I bake cookies, I bake it.	Teresa imitates peer and further expands pretend play theme while maintaining a common focus with peer.	

Source: Wolfberg (1999).

guiding the group and organizing materials for this activity, the teacher arranged for the expert players to sit beside Teresa and model their play for her. Teresa and Keila gradually achieved social coordination in play as they engaged in joint action, sharing, and taking turns with the Play-Doh. This gradually shifted to enacting pretend roles as Keila provided a context for Teresa by pointing out that she was baking cookies. Imitating Keila, Teresa announced that she, too, was baking cookies. In this coordinated event, Teresa showed the capacity for advanced pretend play by transforming Play-Doh into imaginary "cookies" that she planned to bake in the oven.

DIRECTIONS FOR FUTURE RESEARCH

One of the major questions to be addressed by future research pertains to the extent to which speech, language and overall communication skills can be advanced through scaffolded participation in peer play. Although we did observe remarkable improvements in the communicative initiations and/or spontaneous language use of the children included in our case studies, these changes were not specifically addressed in our research. Hopefully, further studies will examine such gains more systematically in a larger sample of children. One phenomenon that deserves special attention pertains to the observed changes in delayed echolalia. Engagement in scaffolded peer play seemed to invite the transformation of nonfocused echoes into more communicative and mitigated forms of echolalia and eventually into true language (for more in-depth discussions of different types of echolalia, see Prizant & Rydell, 1993, and Schuler, 1979). It seemed as if the peer interactions served to remove the literal and rigid edges from the echoing behaviors. By contextualizing delayed echolalic phrases, peers were provided with an incentive to repeat the target phrases and transform them into more functional and less literal forms; slight modifications were modeled in meaningful contexts. A better understanding of this kind of collectively negotiated mitigation process would be most useful to upgrade language intervention practices. What seems to be the special appeal of play is that it allows for almost unlimited contextualization. When compared with the logistics of field trips and incidental training arrangements, there are considerably fewer constraints in the world of make-believe. Although real life scenarios afford only limited opportunities for practice, play allows for almost endless repetition of targeted utterances; participants can play the check-out clerk over and over, as well as take turns being the clerk, incorporating all kinds of script variations and embellishments.

Our own clinical impressions suggest that the participating children with autism became more aware of the presence of others, displaying a greater sensitivity to the perspectives of others. The need to share and negotiate access to toys and to co-construct play scenarios may invite the formation of ToM. Is it possible that those children who learn to play with more competent peers are coaxed into the development of ToM? Future research might examine whether observed gains in both the social and cognitive dimensions of play are paralleled by changes in mentalizing skills. This could be evaluated in a number of different ways, combining quantitative and qualitative measures. Formalized tests specifically designed to assess such mentalizing skills should be supplemented by more naturalistic observations.

A closely related need for further investigation pertains to matters of affect and prosody. Judging from the spontaneous comments of different people asked to review videotapes of our play sessions, the longer the children with ASD are involved in play groups, the more difficult it becomes to tell them apart from their typical peers. Besides the observed gains in conventional object use, the overall affect of the children involved in play groups seems more typical. Positive changes in overall affect seem corroborated by the apparent normalization of the prosodic features of the children's vocalizations. If such changes could indeed be confirmed by future research efforts, one might indeed claim that participation in peer play serves as the ultimate antidote against behavior characteristic of autism.

CONCLUSIONS

This chapter addresses the paucity of play in children with ASD. It is argued that the facilitation of peer play and the related socialization processes are of critical importance. That little progress has been made in the teaching of play is attributed to the prevalence of highly directive intervention techniques that do not invite reciprocity and/or child initiations. We argue that more flexible, child-centered structures should be utilized and that access to peer culture is of critical importance in facilitating play. Features of effective scaffolding and a comprehensive model of intervention are described along with a case illustration. It is hypothesized that gains in play are typically accompanied by collateral improvements in speech, communication, and language as well as affect and that larger-scale future research is warranted to substantiate these claims.

REFERENCES

Baron-Cohen, S., Leslie, A.M., & Frith, U. (1985). Does the autistic child have a theory of mind? *Cognition, 21,* 37–46.

Baumgart, D., Brown, L., Pumpian, I., Nisbet, J., Ford, A., Sweet, M., Messina, R., & Schroeder, J. (1982). Principle of partial participation and individualized adaptations in educational programs for severely handicapped students. *Journal of The Association for the Severely Handicapped,* 7(2), 17–27.

Boucher, J., & Lewis, V. (1990). Guessing or creating? A reply to Baron-Cohen. *British Journal of Developmental Psychology, 8,* 205–206.

Bretherton, I. (Ed.). (1984). *Symbolic play: The development of social understanding.* San Diego: Academic Press.

Brown, A.L., & Campione, J.C. (1990). Communities of learning and thinking, or A context by any other name. *Human Development, 21,* 108–125.

Bruner, J.S. (1975). The ontogenesis of speech acts. *Journal of Child Language, 2,* 1–20.

Bruner, J.S. (1986). *Actual minds, possible worlds.* Cambridge, MA: Harvard University Press.

Castaneda, K.G., Schuler, A.L., & Watanabe, A.K. (1997). *Teachers as researchers: Implications for inclusion.* Workshop presented at the annual meeting of the Council for Exceptional Children, Salt Lake City, Utah.

Corsaro, W.A. (1985). *Friendship and peer culture in the early years.* Greenwich, CT: Ablex Publishing Corp.

Corsaro, W.A. (1988). Routing in the peer culture of American and Italian nursery school children. *Sociology of Education, 61*, 1–14.

Corsaro, W.A. (1992). Interpretive reproduction in children's peer cultures. *Social Psychology Quarterly, 55,* 160–177.

Corsaro, W.A., & Schwarz, K. (1991). Peer play and socialization in two cultures. In B. Scales, M. Almy, A. Nicolopoulou, & S. Ervin-Tripp (Eds.), *Play and the social context of development in early care and education* (pp. 234–254). New York: Teachers College Press.

Curcio, F. (1978). Sensorimotor functioning and communication in mute autistic children. *Journal of Autism and Childhood Schizophrenia, 8,* 181–189.

Dawson, G., & Osterling, J. (1997). Early intervention in autism. In M.J. Guralnick (Ed.), *The effectiveness of early intervention* (pp. 307–326). Baltimore: Paul H. Brookes Publishing Co.

Denzin, N. (1977). *Childhood socialization.* San Francisco: Jossey-Bass.

Dodge, K.A., Schlundt, D.C., Schocken, I., & Delugach, J.D. (1983). Social competence and children's sociometric status: The role of peer group entry strategies. *Merrill-Palmer Quarterly, 29,* 309–336.

Dunn, J. (1991). Understanding others: Evidence from naturalistic studies of children. In A. Whiten (Ed.), *Natural theories of mind.* Oxford, England: Blackwell Publishers, Ltd.

Ervin-Tripp, S. (1991). Play in language development. In B. Scales, M. Almy, A. Nicolopoulou, & S. Ervin-Tripp (Eds.), *Play and the social context of development in early care and education* (pp. 84–97). New York: Teachers College Press.

Fay, W.H., & Schuler, A.L. (Vol. Eds.). (1980). *Emerging language in autistic children.* In R.L. Schiefelbusch (Series Ed.), *Language intervention series* (Vol. 5). Baltimore: University Park Press.

Ferguson, D., & Baumgart, D. (1991). Partial participation revisited. *Journal of The Association for Persons with Severe Handicaps, 16*(4), 218–227.

Garvey, C. (1977). *Play.* Cambridge, MA: Harvard University Press.

Goldstein, H., & Cisar, C.L. (1992). Promoting interaction during sociodramatic play: Teaching scripts to typical preschoolers and classmates with disabilities. *Journal of Applied Behavior Analysis, 25,* 265–280.

Greenspan, S.I., & Wieder, S. (1997). Developmental patterns and outcomes in infants and children with disorders in relating and communication: A chart review of 200 cases of children with autistic spectrum diagnoses. *Journal of Developmental and Learning Disorders, 1*(1), 87–141.

Hadwin, J., Baron-Cohen, S., Howlin, P., & Hill, K. (1997). Does teaching theory of mind have an effect on the ability to develop conversation in children with autism? *Journal of Autism and Developmental Disorders, 27,* 519–539.

Harris, P. (1993). Pretending and planning. In S. Baron-Cohen, H. Tager-Flusberg, & D.J. Cohen (Eds.), *Understanding other minds: Perspectives from autism* (pp. 228–246). New York: Oxford University Press.

Harris, S.L., & Handleman, J.S. (1985). *Preschool education programs for children with autism.* Austin, TX: PRO-ED.

Hartup, W.W. (1979). The social worlds of childhood. *American Psychologist, 34,* 944–950.

Hartup, W.W. (1983). Peer relations. In M. Heatherington (Ed.), *Handbook of child psychology* (pp. 103–196). New York: John Wiley & Sons.

Hartup, W.W., & Sancilio, M.F. (1986). Children's friendships. In E. Schopler & G.B. Mesibov (Eds.), *Social behavior in autism* (pp. 61–80). New York: Plenum.

Hay, D.F. (1985). Learning to form relationships in infancy: Parallel attainments with parents and peers. *Developmental Review, 5,* 122–166.

Heath, S.B. (1989). The learner as cultural member. In M.L. Rice & R.L. Schiefelbusch (Eds.), *The teachability of language* (pp. 333–350). Baltimore: Paul H. Brookes Publishing Co.

Howes, C., Unger, O., & Matheson, C.C. (1992). *The collaborative construction of pretend.* Albany: State University of New York Press.

Howlin, P. (1981). The effectiveness of parent language training with autistic children. *Journal of Autism and Developmental Disorders, 11,* 54–69.

Howlin, P. (1986). The effects of behavioral approaches to language teaching for autistic children. *Australian Journal of Human Communication Disorders, 14*(1), 5–19.

Jarrold, C., Boucher, J., & Smith, P. (1993). Symbolic play in autism: A review. *Journal of Autism and Developmental Disorders, 23,* 281–307.

Kohler, F.W., Strain, P.S., Hoyson, M., & Jamison, B. (1997). Merging naturalistic teaching and peer-based strategies to address the IEP objectives of preschoolers with autism: An examination of structural and child behavior outcomes. *Focus on Autism and Other Developmental Disabilities, 12*(4), 196–218.

Lave, J., & Wenger, E. (1991). *Situated learning: Legitimate peripheral participation.* Cambridge, England: Cambridge University Press.

Leslie, A.M. (1987). Pretense and representation: The origins of "theory of mind." *Psychological Review, 94,* 412–426.

Lewis, V., & Boucher, J. (1988). Spontaneous, instructed and elicited play in relatively able autistic children. *British Journal of Developmental Psychology, 6*(4), 325–339.

Lord, C. (1984). Development of peer relations in children with autism. In F. Morrison, C. Lord, & D. Keating (Eds.), *Applied developmental psychology* (pp. 165–229). San Diego: Academic Press.

Lord, C., & Hopkins, M.J. (1986). The social behavior of autistic children with younger and same-age nonhandicapped peers. *Journal of Autism and Developmental Disorders, 16,* 249–262.

Lovaas, O.I. (1987). Behavioral treatment and normal educational and intellectual functioning in young autistic children. *Journal of Consulting and Clinical Psychology, 55*(1), 3–9.

Lyons, C.A. (1991). Helping a learning-disabled child enter the literate world. In D. DeFord, C.A. Lyons, & G.S. Pinnel (Eds.), *Bridges to literacy: Learning from reading recovery* (pp. 206–216). Portsmouth NH: Heinemann.

McCune-Nicholich, L. (1981). Toward symbolic functioning: Structure of early pretend games and potential parallels with language. *Child Development, 3,* 785–797.

McEachin, J., Smith, T., & Lovaas, O.I. (1993). Long term outcome for children with autism who received early intensive behavioral treatment. *American Journal on Mental Retardation, 97,* 359–372.

McHale, S. (1983). Social interactions of autistic and nonhandicapped children during free play. *American Journal of Orthopsychiatry, 53,* 81–91.

Mundy, P., Sigman, M.D., Ungerer, J., & Sherman, T. (1986). Defining the social deficits of autism: The contribution of non-verbal communication measures. *Journal of Child Psychology and Psychiatry and Allied Disciplines, 27*(5), 657–669.

Mundy, P., Sigman, M.D., Ungerer, J., & Sherman, T. (1987). Nonverbal communication and play correlates of language development in autistic children. *Journal of Autism and Developmental Disorders, 17,* 349–364.

Odom, S.L., & Brown, W.H. (1993). Social interaction skills intervention for young children with disabilities in integrated settings. In C.A. Peck, S.L. Odom, & D.D. Bricker (Eds.), *Integrating young children with disabilities into community programs: Ecological perspectives on research and implementation* (pp. 39–64). Baltimore: Paul H. Brookes Publishing Co.

Odom, S., & Strain, P. (1984). Peer-mediated approaches to promoting children's social interaction: A review. *American Journal of Orthopsychiatry, 54,* 544–557.

Papy, F., Papy, G., & Schuler, A.L. (1995). *La pensée hors langage: A la rencontre d'adolescents autistes* [Thought outside of language: Experiences of autistic adolescents]. Paris: Bayard Editions.

Parker, J.G., & Gottman, J.M. (1989). Social and emotional development in a relational context: Friendship interaction from early childhood to adolescence. In T.J. Berndt & G.W. Ladd (Eds.), *Peer relationships in child development* (pp. 95–131). New York: John Wiley & Sons.

Parten, M.B. (1932). Social participation among preschool children. *Journal of Abnormal and Social Psychology, 27,* 243–269.

Peck, C.A., Schuler, A.L., Tomlinson, C., Thiemer, R.K., & Haring, T. (1984). *The social competence curriculum project: A guide to instructional communicative interactions.* Special Education Research Institute. Santa Barbara: University of California at Santa Barbara.

Pellegrini, A. (1985). Relations between symbolic play and literate behavior: In L. Galda & A. Pellegrini (Eds.), *Play, language and story: The development of children's literate behavior* (pp. 79–97). Greenwich, CT: Ablex Publishing Corp.

Piaget, J. (1962). *Play, dreams, and imitation in childhood.* New York: W.W. Norton.

Prizant, B.M., & Rydell, P.J. (1993). Assessment and intervention considerations for unconventional verbal behavior. In S.F. Warren & J. Reichle (Series Eds.) & J. Reichle & D. Wacker (Vol. Eds.), *Communication and language intervention series: Vol. 3. Communicative alternatives to challenging behavior: Integrating functional assessment and intervention strategies* (pp. 263–297). Baltimore: Paul H. Brookes Publishing Co.

Riquet, C., Taylor, N., Benaroya, S., & Klein, L. (1981). Symbolic play in autistic, Downs and normal children of equivalent mental age. *Journal of Autism and Developmental Disorders, 11,* 439–448.

Roeyers, H. (1996). The influence of nonhandicapped peers on the social interactions of children with pervasive developmental disorder. *Journal of Autism and Developmental Disorders, 26,* 303–321.

Rogoff, B. (1990). *Apprenticeship in thinking.* New York: Oxford University Press.

Rubin, K.H. (1980). Fantasy play: Its role in the development of social skills and social cognition. In K.H. Rubin (Ed.), *Children's play* (pp. 69–84). San Francisco: Jossey-Bass.

Schoenwald, B. (1997). *Structure: A forgotten dimension of inclusion.* Unpublished field study, School of Education, San Francisco State University, San Francisco.

Schuler, A.L. (1979). Echolalia: Issues and clinical applications. *Journal of Speech and Hearing Disorders, 44,* 411–434.

Schuler, A.L. (1995). Thinking in autism: Differences in learning and development. In K. Quill (Ed.), *Teaching children with autism: Methods to enhance communication and socialization* (pp. 11–31). Albany, NY: Delmar Publishers.

Schuler, A.L. (1998). *Facilitating communicative competence: Matters of context and interaction style.* Paper presented at the 20th National Congress of the Spanish Association of Logopedics, Phoniatrics and Audiology, Barcelona, Spain.

Schuler, A.L., Gonsier-Gerdin, J., & Wolfberg, P. (1990). The efficacy of speech and language intervention: Autism. *Seminars in Speech and Language, 11,* 242–251.

Schuler, A.L., Prizant, B.M., & Wetherby, A.M. (1997). Enhancing language and communication: Prelinguistic approaches. In D. Cohen & F. Volkmar (Eds.), *Handbook of autism and pervasive developmental disorders* (2nd ed., pp. 539–571). New York: John Wiley & Sons.

Selmer-Olsen, I. (1993). Children's culture and adult presentation of this culture. *International Play Journal, 1,* 191–202.

Sigman, M., & Ungerer, J.A. (1984). Cognitive and language skills in autistic, mentally retarded, and normal children. *Developmental Psychology, 20,* 293–302.

Smilansky, S. (1968). *The effects of sociodramatic play on disadvantaged preschool children.* New York: John Wiley & Sons.

Smith, F. (1983). *Essays into literacy.* Portsmouth, NH: Heinemann.

Smith, F. (1988). *Joining the literacy club.* Portsmouth, NH: Heinemann.

Smith, P., & Vollstedt. (1985). An empirical study of play and the criteria used to judge play, *Child Development, 56.*

Stanovich, K.E., & Stanovich, P.J. (1996). Rethinking the concept of learning disabilities: The demise of aptitude/achievement discrepancy. In D.R. Olson & N. Torrance (Eds.), *Education and human development: New models of learning, teaching and schooling.* Malden, MA: Blackwell Publishers.

Strain, P.S., & Kohler, F.W. (1995). Analyzing predictors of daily social skill performance. *Behavioral Disorders, 21,* 79–88.

Tomasello, M., Kruger, A.C., & Ratner, H.H. (1993). Cultural learning. *Behavioral and Brain Sciences, 16,* 495–552.

Van Berckelaer-Onnes, I.A. (1994). Play training for autistic children. In J. Hellendoorn, R. van der Kooij, & B. Sutton-Smith (Eds.), *Play and intervention* (pp. 173–182). Albany: State University of New York Press.

Vandell, D.L., & Wilson, K.S. (1982). Social interaction in the first year: Infants' social skills with peers versus mother. In K.H. Rubin & H.S. Ross (Eds.), *Peer relationships and social skills in childhood* (pp. 187–208). New York: Springer Verlag.

Vygotsky, L.S. (1962). *Thought and language* (F. Hanfmann & G. Velar, Trans.). Cambridge, MA: MIT Press. (Original work published 1934)

Vygotsky, L. (1966). Play and its role in the mental development of the child. *Soviet Psychology, 12,* 6–18. (Original work published 1933)

Vygotsky, L.S. (1978). *Mind in society: The development of higher psychological processes* (M. Cole, V. John-Steiner, S. Scribner, & E. Souberman, Eds. and Trans.). Cambridge, MA: Harvard University Press.

Wetherby, A.M., & Prutting, C.A. (1984). Profiles of communicative and cognitive-social abilities in autistic children. *Journal of Speech and Hearing Research, 27,* 364–377.

Wing, L., & Attwood, T. (1987). Syndromes of autism and atypical development. In D.J. Cohen & A.M. Donnellan (Eds.), *Handbook of autism and pervasive developmental disorders* (pp. 3–19). New York: John Wiley & Sons.

Wing, L., & Gould., J. (1979). Severe impairments of social interaction and associated abnormalities in children: Epidemiology and classification. *Journal of Autism and Developmental Disorders, 9,* 11–29.

Wolfberg, P.J. (1995a). Enhancing children's play. In K.A. Quill (Ed.), *Teaching children with autism: Strategies to enhance communication and socialization* (pp. 193–218). New York: Delmar Publishers Inc.

Wolfberg, P.J. (1995b). Supporting children with autism in play groups with typical peers: A description of a model and related research. *International Play Journal, 3,* 38–51.

Wolfberg, P.J. (1999). *Play and imagination in children with autism.* New York: Teachers College Press.

Wolfberg, P.J., & Schuler, A.L. (1993). Integrated play groups: A model for promoting the social and cognitive dimensions of play in children with autism. *Journal of Autism and Developmental Disorders, 23,* 467–489.

Wolfberg, P.J., & Schuler, A.L. (1999). Fostering peer interaction, imaginative play, and spontaneous language in children with autism. *Child Language Teaching and Therapy, 15*(1), 41–52.

12

A Developmental Approach to Difficulties in Relating and Communicating in Autism Spectrum Disorders and Related Syndromes

Stanley I. Greenspan and Serena Wieder

Most developmental and learning disorders, including autism spectrum disorders (ASDs), are nonspecific with regard to etiology and pathophysiology and are therefore best characterized in terms of types and degrees of functional limitations as well as symptoms (which are often only one expression of a functional limitation, e.g., echolalia instead of pragmatic language). Yet, both historically and recently, research has focused on syndromes comprising symptoms and groups of symptoms with only partial emphasis on the broad range of important functional capacities that often underlie symptoms and determine overall adaptation.

Many practitioners, especially speech-language, occupational, and physical therapists and educators, have been using and expanding a functional approach geared to each child's unique characteristics. For example, oral-motor exercises can help with the motor planning and sequencing needed for language development, visuospatial problem-solving approaches can help with the "big picture" thinking necessary for more abstract academic challenges, and auditory discrimination work can facilitate phonemic awareness as a basis for reading. With increasing knowledge about underlying processing capacities and functional abilities, it is timely to further systematize the functional approach and explore more fully its implications for improving assessment and intervention practices.

A functional approach can change not only the way we think about developmental disorders, including ASDs, but also what is included in the re-

This chapter has been adapted by permission from Greenspan, S.I., & Wieder, S. (1999, Fall). A functional developmental approach to autism spectrum disorders. *Journal of The Association for Persons with Severe Handicaps, 24*(3), 147–161.

search base to improve assessment and interventions. Historically, research reviews on autism have been limited to assessment, intervention, or etiologic studies on children with ASD. From a functional perspective, however, the use of a syndrome to define the research base may not be appropriate. Instead, the research base should be defined by the relevant areas of functioning, some of which are impaired in a variety of syndromes or problems. For example, should all studies on improving auditory processing be included when considering interventions for children with receptive language problems (some of whom may also evidence ASD), or should practitioners only look at those language studies that deal with children with autism? Is the general literature on motor planning and sequencing relevant, or is only the motor planning literature on autism relevant? Almost all children with autism have severe motor planning and sequencing problems, but so do lots of other children. In short, should interventionists use the more limited autism literature or the broader literature on various types of functional and processing impairments, which are present in ASDs as well as in many other types of disorders?

Because there is not yet a clearly identified etiologic mechanism or well-described pathophysiologic pathway for autism, assumptions must be modest and assessments and interventions should be based on what is clearly observable and known. What is observable and known about ASDs are the functional limitations in critical areas, including language, motor planning and sequencing, and modulation. Therefore, all relevant research on these functional areas must be used to improve assessments and interventions. In fact, as most clinicians recognize, there are huge differences among children with ASD: One may be relatively strong in visuospatial processing, whereas another in auditory-verbal memory. A given child with ASD may be more similar to a given child with Down syndrome in terms of motor planning or visuospatial processing than to another child with ASD. A functional approach allows for the study of all of the relevant functional impairments in their unique configurations and, in this way, broadens the research and clinical basis for improving assessments and intervention for a range of developmental disorders, including autism.

In a functional approach, assessments and interventions must include all relevant areas of functioning and deal with each child and family in terms of their unique profiles of functional limitations. Since the early 1980s, we have created a developmental approach, the Developmental, Individual-Difference, Relationship-Based (DIR) model, that engages a child at his or her current level of functioning, works with the unique features of his or her nervous system, and utilizes intensive interactive experiences that are part of ongoing relationships to enable him or her to master new capacities (Greenspan, 1992a; Greenspan & Wieder, 1998). The model considers the relevant areas of functioning and helps with the construction of each child's developmental profile.

THE DEVELOPMENTAL, INDIVIDUAL-DIFFERENCE, RELATIONSHIP-BASED MODEL

The DIR model allows developmental disorders to be viewed in a unique way. Traditionally, clinicians have looked at children with disabilities in terms of syndromes and have used the global labels *autism, autism spectrum, pervasive developmental disorder (PDD), mental retardation, Down syndrome,* and so forth. Underlying these assumptions is the belief that children classified as having each syndrome are very similar to each other—more similar than they are different. But as researchers have looked at the development of infants and very young children, the focus has shifted from older children who have lived with these syndromes for years to children from infancy to 3 years old who are just beginning to have difficulties. The field also has formed a different picture of the nature of these challenges. Researchers have found that children who traditionally have been grouped in the same categories are sometimes quite different from each other. In some cases the differences are greater than the similarities.

As we have worked with many different children from the time they were babies until they were 8–10 years old, we have evolved a developmental model for working with them. This approach focuses on helping each child climb the developmental ladder; specifically, it works to help each child master the seven fundamental developmental skills (attention and focus, engaging and relating, nonverbal gesturing, affect cuing, complex problem solving, symbolic communication, abstract and logical thinking) that underlie all intelligence and interactions with the world. The achievement of each of these skills represents a new level, or milestone, of development. These basic skills are not the traditional cognitive skills of identifying shapes, naming letters, and counting. They are not the traditional social skills of taking turns and sitting still. They are more fundamental; they are called *functional emotional processes* because they are based on early emotional interactions and provide the basis for intellect and sense of self as well as the basis for such familiar skills as counting and taking turns.

Three aspects of the child's world come together to influence how well he or she masters these functional emotional milestones. The first is the child's biology, the neurological potential or challenges that enhance or impede his or her functioning. The second is the child's own interactive patterns with his or her parents, teachers, grandparents, and others. The third is the patterns of the family, the culture, and the larger environment. In the DIR model, these three areas are worked with as part of the assessment and intervention process. The basic categories in the DIR model include the functional developmental level; motor, sensory, and affective patterns; and relationship and affective interaction patterns.

Functional Developmental Level

The functional developmental level looks at how the child integrates all of his or her communicative, cognitive, and emotional capacities to meet meaningful goals. These include the capacities for shared attention, engagement, nonverbal gestural and affective communication, complex problem-solving interactions, the purposeful and meaningful use of ideas, and building logical connections between these ideas. The support for these functional developmental levels is reviewed elsewhere (see Greenspan, 1979b, 1989, 1992a, 1997). These core functional capacities include the following:

1. *The dual ability to take an interest in the sights, sounds, and sensations of the world and to calm oneself:* This capacity includes attending to multisensory affective experience and at the same time organizing a calm, regulated state and experiencing pleasure.
2. *The ability to engage in relationships with other people:* This ability includes engaging with and evidencing affective preference and pleasure for a caregiver.
3. *The ability to engage in two-way communication with gestures:* This kind of communication includes imitating and responding to two-way presymbolic gestural communication.
4. *The ability to create complex gestures or to string together a series of actions into an elaborate and deliberate problem-solving sequence:* These actions involve organizing chains of two-way communication (opening and closing many circles of communication in a row), maintaining communication across space, integrating affective polarities, and synthesizing an emerging prerepresentational organization of self and other.
5. *The ability to create ideas:* This capacity includes representing (symbolizing) affective experience (e.g., pretend play, functional use of language). It should be noted that this ability calls for higher-level auditory and verbal sequencing ability.
6. *The ability to build bridges between ideas to make them reality based and logical:* This ability includes creating representational (symbolic) categories and gradually building conceptual bridges between these categories, thus providing a foundation for such basic personality functions as reality testing, impulse control, self–other representational differentiation, affect labeling and discrimination, stable mood, and a sense of time and space that allows for logical planning. It should be noted that this ability rests not only on complex auditory and verbal processing abilities but also on visuospatial abstracting capacities.

Motor, Sensory, and Affective Patterns

This category in the DIR model concerns the degree to which the infant or child is over- or underreactive to sensations in each sensory modality such as touch, movement, sound, sight, and so forth, including auditory processing, visuospatial processing, and motor planning and sequencing. The biologically based individual differences are the result of genetic, prenatal, perinatal, and maturational variations and/or deficits and can be characterized functionally as follows (see Chapter 7 for further discussion):

1. Sensory modulation, including hypo- and hyperreactivity in each sensory modality
2. Sensory processing in each sensory modality (e.g., the capacity to decode and comprehend sequences, configurations, and/or abstract patterns)
3. Sensory-affective processing in each modality (e.g., the ability to process and react to affect, including the capacity to connect "intent" or affect to motor planning and sequencing, language, and symbols). This processing capacity may be especially relevant in ASDs (Greenspan & Wieder, 1997, 1998).
4. Motor planning and sequencing, including the capacity to sequence actions, behaviors, and symbols (e.g., thoughts, words, visual images, spatial concepts)

Relationship and Affective Interaction Patterns

This area of inquiry concerns whether the parents, caregivers, and others who interact with the child understand his or her functional level and individual differences. This includes existing caregiver, parent, and family patterns. Interaction patterns between the child and caregivers and family members bring the child's sensory and motor needs and sensitivities into the larger developmental picture and can contribute to the negotiation of the child's functional developmental capacities.

Developmentally appropriate interactions mobilize the child's intentions and affects and enable the child to broaden his or her range of experience at each level of development and to move from one functional developmental level to the next. In contrast, interactions in which caregivers or others do not consider the child's functional developmental level or individual differences undermine progress. For example, if a caregiver is aloof and an infant is underreactive and self-absorbed, then that caregiver may not help the child become engaged. Our clinical experience has shown that depressed caregivers will often talk to their child in a slow rhythm with much longer pauses than expected. Sometimes a child becomes preoccupied and self-absorbed because of a combination of auditory processing problems and caregiver patterns that are not sufficiently interactive to compensate for the processing difficulties. An intrusive caregiver may overwhelm an infant, especially if the infant is overly sensitive to touch and sound; such intrusion may lead to withdrawal or unpurposeful, chaotic behavior. A disorganized family may throw so many meanings (both in language and in ambiguous nonverbal affect) at a child that they undermine an emerging capacity for emotional thinking and sense of reality, especially if the child has difficulties with auditory-verbal or spatial sequencing. (See Chapter 15 for a discussion of challenges facing families.)

Autism, Autism Spectrum Disorders, and Pervasive Developmental Disorders

As indicated previously, the DIR model takes into account all of a child's developmental capacities in the context of his or her unique biologically based processing profile, family relationships, and interactive patterns. As a functional approach, DIR uses the complex interactions between biology and experience to understand behavior. An appropriate assessment of all of the relevant functional areas requires a number of sessions with the child and family, which must begin with discussions and observations. Structured tests, if indicated, should be implemented later to further understand specific functional areas. (See Greenspan, 1992a, and Greenspan & Wieder, 1998, for details on this approach to assessment.)

The functional assessment leads to an individualized functional profile that captures each child's unique developmental features and serves as a basis for creating individually tailored intervention programs (i.e., tailoring the program to the child rather than fitting the child to a general program). The profile describes the child's functional developmental capacities and contributing biological processing differences and environmental interactive patterns, including the different interaction patterns available to the child at home, at school, with peers, and in other environments. The profile should include all areas of dysfunction, not simply the ones that are more obviously associated with pathologic symptoms. For example, a preschooler's lack of ability to symbolize a broad range of emotional interests and themes in either pretend play or talk is just as important to note, if not more important, than the same preschooler's tendency to be perseverative or self-stimulatory. In fact, clinically we have often seen that as a child's range of symbolic expression broadens, perseverative and self-stimulatory tendencies decrease.

It is important to reiterate that because the profile captures the child's individual variations, children with the same diagnosis (e.g., ASD) may have very different profiles and children with different diagnoses may have similar profiles. A child evidencing perseveration, self-stimulation, and partial self-absorption may be oversensitive to sound and touch, with relative strengths in visuospatial processing and moderate degrees of impairment in auditory processing. Such a child may be capable of some engagement and preverbal communication and islands of symbolic communicating. His or her family may work hard to engage and communicate. Another child sharing the ASD diagnosis and symptoms of perseveration, self-stimulation, and social isolation may evidence quite a different pattern, such as underreactivity to sensation and craving of sensory input, relatively weak visuospatial processing, severely impaired auditory processing, an inability for even the most rudimentary patterns of engagement or symbolic communication, and a family pattern characterized by little else than attempts at restraining the child from episodic aggression. A third child diagnosed with mental retardation requiring intermittent to limited support may share the profile of the first child, with the exception of being more engaged because of somewhat less sensory overreactivity. A fourth child with mental retardation who also has some capacity to engage with caregivers may resemble more closely the second child.

In the functional approach, the child's profile captures his or her unique features and orients the clinician toward the proper assessment and intervention plan. In addition, the developmental profile, which highlights particular biologically based processing patterns, may relate to underlying biological mechanisms more readily than syndromes with differing processing patterns (which have thus far been nonspecific in terms of underlying biological mechanisms). The functional profile is updated with continuing clinical observations as part of the intervention. These ongoing observations and updated profiles then serve as a basis for revising the child's intervention program. The functional approach, therefore, provides a broad and yet highly individualized perspective in which new research findings can be interpreted.

The functional approach enables the clinician to consider each functional impairment separately, explore different explanations, and resist the temptation to assume that impairments are necessarily tied together as part of a syndrome (unless all alternative explanations have been ruled out). For example, hand flapping often is related to motor problems and is seen when children with a variety of motor problems become excited or overloaded. Many conditions, including cerebral palsy, autism, hypotonia, and dyspraxia, involve motor problems and, at times, hand flapping. Yet this symptom is often assumed to be uniquely a part of ASDs. Similarly, sensory over- or underreactivity is present in many disorders and developmental variations yet is also often assumed to be a unique part of autism. The functional approach does not detract from an understanding of existing syndromes. In fact, over time it may clarify which symptoms are unique to particular syndromes, lead to new classifications, and further tease out biological and functional patterns. Constructing the child's profile of functional capacities through appropriate clinical assessments enables the clinician to tailor the intervention program to the child's and family's unique features rather than to make the child fit the program, based on some broad, but nonspecific, diagnostic criteria.

For reasons not yet entirely clear (but that may go beyond improvements in early identification services), programs that serve infants and young children and their families report an increasing number of children with severe relationship and communication problems. Very often these children seemed to be making reasonable progress until 12–24 months of age. Parents recall that their child enjoyed hugging and cuddling and began purposeful gesturing "on time," and family videotapes often document these observations. But between the ages of 12 and 15 months, the preverbal, gestural system of communication had begun to stop developing. The toddler did not, for example, grab her father's hand, lead him to the kitchen, and vocalize or gesture for a certain food. At the same time, the child began showing (or intensifying existing) oversensitivity, or became more reactive, to certain sounds or kinds of touch. The child no longer seemed to understand even simple words or gestures, and language stopped developing. Gradually parents noticed that their child was increasingly withdrawn and aimless and was engaging more often in repetitive behavior.

Many of these behaviors, however, do not fully fit the original description of autism coined in 1943 by Leo Kanner, a child psychiatrist. According to Kanner, the child with autism's "outstanding fundamental disorder" is the "inability to relate . . . from the beginning of life . . . an extreme aloneness that . . . disregards, ignores, shuts out anything . . . from the outside." These behaviors are systematized in the American Psychiatric Association's *Diagnostic and Statistical Manual of Mental Disorders, Fourth Edition* (DSM-IV; 1994), in the category of PDD or ASD. PDD has a number of subtypes, including autistic disorder (the more classic and severe form) and pervasive developmental disorder-not otherwise specified (PDD-NOS), a more general type diagnosed when there is a basic impairment in relating and communicating but when all of the formal criteria for autistic disorder are not met.

As more children are diagnosed with ASD at younger ages, clinical features challenge the existing conceptual framework. Children's patterns of relating, communicating, and expressing emotions seem to fall along a continuum (e.g., from somewhat interactive and related to self-absorbed and perseverative) rather than into one distinct type. Because of the lack of more appropriate diagnostic categories, clinicians use the diagnosis of PDD-NOS for many children who have various combinations of social, language, and cognitive dysfunctions, even when they show varying degrees of social relatedness. Most parents, however, are aware that autism and PDD-NOS are part of the same broad PDD category (see Chapter 2 for further discussion of early identification and diagnosis).

For many children, according to a review of 200 cases (Greenspan & Wieder, 1997), the relationship problem is not clearly in evidence in the first year of life, as thought by Kanner (1943), but appears in the second and third years, in connection with difficulties with processing sensations. In contrast to other studies, we have found that the majority of children first develop clear symptoms in the second and third years of life. Furthermore, each child has his or her own unique profile for processing sensations. These profiles vary in sensory reactivity (e.g., tactile, auditory, visual), sensory processing (e.g., auditory-verbal, visuospatial), muscle tone, and motor planning or sequencing. Also, the assumption that children with PDD tend to remain relatively unrelated to others and to be rigid, mechanical, and idiosyncratic (as stated in the DSM-IV) is not supported by our clinical experience. With early diagnosis and a comprehensive, integrated, and developmental, relationship-based treatment approach, many children originally diagnosed with PDD are learning to relate to others with warmth, empathy, and emotional flexibility (Greenspan & Wieder, 1997). We have worked with a number of children who were diagnosed with autism or PDD-NOS between the ages of 18 and 30 months and who, now older, are fully communicative (using complex sentences adaptively), creative, warm, loving, and joyful. They attend typical schools, are mastering early academic tasks, enjoy friendships, and are especially adept at imaginative play. Although many children make very slow progress and some make almost no progress, it is important to document and further understand the large range of developmental paths that different children with ASD can take (Greenspan & Wieder, 1997). The term *multisystem developmental disorder* has been introduced (ZERO TO THREE/National Center for Clinical Infant Programs, 1994) to characterize children who have communication problems and are perseverative but who can relate or have the potential for relating with joy and warmth. The capacity to become comfortable with intimacy and dependency and to experience joy often appears to be attainable early in the treatment program. In addition, cognitive potential cannot be explored until interactive experiences are routine.

The traditional pessimistic prognosis for most children with ASD is based on patterns of experience with children whose treatment programs tend to be mechanical and structured rather than based on individual differences, relationships, affect, and emotional cuing. Approaches that do not pull the child into *spontaneous,* joyful relationship patterns may intensify rather than remediate the difficulty. We have observed that even with older children with ASD-type patterns, as more spontaneous affect based on emotionally robust gestural or verbal interactions appears, perseveration and idiosyncratic behavior decrease and relatedness increases.

The existence of many types of relationship and communication problems, of significant individual differences among children, and of greater potential for intellectual and emotional growth than formerly thought forces practitioners to reconsider long-held assumptions about ASDs. It is especially important to reconsider the notion of a fixed biological deficit that prevents people from relating to others and experiencing joy, happiness, and, eventually, empathy. Evidence suggests that biological processing deficits can be dealt with by the child in different ways and that certain types of intervention can enhance adaptive outcomes, including joy and creativity.

UNIQUE FUNCTIONAL IMPAIRMENT UNDERLYING AUTISM SPECTRUM DISORDERS

Looking at how certain functional capacities do or do not arise may help practitioners understand important features of ASDs and at the same time illustrate why a functional approach helps us understand the relationship between adaptive capacities and pathologic symptoms and sets the stage for creating an appropriate intervention. For example, if an infant, toddler, or preschooler has auditory-verbal, visuospatial, and/or perceptual-motor processing difficulties, these difficulties may make ordinary relating and communication challenging. The people in the child's immediate environment often will not be able to find some special way to engage and interact with him or her. Without appropriate interaction, vital social learning may not occur during important periods of development. For example, critical social skills (e.g., reciprocal affective and motor gesturing and comprehending the "rules" of complex social interactions) as well as patterns of recognition, a sense of self, and early forms of thinking are learned at an especially rapid rate between 12 and 24 months of age. A deficit in these skills could easily look like a primary deficit rather than a reaction to underlying biologically based processing difficulties. By the time these children come to professional attention, their challenging interaction patterns with their caregivers may be intensifying their difficulties. They are likely to perplex; confuse; frustrate; and undermine purposeful, interactive communication of even very competent parents. Parents often rely as much on the child's communicative signals as the child relies on the parents' signals. Parents are not prepared for a toddler who looks away or withdraws from touch. Losing engagement and intentional, interactive relatedness to key caregivers, a child may withdraw more idiosyncratically into his or her own world.

This hypothesis suggests, therefore, that there are biologically based processing (regulatory) difficulties that contribute to but are not decisive in determining relationship and communication difficulties. When problems are perceived early, caregivers and children can learn, with appropriate professional help, to work around the regulatory dysfunctions and their associated relationship and communication difficulties and form varying degrees of warm, empathetic, and satisfying relationships.

Our observations further suggest that children at risk for ASD may have a unique type of biologically based processing deficit involving the connection of affect or intent to motor planning and sequencing capacities and auditory processing and language capacities (Greenspan & Wieder, 1997). A child uses his or her *intent* or affect to provide direction for actions and meaning for his or her words. Typically, during the second year of life, intentional problem-solving behavior emerges, and later meaningful use of language develops, based in part on the child's ability to connect *intent* to his or her motor sequencing and emerging capacity to form symbols (Greenspan, 1997). Our hypothesis (i.e., the affect diagnosis hypothesis) is that when these critical connections are not formed, the child is vulnerable to aimless or repetitive use of behavior and/or words rather than intentional use of behavior and/or words and that the level of functioning in many of the components of the central nervous system that are not under intentional control, such as auditory memory, may determine the different symptoms and presence or absence of splinter skills (e.g., rote recall of entire books).

THE DEVELOPMENTAL, INDIVIDUAL-DIFFERENCE, RELATIONSHIP-BASED MODEL INTERVENTION PROGRAM

The DIR mobilizes the child's emerging developmental capacities and is based on the thesis that affective interaction can harness cognitive and emotional growth (Feuerstein, Rand, Hoffman, & Miller, 1979; Feuerstein et al., 1981; Greenspan, 1979a, 1979b, 1989, 1997; Klein, Wieder, & Greenspan, 1987). The following principles guide caregiver–child interactions so that they are developmentally appropriate in the fullest sense. These principles also guide the work of the therapeutic team so that the speech-language and occupational therapy, in addition to their traditional goals, mobilize fundamental developmental processes. The primary goal of the DIR intervention is to enable children to form a sense of themselves as intentional, interactive individuals and to develop cognitive language and social capacities from this basic sense of intentionality.

Because children with severe problems in relating and communicating often lack the most basic foundation for interpersonal experiences (i.e., they often are not interactive in the purposeful way that ordinary 8-month-olds are), much of the experience that they might use to abstract a sense of their own personhood is not available to them. Therefore, for these children, the earliest therapeutic goals often must be geared to the first steps in the developmental progression, that is, to foster focus and concentration (shared attention), engagement with the human world, and two-way intentional communication (and then symbolic communication) to create the interactive experiences the child can use to abstract a sense of self and form higher-level cognitive and social capacities. As noted previously, mobilizing these basic developmental processes is especially important because our observations further suggest that children at risk for ASD may have a unique type of biologically based processing deficit involving the connection of affect or intent to motor planning and sequencing capacities and auditory processing and language capacities (Greenspan & Wieder, 1997).

A comprehensive treatment program for an infant, toddler, or preschooler with these problems involves helping the child reestablish the developmental sequence that went awry, with a special focus on helping the child become more affectively connected and intentional. This means determining which of the six fundamental developmental processes outlined previously (shared attention, engagement, reciprocal gesturing, preverbal problem solving, creating ideas, and building bridges between ideas) have been mastered fully, partially, or not at all and using understanding of the child's biological differences to establish a relationship that creates interactive, affective opportunities to negotiate the partially mastered or unmastered developmental process. Rather than focus only on isolated behaviors or skills, the DIR approach focuses on the fundamental functional developmental processes, which underlie particular symptoms or behaviors. For example, rather than trying to teach a child who is perseveratively spinning the wheels on a car to play with something else or to play with the car appropriately, a practitioner using the DIR approach would draw on the child's interest and, warmly smiling, spin the wheels in the opposite direction to get reciprocal, affective interaction started.

The DIR approach, therefore, includes an emphasis on the following: 1) affect, intent, and relationships; 2) the child's developmental level; and 3) individual differences in motor, sensory, affective, cognitive, and language functioning. This group of interactive experiences (sometimes referred to as *floor time*) at home often ranges from 2 to 5 hours a day. Also, family patterns, feelings, and coping efforts are addressed continually (Greenspan, 1992a, 1992b; Greenspan & Wieder, 1998).

In addition, a comprehensive program often includes interactive speech-language therapy (three to five times per week), occupational therapy (two to five times per week), and consultation to parents for floor time interactions and family support. During the preschool years, an important component of such a program is an inclusive preschool (i.e., one quarter of a class is children with disabilities, and three quarters of the class is children without disabilities) that has teachers especially gifted in interacting with challenging children and working with them on interactive gesturing and affective cuing and early symbolic communication. The DIR model enables children with disabilities to interact with children who are interactive and communicative (e.g., as a child reaches out for relationships and communication, there are peers who reach back).

All the elements in the DIR model have a long tradition, including speech-language therapy, occupational therapy, special and early childhood education, and floor time–type interactions with parents (which is consistent with the developmentally appropriate practice guidelines of the National Association for the Education of Young Children and pragmatic speech-language therapy practices, both of which attempt to foster preverbal and symbolic communication and thinking). The DIR model, however, contributes to these traditional practices by further defining the child's developmental level, individual temperament, and processing differences and the need for certain types of interactions in terms of a comprehensive program in which all the elements work together toward common goals.

In this model, the therapeutic program must begin as soon as possible so that the children and their parents are reengaged in emotional interactions that use the children's emerging but not fully developed capacities for communication (often initially with gestures rather than words). The longer such children remain uncommunicative and the more parents lose their sense of their child's relatedness, the more deeply the children tend to withdraw and become perseverative and self-stimulatory.

Such an intensive approach, however, is not intended to overwork or stress a child. The child's state of mind is considered and the interactive activities that are recommended are part of playful interactions in which the child's interests and initiative are followed and opportunities are created for joyful, soothing, and pleasurable interactions. When the child is tired, the playful interactions might involve the child's showing the parents or verbalizing to the parents where it is best to rub his or her back or feet. Passive television watching (except for half an hour per day) and rote memory exercises such as memorizing letters or numbers are not recommended.

The DIR interventions are fundamentally different from behavioral skill building, play therapy, or psychotherapy. The primary goal of the DIR intervention program (floor time) is for children to form a sense of themselves as intentional, interactive individuals; develop cognitive language and social capacities from this basic sense of intentionality; and progress through the seven functional milestones.

STEPS IN THE THERAPEUTIC PROCESS

As one fosters focus and engagement, one must pay attention to the child's regulatory profile, as described previously. For example, if the child is overreactive to sound, talking to him or her in a normal voice may lead him or her to become more aimless and withdrawn. If the child is overreactive to sights, then bright lights and even very animated facial expressions may be overwhelming. If the child is underreactive to sensations of sound and visuospatial input, however, talking in a strong voice and using animated facial expressions in a well-lit room may help him or her attend. Similarly, in terms of receptive language skills, if the child can already decode a complex rhythm, then making interesting sounds in complex patterns may be helpful. On the other hand, if the child can only decode very simple, two-sequence rhythms and perhaps understands single words, then using single words (not as symbolic communication, but as gestural communication) and using simple patterns of sound may help him or her engage.

One may find that the child remains relatively better focused while in motion, such as while being swung. Certain movement rhythms may be more effective than others. For some children, fast rhythms, such as one swing per second, may be ideal. For others, slow rhythms, such as one swing every 4–6 seconds, may be better. Different kinds of tactile input, such as firm pressure on the back or the arms or the legs, may foster concentration and focus. Large motor movement and joint compressing (e.g., jumping on a bed, any trampoline-like motion) may also foster attending. Each infant and child is unique.

Fostering a sense of intimacy is especially difficult. Therefore, as one helps a child attend and engage, taking advantage of the child's own natural interests is of critical importance. It is most helpful to follow the child's lead and look for opportunities for that visceral sense of pleasure and intimacy that leads him or her to *want* to relate to the human world. Intimacy is further supported as one works on forming simple, and then more complex, gestural communications.

For example, the father of a very withdrawn child was only verbalizing to his child. The therapist suggested trying simple gestural interactions first. The father put his hand on a toy car very gently as his son was exploring it and pointed to a particular part, as though to say, "What's that?" But, in pointing, the father actually moved the car, so the son felt the car moving in his hands and noticed his father's involvement without becoming upset. The son took the car back but looked at where the father had touched it with his fingers. This more physical, gestural communication seemed to be at least a faint circle of communication—the son's interest in the car and the father's pointing to a spot on the car and moving it a little opened a circle of communication. The son's looking at that particular spot and taking the car back closed a circle of communication. These opening and closing circles of communication create a foundation for subsequent communication.

After this minimal interaction, as the son was moving the car back and forth, the father got another car and started moving it back and forth next to his son. The father and his car moved toward his son's car but did not crash into it. The son initially pulled his car out of the way but then moved his car as fast as his father had, toward his father's car. Now three or four circles of communication in a row were closed, and a real interaction was beginning.

After gestural interaction becomes complex, for example, with the father hiding his son's car and his son pointing, searching, and vocalizing to find it, one fosters the movement from gestures to symbols. As father and son were using the car for simple and complex gestures, the father started to describe his own action. When he moved the car fast, he said, "Fast," and when he moved it slowly, he said, "Slow." After four or five repetitions, the boy crashed his car into his father's car and said the word *fast,* although he did not pronounce it clearly. The father beamed. He was amazed that his son could learn a new word and use it appropriately so quickly. Although in this case symbols came quickly, in many cases it is a long and slow process with lots of work occurring first at presymbolic levels. Words and symbols are more easily learned, however, when they are related to the child's actual experiences and built on the child's affective gestures. Words in isolation or as imposed labels have little meaning for the child.

A major challenge is a child's tendency to perseverate. One child would only open and close a door. Another would only bang blocks together. The key is to transform the perseveration into an interaction. We use the child's intense motivation to his or her advantage to open and close gestural circles of communication. For example, we get stuck in the child's door or catch our hands between his or her blocks. We are gentle and playful as he or she tries to get us out of the way (like a cat-and-mouse game). As gestural interactions occur, behavior becomes purposeful and affective. We modulate the child's feelings of annoyance and help soothe and comfort as well, though often he or she finds our "playful obstruction" amusing.

As the child becomes more purposeful, we have found that he or she can imitate gestures and sounds more readily and can copy feeding a doll or kissing a bear. With continuing challenges to be intentional, the child copies complex patterns and imitates sounds and words, often gradually beginning to use words and pretend on his or her own. Another challenge, as intervention moves toward more representational or symbolic elaboration, is for the clinician to help the child differentiate his or her experience. The child needs to learn cause-and-effect communication at the level of ideas and to make connections between various representations or ideas.

Because most children with ASD have difficulty with receptive language (i.e., auditory processing) and some also have difficulty with visuospatial processing, it is much easier for them to pay attention to their own ideas rather than to the ideas of others. A child categorizes his or her experiences at the level of symbols or representations through interaction, which involves opening and closing symbolic circles. The parent becomes the representative of what is outside the child and the foundation for reality. The clinician's or parent's ability to enter the child's symbolic world becomes the critical vehicle for fostering emotional differentiation and higher levels of abstract and logical thinking. During pretend play, for example, when the child ignores the therapist's inquiry about who sits where at the tea party, the therapist brings the child back to the comment or question until the child closes the symbolic circle. The adult might "play dumb" and bring the child back to the point of confusion. For example, when the child has a puppet biting the head off a cat, the parent may say, "Ouch, you hurt me." Then, if the child looks at the tree outside, the parent might ask, "I see the tree you are looking at, but what about the cat? What about his ouch?" If the child then says, "I'll give another ouch," and bites the cat with the puppet, the child has closed the symbolic circle of communication. If the parent then says as the child looks back at the tree, "Do you want to talk about the tree or the cat?" and the child says, "Let's look at the tree," the child has closed yet another circle and also created a logical bridge from one set of ideas to the other. As the parent or therapist helps the child create such bridges and always follows the child's lead, the child becomes more representationally differentiated. If the parent either lets the child become fragmented or becomes too rigid and controlling, however, differentiation may become compromised.

Relating to the child when he or she is displaying strong affect is critical. He or she is connecting words and movements to underlying affect that gives them purpose and meaning. When a child is motivated, for example, to negotiate for a certain kind of food or to go outside, there is often an opportunity to open and close many symbolic circles. The child who is trying to open the door because he or she wants to go outside and is angry that he or she cannot may, in the midst of the situation, open and close 20 circles of communication if the adult soothingly tries to find out what the child wants to do outside and so forth.

Children with ASD often find it especially difficult to shift from concrete modes of thinking to more abstract ones, in part because they do not easily generalize from a specific experience to other similar experiences. There is a temptation to teach the child answers and to repeat the same question by scripting the dialogue, but the child can only learn to abstract and generalize through active, emotionally meaningful experience. Most helpful are long conversations with debates or ones in which the child gives his or her opinions (e.g., "I like juice because it tastes good") rather than memorized elaboration of facts.

As the child progresses through the seven functional emotional milestones, the therapeutic program works on mobilizing all seven levels at the same time in each and every interaction. The therapeutic program often evolves to a point where the child and family are involved in three types of activities: 1) spontaneous, creative interactions (floor time); 2) semistructured, problem-solving interactions to learn new skills, concepts, and master academic work (e.g., negotiating for cookies, mastering spatial concepts such as *behind* and *next to* by discovering where a favorite toy is located); and 3) motor, sensory, and spatial play to strengthen fundamental processing skills.

ELEMENTS OF A COMPREHENSIVE INTERVENTION PROGRAM

A comprehensive DIR program often involves the following components.

Home-Based Interactions and Practices

This developmentally appropriate floor-time program includes three levels. Because the demands of this home-based program are considerable, it is important to schedule the time and bring in other family members and people (e.g., graduate students, volunteers) to help implement the program. All should learn about floor time and be familiar with its principles.

Spontaneous, Follow-the-Child's-Lead Floor Time

These spontaneous sessions focus on encouraging the child's initiative and purposeful behavior, deepening engagement, lengthening mutual attention, and developing symbolic capacities through pretend play and conversations. The length of the sessions will vary depending on how long it takes the child to "warm up" and become fully engaged, as well as on how long it takes the child to create and expand on new ideas. It is recommended that 4 or more hours per day (20- to 45-minute sessions eight or more times per day) be devoted to this effort.

Semistructured Problem Solving

Semistructured sessions involve setting up challenges for a child to solve so that he or she learns something new (e.g., concept, word, gesture, sign). The challenges can be set up as selected learning activities that are meaningful and relevant to the child's experiences. The child may encounter the challenges spontaneously in the environment when he or she desires something or confronts something different from what he or she expects and, therefore, must solve a problem to get what he or she wants. The challenges can be created when it becomes evident the child may want something; a problem is set up for the child to obtain the desired object.

Problem solving can take different forms and multiple interactions, such as expressing a new word or gesture, learning a new concept, manipulating an object (motor planning), sequencing a series of steps to obtain an objective, or negotiating a turn or a trade. An example is putting a child's favorite toy outside the door and saying, "Open," or, "Close," to help him learn what *open* is and to say, "Open," when he's feeling a strong desire (affect) to open the door. Purposeful gestures, words, concepts, and the use of pictures and signs can all be taught through creating problem-solving interactions (e.g., the child uses pictures, signs, and, gradually, words to convey *open, juice,* or *more*).

The amount of time spent on semistructured problem solving will vary depending on the developmental level of the child; how purposeful he or she is; and specific areas of need such as the need to increase gestural communication, language, concepts, motor planning, and so forth. Children requiring more semistructured activities should do 2 or more hours per day (15 minutes or more, five to eight times per day).

Problem-solving interactions can occur in the course of daily routines if enough time is allowed for extended interactions. Problem solving also can be added to activities such as fingerplays and songs (e.g., "If You're Happy and You Know It"), social games (e.g., Duck, Duck, Goose), listening-auditory games (e.g., Telephone), board games (e.g., Memory, Connect Four), storytelling, and so forth. The key is to challenge the child to solve a problem generated by the game.

For children who are unable to imitate, more structured learning and behavioral approaches (e.g., TEACCH [Treatment and Education of Autistic and related Communications Handicapped Children], discrete trial, special education) can be implemented to teach imitation, motor planning, and problem-solving patterns. Once a child can imitate and problem-solve, dynamic challenges should be used to teach new skills.

Sensorimotor, Sensory Integration, Visuospatial, and Perceptual Motor Activities

Various sensorimotor activities are geared to address the child's individual differences and regulatory patterns; build basic processing capacities; and support the child to become engaged, attentive, and regulated during interactions with others. For example, an underreactive child with low muscle tone will benefit from proprioceptive (e.g., jumping on a trampoline) or vestibular (e.g., swinging) activities to increase arousal, attention, and intentionality. Another child needs calming and organizing activities that build awareness of his or her body in space, require bilateral movements, and reduce tactile defensiveness. Some children try to find their own "solutions," evident in such behaviors as constant running and jumping or lying on the floor for more support.

To understand a child's sensorimotor and regulatory profile and organize a home program, it is useful to organize specific recommendations from all therapists (e.g., occupational therapist, physical therapist, sensorimotor or movement therapist, developmental optometrist, speech-language and oral-motor therapist, music therapist, art therapist). These activities can be used to help children get ready for floor time and semistructured activities, to reorganize, to increase arousal ("rev up"), or to calm down and focus, as well as to strengthen basic processing abilities.

Children will need different amounts of time participating in these activities depending on their individual needs, ranging from 1 or 2 to more hours with 15- to 20-minute intervals interspersed throughout the day. For children at early developmental levels, who need to become more fully engaged and purposeful, these activities may be used a great deal because they are "fun" and increase the pleasurable interactions with a child. They also increase communication because a child can be taught to gesture or use picture communication to indicate what he or she wants (e.g., more or less, slower or faster). They can also be used for problem-solving interactions and sequencing (e.g., obstacle courses, other motor planning activities).

At more advanced developmental levels, activities may focus on practice in specific abilities such as visual pursuit and motor planning (e.g., flashlight games, bilateral drawing activities, construction). The activities can also be integrated with symbolic ideation such as "flying to outer space" on the swing, "steering clear of sharks and pirates" on the platform swing, Peter Pan fighting Hook with foam swords (eye–hand coordination), making jungle safaris in search of wild animals, and constructing forts. At all levels, children will benefit from regulatory games and practicing basic visual-motor and visuospatial skills. These activities may overlap with some of the semistructured activities described above.

The basic areas of functioning that should be addressed during these activities include the following:

- *Sensory and motor modulation and integration:* Games and activities to improve sensory and motor modulation and integration include start–stop activities, running and changing direction, Red Light–Green Light, jumping on a mattress or trampoline, spinning, swinging, gentle roughhousing or wrestling, and Musical Chairs with changing speeds.
- *Perceptual motor challenges:* Activities to sharpen perceptual motor skills include looking and playing games and activities involving destinations,

such as throwing and catching; reaching for a desired object moving on a string to the left, right, and across the midline; kicking and hitting a big Nerf ball; walking on or over balance beams; playing Dodge Ball; and flashlight tracking. Fine motor and graphomotor activities include going through pencil-and-paper mazes, completing dot-to-dot puzzles, copying designs, playing with Legos or Lite Brite, cutting and pasting, painting, and coloring.

- *Visuospatial processing activities:* Tasks to foster visuospatial processing abilities include going on treasure hunts; completing obstacle courses; playing Hide-and-Seek and What's Missing?; and using board games such as Connect Four, Guess Who? and Othello.
- *Tactile discrimination:* Activities to strengthen tactile discrimination include finding objects hidden in materials of different textures (e.g., rice, beans, birdseed); finger painting in pudding, paints, or shaving cream; and identifying objects and toys hidden in a pillowcase (with verbal clues or categories added).
- *Peer play with one other child:* Once a child is fully engaged and interactive, he or she should begin to play with one other peer, with parents providing mediation to encourage engagement and interaction between the children. It is best to invite a child who is interactive and verbal and can reach out and encourage as well as model for the child with a disability. Play dates should be increased to three or four times a week as soon as possible.

Speech-Language and Oral-Motor Therapy

In addition to home-based interaction, comprehensive DIR intervention includes speech-language and oral-motor therapy; three or more 30- to 60-minute sessions per week are optimal. In addition, a daily home program should be prescribed, part of which can be incorporated into floor time and semistructured problem-solving activities.

Sensory Integration Occupational Therapy and/or Physical Therapy

Comprehensive intervention also includes occupational and/or physical therapy two or more times per week for 30–60 minutes. In addition, a daily home program should be prescribed and included as part of the home-based interaction program described previously.

Educational Program

For children who can interact and imitate gestures and/or words and engage in preverbal problem-solving, either an inclusive program or a typical preschool program, with an additional teacher or aide if needed, is recommended. The aide may also help the teacher with various preparation tasks to free the teacher to facilitate interaction with other children. An inclusion consultant should be brought in to address needs of the child with ASD as well as those of the other children in the class. For children not yet able to engage in preverbal problem solving or imitation, a special education program is recommended, in which the major focus is on engagement; preverbal purposeful gestural interaction; preverbal problem solving (a continuous, two-way flow of communication); and learning to imitate actions, sounds, and words.

Transition education programs with typical peers are recommended to augment primary educational programs or prior to enrollment in preschool. These programs include classes in movement or gymnastics, music, creative drama, therapeutic riding, art, swimming, and parent–child groups. Parents are usually included and can facilitate participation and interaction. Groups should be selected to match developmental rather than chronological age.

Biomedical Interventions

Comprehensive DIR intervention may also involve biomedical interventions, such as medication to enhance motor planning and sequencing, self-regulation, concentration, and/or auditory processing and language. Also necessary are a consideration of nutrition and diet and of technologies geared to improve processing abilities, including auditory processing, visuospatial processing, sensory modulation, and motor planning. For more on the DIR model, see the appendix at the end of this chapter.

CHARACTERISTICS ASSOCIATED WITH DIFFERENT PATTERNS OF PROGRESS

In working clinically with a large number of individuals, we have observed patterns that have permitted us to form hypotheses on the relationship between presenting patterns and different types of progress. We have found that the severity of symptoms such as perseveration or self-stimulation is not a good predictor of a child's potential for progress. The way in which the child responds to the early phases of the intensive DIR intervention program, in contrast, can be a useful indicator of progress. Two related features enable a child to respond quickly to the intervention program. One is the ability to sequence actions (i.e., motor planning) and use this sequence to form complex reciprocal problem-solving interactions, and to learn to imitate. Complex intentional behavior and imitation then leads to symbolic communication and imaginative play. Banging a block is a one-step sequence, whereas putting a toy car in a garage, taking it out, and zooming it is a three-step sequence. Children with little or no progress were four times more likely to have severe motor planning difficulties than were children who made consistent and/or good progress (Greenspan & Wieder, 1997).

The other feature associated with rapid progress is the availability of a great deal of interactive opportunities geared to the child's developmental level and individual differences. These opportunities often involve eight or more 20- to 30-minute developmentally appropriate, interactive (floor time) sessions each day rather than periods of time during which the child is allowed to be self-absorbed, to perseverate, to self-stimulate, or to watch television and a comprehensive intervention program involving speech therapy, occupational therapy, psychological and/or psychiatric consultation, and early and/or special education. When these two conditions are present, some children make rapid progress and shift from varying degrees of self-absorption and avoidance into patterns of engagement, preverbal reciprocal interaction, and, eventually, symbolic communication and imaginative play.

The children in the group who make the most progress are able to learn to be warm, emotionally expressive, flexible, empathetic children with a sense of humor, solid abstract thinking skills, and age-appropriate academic capacities. They are eventually able to go to typical schools and have many friends. In our review of 200 individuals (Greenspan & Wieder, 1997), more than 50% of the children were able to progress to this level. It should be pointed out, however, that our cases were not a representational sample of children with ASD diagnoses, and, therefore, the percentage should only indicate that there appears to be a subgroup capable of significant progress.

We compared 20 children diagnosed with ASD who made outstanding progress, 14 typically developing school-age children, and 12 children with continuing difficulties. We used the Functional Emotional Assessment Scale (FEAS; DeGangi & Greenspan, in press; Greenspan, 1992a) and the Vineland Adaptive Behavior Scales (Sparrow, Balla, & Cicchetti, 1984) to describe the children's functioning. The FEAS reliably measures subtle aspects of emotional and social functioning through the analysis of videotaped interactions between the child and his or her caregiver. Both the outstanding progress group and the typically developing group evidenced age-appropriate emotional, social, and cognitive capacities. There were no significant differences between these groups (Greenspan & Wieder, 1997). The group with continuing difficulties, in contrast, evidenced low functioning on these scales.

A number of studies have investigated outcomes with intensive interventions for children with ASD. Interestingly, many of the studies report that roughly 50% of the children become verbal, academically able (at age and grade level), and social (Bondy & Peterson, 1990; Lovaas, 1987; Miller & Miller, 1992; Rogers, Herbison, Lewis, Pantone, & Reis, 1988; Rogers & Lewis, 1989; Strain & Hoyson, 1988; Strain, Hoyson, & Jamison, 1983). These studies, however, do not use representative samples. In the Lovaas (1987) study, for example, all of the children who enrolled had developmental quotients at least in the 10- to 12-month age level. They could carry out some early types of imitation and reciprocal interactions. The families were motivated and relatively well-organized. In addition, their outcome evaluations did not look closely at the emotional range, depth, and flexibility or creativity of the children. In our chart review of 200 individuals (Greenspan & Wieder, 1997), we saw children whose parents were highly motivated and often traveled great distances to seek extra help. Although there was no exclusion criteria, and some of the children began their intervention while functioning at the 6- to 8-month developmental level, parents may have seen behaviors in their children that gave them reason to be especially hopeful.

That some children can do especially well, however, does not suggest that significantly improving the functioning of many children with ASD is possible. Many children with ASD do not show rapid gain. Working with children for 6–12 months before making a definitive diagnosis (a provisional diagnosis may be made in the interim) can help the clinician determine the type of developmental pattern that is likely. It is important for clinical researchers to further develop criteria to determine the type of progress a child will likely make.

Clinical Implications for Goals of Speech-Language and Communication Therapy

Speech-language pathologists have been at the forefront of using dynamic affect-based interactions to promote language and thinking. Following are a few clinical observations that may contribute to the strategies that can be employed. We have found that the quicker a child can harness preverbal and verbal communication patterns in connection with strong states of affect (i.e., intent), the better. For example, a parent's repeating, "Open," while a child is trying to open the pantry door to get a favorite cookie on the other side is far more useful than simply having the child imitate "Open," without the strong affect or than having the child look at a picture and use a word to label it. As soon as a child can repeat the word in connection with an emotionally motivated action, it is especially helpful to challenge the child to think and, for example, to say, "Open," or, "Close," rather than to just repeat both words. If the child says, "Open close," then we show the child the open door and the closed door and, with even more emphasis, challenge him or her with a multiple choice "Open? . . . Or close?" Eventually, because of strong motivation, the child thinks it through and repeats the first rather than the second word and comes to understand the concept *open.* The affect and motivation coupled with solving a problem appear to speed up the learning process considerably.

As part of mobilizing the child's affect, we also have found that children's grammar and, more generally, pragmatic language is mobilized quickest when we help children open and close many preverbal and verbal circles in a row. The key is long interactive dialogues using gestures and, when possible, words. For example, if the child said, "Out," we would say, "Do what?" If the child said, "Play outside," we would say, "What do you want to play?" If the child was stymied, we might offer a few choices: "Play with swing or a chase game?" We would try to get long sequences rather than to focus on full sentences. Rather than have the child imitate, "I want to go outside," for example, we would focus on the number of circles of communication, even if each circle only contained one or two words or a short phrase. Similarly, even if the child confused pronouns and said, "You want to go outside," when the child meant he or she wanted to go outside, we would go after the affect (intent) rather than model the correct response to the child. We might playfully, for example, say, "Okay, I'll go outside" and then ask again, "Who wants to go outside?" If the child said, "You go outside," we might say, "I am outside" and ask the child whether he or she wants to go outside, emphasizing "you" and then maybe use his or her name: "Johnny, want to go outside?" Although this may sound similar to a little bit of the old Abbott and Costello "Who's on first?" routine, if done with a gleam in the eye and a light-hearted attitude, we find that the child actually learns pronouns more quickly and frequently will start off with "Johnny go outside" and then eventually get the idea that "I" refers to Johnny. More important, in this view, than long, grammatically correct sentences is the reciprocal use of speech, motivated and initiated through connections with strong affect. In a sense, the affect creates the proper verb–noun relationships and eventually helps organize the pronouns as well. The goals of this approach are the same as approaches that would use a little more modeling in place of this much interaction. We find that the more you can use interaction with some modeling to help the child formulate the relevant utterances, the better.

Using the same principles, we would approach a child who is echolalic or who is repeating scripts or lists of nouns in a seemingly meaningless way. We would create opportunities for interaction based on strong affect. For example, we might hide a toy in our hand that the child really wants and, as he grabs for it, help him find the word either to label the toy or to say, "Mine," or, "Give it to me." The affect combined with action quickly pulls the child out of the echolalic, scripted, or repetitive word patterns and into a meaningful gestural and verbal dialogue. The action and affect combined provide the organizational structure, or the "roadway," for the meaningful use of words. What we are doing is working at the earlier affect/gestural/action level, which is compromised in many children with developmental problems, at the same time that we are working on the verbal/symbolic level (see Chapters 9 and 10 for further discussion of enhancing preverbal and verbal communication abilities).

CONCLUSIONS

This chapter presents a model to help systematize functional understanding of processing and developmental challenges in ASDs and discusses the implications of this model for assessment and intervention. The DIR model provides conceptual tools for the clinician to use to form a profile of each child's strengths and challenges and to formulate interventions to promote developmental progress in the most critical areas of functioning. The DIR model enables the therapeutic team to create a program based on the child's unique developmental profile and enables parents and therapists to harness in an integrated, more developmentally appropriate manner many of the therapeutic elements traditionally found helpful.

REFERENCES

American Psychiatric Association. (1994). *Diagnostic and statistical manual of mental disorders (DSM-IV)* (4th ed.). Washington, DC: Author.

Bondy, A.S., & Peterson, S. (1990). *The point is not to point: Picture exchange communication system with young students with autism.* Paper presented at the Association for Behavior Analysis conference, Nashville.

DeGangi, G., & Greenspan, S. (in press). *The Functional Emotional Assessment Scale Manual.* San Antonio, TX: The Psychological Corporation.

Feuerstein, R., Rand, Y., Hoffman, M., & Miller, R. (1979). Cognitive modifiability in retarded adolescents: Effects of instrumental enrichment. *American Journal of Mental Deficiency, 83,* 539–550.

Feuerstein, R., Miller, R., Hoffman, M., Rand, Y., Mintsker, Y., Morgens, R., & Jensen, M.R. (1981). Cognitive modifiability in adolescence: Cognitive structure and the effects of intervention. *Journal of Special Education, 150,* 269–287.

Greenspan, S.I. (1979a). Intelligence and adaptation: An integration of psychoanalytic and Piagetian developmental psychology [Monograph]. *Psychological Issues, 47*(Serial No. 68). Madison, CT: International Universities Press.

Greenspan, S.I. (1979b). *Psychopathology and adaptation in infancy and early childhood: Principles of clinical diagnosis and preventive intervention.* In ZERO TO THREE: National Center for Clinical Infant Programs (Ed.), *Clinical Infant Reports* (Vol. 1). Madison, CT: International Universities Press.

Greenspan, S.I. (1989). *The development of the ego: Implications for personality theory, psychopathology, and the psychotherapeutic process.* Madison, CT: International Universities Press.

Greenspan, S.I. (1992a). *Infancy and early childhood: The practice of clinical assessment and intervention with emotional and developmental challenges.* Madison, CT: International Universities Press.

Greenspan, S.I. (1992b). Reconsidering the diagnosis and treatment of very young children with autistic spectrum or pervasive developmental disorder. *ZERO TO THREE Bulletin, 13,* 1–9.

Greenspan, S.I. (1997). *The growth of the mind and the endangered origins of intelligence.* Reading, MA: Addison Wesley Longman.

Greenspan, S.I., & Wieder, S. (1997). Developmental patterns and outcomes in infants and children with disorders in relating and communicating: A chart review of 200 cases of children with autistic spectrum diagnoses. *The Journal of Developmental and Learning Disorders, 1,* 87–141.

Greenspan, S.I., & Wieder, S. (1998). *The child with special needs: Intellectual and emotional growth.* Reading, MA: Addison Wesley Longman.

Kanner, L. (1943). Autistic disturbances of affective contact. *Nervous Child, 2,* 217–250.

Klein, P.S., Wieder, S., & Greenspan, S.I. (1987). A theoretical overview and empirical study of mediated learning experience: Prediction of preschool performance from mother–infant interaction patterns. *Infant Mental Health Journal, 8,* 110–129.

Lovaas, O.I. (1987). Behavioral treatment and normal educational and intellectual functioning in young autistic children. *Journal of Consulting and Clinical Psychology, 55,* 3–9.

Miller, A., & Miller, E. (1992). *A new way with autistic and other children with pervasive developmental disorder* [Monograph]. Boston: Language and Cognitive Center.

Rogers, S. J., Herbison, J.M., Lewis, H., Pantone, J., & Reis, K. (1988). An approach for enhancing symbolic, communicative, and interpersonal functioning of young children with autism and severe emotional handicaps. *Journal of the Division of Early Childhood, 10*(2), 135–145.

Rogers, S.J., & Lewis, H. (1989). An effective day treatment model for young children with pervasive developmental disorders. *Journal of the American Academy of Child and Adolescent Psychiatry, 28,* 207–214.

Sparrow, S.S., Balla, D.A., & Cicchetti, D.V. (1984). *Vineland Adaptive Behavior Scales.* Circle Pines, MN: American Guidance Service.

Strain, P.S., & Hoyson, M. (1988). *Follow-up of children in LEAP.* Paper presented at the meeting of the Autism Society of America, New Orleans.

Strain, P.S., Hoyson, M., & Jamison, B. (1983). Normally developing preschoolers as intervention agents for autistic-like children: Effects on class, department, and social interaction. *Journal of the Division of Early Childhood, 9,* 105–119.

ZERO TO THREE/National Center for Clinical Infant Programs. (1994). *Diagnostic Classification: 0–3 Diagnostic classification of mental health and developmental disorders of infancy and early childhood.* Arlington, VA: Author.

Appendix

A Generic Model of Intervention

The Developmental Pyramid

The approaches described in Chapter 12 are examples of ways to create experiences that help a child to master the processes essential to relating; communicating; attending, engaging, and sending and responding to gestures and affect; problem solving; using ideas; and thinking. Experiences that support these processes need to be part of any intervention effort.

Intervention efforts often only deal with a few of the essential developmental needs of children such as certain motor, language, cognitive, or social skills. The Developmental, Individual-Difference, Relationship-Based (DIR) model, a developmentally based functional approach, deals with a number of components essential for mobilizing core functional capacities, overcomes symptoms and problems, and can be conceptualized as a pyramid (see Figure 12.1).

At the foundation of the intervention pyramid are the stable, nurturing, developmentally supportive, and tailored family patterns that all children require, especially children with developmental disabilities. This foundation includes physical protection and safety and an ongoing sense of security. Some families require a great deal of support and/or therapy to stabilize and organize these basic family functions. The family may be dealing with extreme poverty and chronic states of fearfulness. Relationships within the family may be abusive, neglectful, or fragmented. Intervention programs need staff who are trained to assess family needs, develop alliances, problem-solve, advocate (including for social and economic support), and provide family counseling and personal therapy when indicated.

At the second level of the pyramid are the ongoing and consistent relationships that every child requires. Typically developing children require nurturing relationships to have a chance for emotional and cognitive competency. Children with disabilities, who often already have compromises in their capacities to relate, are in even greater need of warm, consistent caregiving. Their caregivers, however, often face challenges to sustaining intimate relationships because misperceiving their child's intentions is so easy. Understanding these children's behavior as attempts to cope with difficulties or as signs that they are overwhelmed by their difficulties often can help caregivers overcome these misperceptions and move toward more creative and empathetic ways of relat-

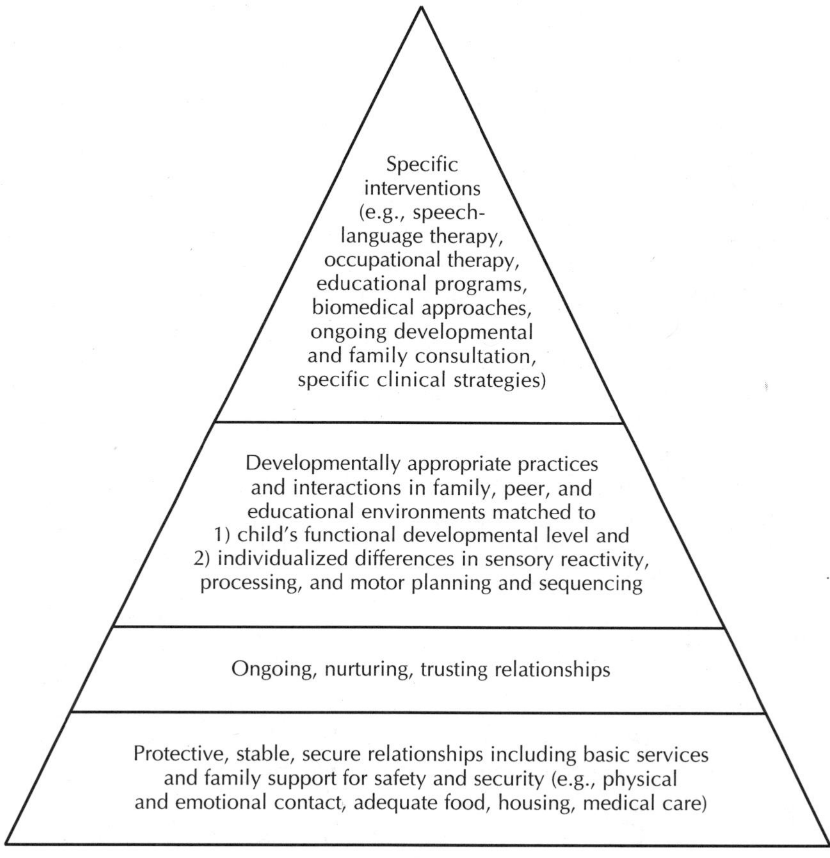

Figure 12.1. Intervention pyramid for children with disabilities.

ing to their children. For example, children who are hypersensitive to touch may not be rejecting the parents' comfort and care when they cry. When holding such children, it may be important to avoid light touch and to use deep pressure to help them feel more comfortable. Or, a child who jumps on a toddler who is crying may not be primarily aggressive but may be so sensitive to the sound frequency of the cry that he or she panics and wants the noise to stop. Similarly, a child who has difficulty comprehending words may become confused and avoid communication. He or she may benefit from pictures or gestural signs to understand the environment and predict what will happen next in interactions with caregivers. A child who is generally avoidant or self-absorbed and appears to prefer to play alone may be giving a signal. He may be underreactive to sensations, with low muscle tone, and may need greater attention to get beyond his self-absorption.

To support the child's ability to relate requires a lot of time, consistency, and understanding from caregivers, educators, and clinicians. Family difficulties or frequent turnover among child care staff or teachers may compromise the requirement for consistency in a child who is just learning how to relate to others.

At the third level of the pyramid lie consistent relationships that have been adapted to individual differences and needs of each child. Caregivers need to learn a variety of strategies, including giving extra attention to an underreactive child with low tone; protecting and soothing the overreactive, easily fragmented child; and slowing down and making auditory communication more deliberate and visuospatial communication more clear to a child with severe auditory processing difficulties.

At the fourth level of the pyramid model, relationships and the emotional interactions that flow from them are geared to the appropriate functional developmental capacities and levels of the child as a starting point for mobilizing growth. Children will vary—some do not relate to others, are unpurposeful, and require work on engaging and intentional communication; others are purposeful but require extra help in using symbols. Still others are using symbols or ideas in a fragmented way and need to learn how to be logical and more abstract. For each developmental level, special types of interactions can enable a child to master that level and its related capacities.

Interactions that are geared to the child's functional developmental capacities and individual differences can be thought of as *developmentally appropriate practices* (DAPs) for the child with disabilities. These DAPs must characterize family time and educational programs and must be integrated into the different therapies.

At the apex of the pyramid are specific therapeutic or educational techniques to promote development in children facing particular challenges. In this model, specific therapies, however, must build on a foundation of developmentally based family, relationship, and interactive approaches. Biological interventions to improve attention, processing skills, and affect regulation also can be considered, as can emerging educational, auditory processing, and nutritional approaches.

The integrated, pyramidal model encompasses certain fundamental experiences that any child, especially a child with special needs, requires. These core experiences enable a child to become a warm, loving, communicative, and creative individual. To become such a fully communicative person, the child must connect his or her emerging abilities to an underlying sense of self-purpose, that is, to his or her affect, wishes, and desires. In the DIR model, therefore, specific interventions must be a part of or built on interactions that bring new skills into an integrated sense of purpose and self.

13

Understanding and Intervening with Children's Challenging Behavior

A Comprehensive Approach

Lise Fox, Glen Dunlap, and Pamelazita Buschbacher

Challenging behavior exhibited by children with autism is often a major barrier to inclusive education, community participation, and opportunities to develop friendships with peers. Families report that such behavior negatively affects many elements of their lifestyle including relationships between siblings, relationships with extended family members, community participation, participation in religious activities, and the quality of home routines (Hart, 1995; Turnbull & Ruef, 1997). Personal accounts from family members offer poignant descriptions of the chronicity and intensity of challenging behavior and the struggle of the family to maintain balance in their lives (Featherstone, 1980; Turnbull & Ruef, 1996, 1997; Turnbull & Turnbull, 1996).

For many families of children with autism, interactions within and outside the family are often altered to accommodate the child's challenging behavior and support needs (Turnbull & Ruef, 1996). Child care is often a problem. Some parents may have given up employment opportunities because of the energy and time needed to attend to the child with challenging behavior. Some families can no longer attend religious services, a potential source of social and emotional support, because of the difficulties in accommodating the child's behavior. Parents and siblings fear embarrassment or criticism in their communities. Siblings may avoid inviting their friends over for fear that the child with challenging behavior may have an outburst. The child's behavior has the potential of disrupting meals, vacations, and family outings (Bristol &

Preparation of this chapter was supported in part by a grant from an outreach project for young children with disabilities (Grant No. H024D70040) from the Office of Special Education and Rehabilitative Services, U.S. Department of Education. The content and opinions expressed herein do not necessarily reflect the position or policy of the U.S. Department of Education, and no official endorsement should be inferred.

Schopler, 1983; Moes, 1995; Turnbull & Ruef, 1996). Disruptive behavior, such as aggression, tantrums, and property damage, not only may disrupt family life but also may exclude the family from typical and inclusive school and community environments (Horner et al., 1990; Turnbull & Ruef, 1997).

This chapter describes an empirically and socially valid process for understanding and developing interventions for children's challenging behavior that is focused on the context of family life. The process includes assessment and intervention designed to result in comprehensive applications of *positive behavioral support* across all activities and domains of family life. The application of positive behavioral support within the context of family life is a departure from the traditional perspective of intervention programs focused solely on the instructional and developmental needs of children. Positive behavioral support provides an approach to supporting children with autism within all of their daily activities and environments. In this chapter we present the theoretical and empirical basis for the use of positive behavioral support within early intervention and other instructional approaches.

Positive behavioral support is a process for understanding the purpose of challenging behavior and developing a plan that promotes the development of new skills while reducing the individual's need to engage in challenging behavior (Dunlap, Vaughn, & O'Neill, 1998; Koegel, Koegel, & Dunlap, 1996). This approach considers the broad context of the family, the interactions of caregivers with the child, and the need to develop intervention strategies that will be used effectively in all environments. Most important, positive behavioral support is designed to result in meaningful lifestyle outcomes for both the child with challenging behavior and the family.

THE CRITICAL IMPORTANCE OF THE FAMILY CONTEXT

The passage of the Individuals with Disabilities Education Act (IDEA) of 1990 (PL 101-476) and its amendments of 1991 and 1997 (PL 102-119 and PL 105-17, respectively) emphasized the shift of early intervention service delivery from "child-focused" toward "family-centered services" (Beckman, 1996; Colarusso & Kana, 1991; Garland, 1993; Griffer, 1997). This more ecological, or systems, perspective (Bronfenbrenner, 1979) is justified by the belief that the child transacts with the family, that the family transacts with the child, and that both are embedded within and transact with communities (Bailey & Wolery, 1992; Beckman, 1996; Sameroff & Chandler, 1975).

There are at least two goals in providing family-centered supports (Dunst & Trivette, 1987; Mahoney & Wheeden, 1997; McGonigel, Kaufmann, & Johnson, 1991). One goal is to support family members as the primary and most constant care providers in a child's life. In doing so, intervention programs provide support to the family system so that issues that may stress the family unit (including social, financial, physical, psychological issues) and thus affect a family's ability to support their child with disabilities are mitigated as much as possible (Mahoney & Wheeden, 1997). The second goal of family-centered intervention is to support families in strengthening their abilities to influence their child's development and well-being (Dunst, Trivette, & Deal, 1988). Family-centered intervention represents a shift from a deficit-oriented model of intervention that provides child "treatment" to a model that recognizes the unique contributions, strengths, and needs of each family member and is focused on supporting families as they embark on the journey of caring for their child with disabilities.

The provision of family-centered intervention that includes positive behavioral support is important for children with autism who have challenging behavior for three reasons. First, the impact of challenging behavior on family life can be highly disruptive and pervasive, affecting all family members and family lifestyle (Turnbull & Ruef, 1996). Positive behavioral support is a comprehensive approach that can be arranged to benefit the full family system. Second, a highly effective approach to changing persistent challenging behavior is to use a communication-based approach to teaching new patterns of communication and social interaction (Carr et al., 1999; Koegel et al., 1996; Reichle & Wacker, 1993). The development of functional communication is an integral ingredient in positive behavioral support. Finally, effective behavioral support is enhanced by the development of partnerships with the people who are most intimately involved with the individual who has challenging behavior (Albin, Lucyshyn, Horner, & Flannery, 1996). Positive behavioral support explicitly incorporates collaboration in its development and implementation.

The following sections of this chapter provide the rationale for providing comprehensive, communication-based interventions to children with autism and challenging behavior within the context of the family. The need for comprehensive interventions is addressed, and a model of family-centered intervention that provides supports to children with autism and challenging behavior is described.

THE COMMUNICATIVE PURPOSE OF CHALLENGING BEHAVIOR

A growing body of research provides support for understanding challenging behavior as purposeful or functional for the individual with disabilities. Challenging behavior is purposeful in that it is often an adaptive response that results in gaining a desired action or effect (Carr et al., 1994). The recognition that challenging behavior is functional for the individual with autism has dictated a radical shift in the development of behavior intervention approaches. In the early 1980s, researchers in applied behavior analysis began to explore methods for understanding the function of challenging behavior and the design of interventions that were linked to the identification of function (Carr & Durand, 1985; Donnellan, Mirenda, Mesaros, & Fassbender, 1984; Durand, 1982; Touchette, MacDonald, & Langer, 1985). Previously, challenging behavior usually was regarded as maladaptive and interventions were focused on behavior reduction without recognition that challenging behavior may serve a communicative function. Interventions were often selected on the basis of the behavior topographies (e.g., interventions for biting) rather than on the bases of an understanding of the individual and the context in which challenging behavior occurs.

Understanding the Purpose of Challenging Behavior

Children with autism are at an increased risk for the development of challenging behavior because of their difficulties with social interactions and communication skill development. Autism is characterized by the failure to develop and use language in a typical manner and by difficulty in attending to social stimuli (Dawson & Osterling, 1997; Klinger & Dawson, 1992).

As typical children develop, first forms of communication (e.g., gestures, eye gaze, vocalizations) include challenging behavior (e.g., crying, having tantrums). As children learn more conventional patterns of communication and understand that adults will be responsive to their communicative acts, challenging behavior becomes a less effective and efficient form of communication. For example, a child who cries to be picked up learns through interactions with adults that raising his or her arms and looking at the adult will mean that he or she will be picked up more quickly than when crying, which requires more physical effort. Communication in children with autism, however, does not develop in a typical manner. These children often use less conventional means for communication and have atypical development in social reciprocity (Wetherby, 1986; Wetherby & Prutting, 1984; see also Chapter 6). It is common to see young children with autism use challenging behavior to regulate the behaviors of others for requesting and protesting.

Functions of Challenging Behavior

Many studies have demonstrated that challenging behavior may be used to control the social environment by gaining attention (Carr & Durand, 1985; Carr & McDowell, 1980; Durand & Carr, 1991; Hagopian, Fisher, & Legacy, 1994; Taylor & Carr, 1992), escaping from demands or undesired events (Carr & Newsom, 1985; Carr, Taylor, & Robinson, 1991; Durand & Carr, 1991; Horner & Day, 1991; Piazza, Moes, & Fisher, 1996), or gaining access to objects or activities (Billingsley & Neel, 1985; Durand & Crimmins, 1988; Horner & Budd, 1985). In addition, research has demonstrated that an individual may use the same set of challenging behaviors to serve multiple functions (Carr & Carlson, 1993; Day, Horner, & O'Neill, 1994; Durand, 1982; Durand & Carr, 1991; Prizant & Duchan, 1981).

The function or purpose of challenging behavior is identified by examining the context in which behavior occurs. Researchers have observed or created antecedent conditions and examined or provided consequences to determine the possible function of the behavior. For example, a researcher may observe a child having a tantrum after the parent asks the child to sit at the dinner table. After several seconds of crying, the child bangs his or her head on the table and the parent allows the child to leave the table. The child moves away from the table and stops crying. The antecedent of requesting the child to sit at the table and the consequential response of the parent provides a framework for understanding why the child was crying. Because the challenging behavior stopped once the child was released from the table, the researcher may hypothesize that the function of the behavior was to escape.

Setting Events

An assessment of proximally related contextual variables may reveal the predictors and function of a child's challenging behavior. There may be occasions, however, when events that do not immediately precede challenging behavior influence the occurrence of challenging behavior (Horner, Vaughn, Day, & Ard, 1996). For example, a child who did not sleep during the night may be more likely to have challenging behavior the next morning. These more distally related events, called *setting events* (Bijou & Baer, 1961) or *establishing operations* (Michael, 1982), set the occasion for a higher probability of challenging behavior but do not directly cause it. Examples of these events are allergies, fatigue, hunger, problematic interactions, medication, sensory overload, environmental irritants (e.g., heat, crowded areas, noise), and chronic illness (e.g., otitis media, upper respiratory infections).

The process of positive behavioral support requires developing an understanding of the ecology of the child and the social contexts in which challenging behavior occurs. Interventions that are designed through the process of positive behavioral support address a multitude of factors based on the information gained from understanding the setting events, predictors, purpose, and consequences of challenging behavior. Because challenging behavior is perceived as being communicative, support plans are developed to focus on enhancing the child's ability to communicate effectively and arranging environments that are responsive to the child's communicative attempts.

Communication-Based Interventions

A communication-based approach to resolving challenging behavior has been developed from the assumption that if a child is taught relevant communication skills that serve the same function as challenging behavior, then challenging behavior may be replaced or eliminated (Carr et al., 1994; Durand, 1990). The effectiveness of this approach has been demonstrated consistently in research on communication-based approaches or functional communication skill training (Billingsley & Neel, 1985; Bird, Dores, Moniz, & Robinson, 1989; Durand & Carr, 1992; Horner & Day, 1991; Lalli, Casey, & Kates, 1995).

For example, in a study conducted by Durand and Carr (1992), the effectiveness of a communication-based approach to reduce challenging behavior and maintain the behavior reduction was demonstrated for children with severe disabilities including autism. Twelve children with challenging behavior were randomly assigned to two intervention approaches following a determination of the purpose of their challenging behavior through functional assessment. One group of children received functional communication skill training, whereas a consequence strategy of time-out for attention-getting behavior was used for the comparison group. The children who received functional communication training were taught to request attention using verbal behavior and to extend their ability to work independently without adult attention. The challenging behavior of both groups of children was effectively reduced, although increases in unprompted communication were only seen with the functional communication training group. More important, the long-term maintenance of challenging behavior reduction was achieved only with the group that received functional communication training. The children who received the time-out intervention resumed their challenging behavior when in the presence of teachers who were unaware of the child's intervention history.

Comprehensive Applications

Most of the published research on behavioral support applications and communication-based interventions has been conducted within clinical or instructional contexts with strategies being implemented by researchers or professionals. Researchers have more recently focused on the application of positive behavioral support within the natural routines of family life (Fox, Dunlap, & Philbrick, 1997; Lucyshyn, Albin, & Nixon, 1997; Vaughn, Dunlap, Fox, Clarke, & Bucy, 1997). The focus on applications of positive behavioral support within the context of family life comes from a recognition that effective intervention practices are driven by family needs and are designed to build the capacity of families to nurture their child's development.

In positive behavioral support, researchers have called for comprehensive applications of a communication-based approach to behavior intervention (Carr et al., 1994; Fox, Dunlap, et al., 1997; Horner & Carr, 1997; Meyer & Evans, 1989). Interventions are comprehensive when they are based on a functional assessment of challenging behavior and result in support plans that address all challenging behavior through the use of multiple intervention procedures that are applied throughout the day and are consistent with the values and resources of the people providing behavioral support (Horner & Carr, 1997). Comprehensiveness is a critical concept in the application of effective behavioral support. The goal of positive behavioral support is to achieve lifestyle change outcomes for the individual with challenging behavior. Those outcomes are individually determined but may include gaining access to new environments and activities and developing meaningful and reciprocal social relationships. These outcomes are ambitious and are only likely to be achieved through a sustained effort of behavioral support that is applied in all environments by the individuals who are most likely to interact with the person who has challenging behavior.

Contextual Fit

It is essential that behavioral support plans be designed so that the family and other care providers can implement strategies in all of the child's routines and environments. The concept of *contextual fit* has been described as the design of behavioral support plans that are compatible with the individual for whom the plan is designed, factors associated with the people implementing the plan, and the environment in which the plan will be implemented (Albin et al., 1996). When the contextual fit of a support plan is good, the plan will be implemented with fidelity. If the contextual fit is poor, then the plan may not be implemented consistently and behavior change will not result. From this perspective, attention to contextual fit has been a key element in successful applications of comprehensive behavioral support with families and their children with severe challenging behavior (Fox, Vaughn, Dunlap, & Bucy, 1997; Lucyshyn et al., 1997; Vaughn et al., 1997).

The emphasis on contextual fit recognizes the critical importance of understanding the broader ecology of the child in the application of positive behavioral support. It is possible to develop a behavioral support plan that is technically sound but that does not fit with the values, routines, and lifestyle patterns of a family (Albin et al., 1996). The development of a plan with contextual fit requires the acknowledgment of the important roles the family and other caregivers have in the development and implementation of the behavioral support plan.

The concept of contextual fit comes from the early intervention literature on "goodness of fit" that has been applied in the development of family-centered early intervention supports (Bailey et al., 1990). Although little research has been conducted on defining how contextual fit is achieved, the following practices and strategies are common to intervention efforts that have been applied successfully in partnership with families (Fox, Vaughn, et al., 1997; Lucyshyn et al., 1997; Vaughn et al., 1997).

To achieve contextual fit, a support plan should be developed through collaborative teaming with the family and other caregivers. These are the people who are most familiar with the child and the child's activities and routines and who will be ultimately responsible for consistent plan implementation across the day. During the assessment process, the interventionist should pay attention not only to variables that affect the child but also to the ecology of the family system. Attention should be paid to the patterns and routines of family life, the ways in which the family has responded to and accommodated challenging behavior, and the resources and sources of stress that affect the family (Albin et al., 1996). Interventionists should work in partnership with families in identifying strategies that will effectively reduce challenging behavior and teach the child new skills that also fit with the values and lifestyles of the family. Once a plan of behavioral support has been developed, ongoing dialogue and assessment of the success of the plan should occur to identify plan components that must be modified or changed. The critical concern in creating contextual fit is the development of strategies that are effective and feasible for implementation by all of the people who interact with the child.

THE IMPLEMENTATION OF COMPREHENSIVE, POSITIVE BEHAVIORAL SUPPORT

The implementation of comprehensive, positive behavioral support provides a process for developing intervention that focuses on communication skill development, challenging behavior reduction, and family support. The process of positive behavioral support begins with functional assessment, person-centered planning, the development of behavioral hypotheses, and support plan development. Once a support plan is developed, caregivers across environments implement, evaluate, and adjust the plan of support. We have applied and evaluated the impact of positive behavioral support through the Individualized Support Project, a model of early intervention support that provides comprehensive support to young children with autism and challenging behavior and their families (Dunlap & Fox, 1996; Fox, Dunlap, et al., 1997). This model was designed during the 1990s with the goal of responding to the unique needs of this population of children and families (Dunlap & Robbins, 1991; Dunlap, Robbins, Morelli, & Dollman, 1988). The following processes and methods describe the fundamental procedures of positive behavioral support and how positive behavioral support may be provided in partnership with the family.

The Process of Functional Assessment

As discussed previously, clinicians and researchers have made considerable gains in understanding the ways that challenging behavior is related to the environment. Functional assessment is the process used to acquire that understanding. The goal of functional assessment is to develop hypotheses about the purpose or function of challenging behavior. The functional assessment should result in the following: 1) clear description of the challenging behavior, 2) identification of events that predict when problems will and will not occur, 3) identification of the consequences that maintain challenging behavior, 4) development of behavioral hypotheses that provide purpose statements about the function of challenging behavior, and 5) direct observations that support the behavioral hypotheses (O'Neill et al., 1997).

Person-Centered Planning

The functional assessment process should follow an effort to understand the child, the family system, and the vision for the future of the child that people in the child's life hold. Person-centered planning processes, such as Personal Futures Planning (Mount & Zwernik, 1988) or group action planning (Turnbull & Turnbull, 1996), are mechanisms for bringing together the people in a child's life who wish to support the child and his or her family in achieving an optimal lifestyle. Because positive behavioral support is targeted at developing lifestyle change, person-centered planning processes have come to be regarded as essential to the functional assessment process. Lifestyle change can only occur with a deep understanding of the child and family members and their vision for the child's future.

In person-centered planning processes, the people who wish to provide support or who care about the individual with disabilities come together to reflect on the child's lifestyle and to develop a vision for the child's immediate future (Fox, Dunlap, et al., 1997). Person-centered planning meetings are informal gatherings that establish a sense of community and collaborative problem solving. Through person-centered planning, professionals become partners with the people who are important in a child's life and develop a deeper understanding of the child within the context of his or her family and community.

As the support provider begins functional assessment, it is critical that information is shared with the family about the purpose of the process and how information will be used in the development of a behavioral support plan. Families should always be regarded as partners within the assessment and intervention process. Ultimately it is desirable that families use positive behavioral support without the guidance of professionals as their child develops new skills and gains access to new environments.

Gathering Information

There are two steps of a complete functional assessment. The first step is to talk to the family and other care providers who have direct knowledge of the child and the challenging behavior. The Functional Assessment Interview developed by O'Neill and colleagues (1997) offers a structured format for systematically collecting information about the nature of the challenging behavior. A structured interview is desirable because it provides a framework for sorting through information that may seem overwhelming. The structured interview allows the clinician to collect information on the nature of the challenging behavior, setting events that may occasion the behavior, predictors of the behavior occurrence and nonoccurrence, responses that may maintain challenging behavior, the child's communication abilities, and the history of previous intervention efforts.

The second step of the functional assessment process is to observe the child within the environments and activities in which challenging behavior is likely to occur. Observations are conducted to validate and/or to supplement the information gained from the functional assessment interview. Observations should provide information on the nature and intensity of the challenging behavior, antecedents or predictors of the challenging behavior, and the ways in which others respond to challenging behavior. Direct observation data may be collected using anecdotal recording, incident reports or crisis logs, frequency counts, duration recording, time-sampling techniques, and antecedent-behavior-consequence (ABC) analysis (Horner, O'Neill, & Flannery, 1993; O'Neill et al., 1997; O'Neill, Vaughn, & Dunlap, 1998). In addition, researchers have developed structured methods for collecting direct observation data to facilitate the identification of the behavioral function. Carr and his colleagues (1994) provided a format to collect ABC information using index cards that may be sorted by hypothesized behavioral function. The observer records information on the social context of challenging behavior, a description of the behavior, and the social response to the behavior on index cards. The cards are then evaluated and sorted by proposed behavioral function. The scatter plot (Touchette et al., 1985) was designed to provide a mechanism for examining when and where behavior occurs. The scatter plot provides a visual display of the activities and times of day during which challenging behavior occurs more frequently. The Functional Assessment Observation Form (FAO; O'Neill et al., 1997) offers a way to examine behavior occurrences that combines features of ABC analysis and the scatter plot. The FAO provides a means for tracking the occurrence of challenging behavior, the relevant antecedents and consequences, and the perceived function of the behavior.

Families as Partners

Families are essential partners in the functional assessment process. No one has better knowledge of the events that precede and follow a child's challenging behavior than family members who provide daily care to the child. Families are more likely to reveal information to service providers when there is rapport and a trusting relationship (Fox, Vaughn, et al. 1997). The value of a trusting relationship should not be underestimated. Family members have reported that they often feel judged when their children have challenging behavior and may be reluctant to share information that makes them feel vulnerable or exposed to criticism. The functional assessment interview may yield more complete information once rapport has been established between the clinician and the family. The family may also be more willing to allow observations within difficult contexts once they feel assured that service providers are family centered and supportive.

Families become partners in the functional assessment process by identifying the environments and activities in which the child is most likely to have challenging behavior and by assisting the professional in conducting and interpreting observations (Albin et al., 1996). Families may also collect information that is relevant for identifying setting events. For example, the child may appear to have more challenging behavior following nights when he or she has little sleep. The family may also suspect that days when there is a high pollen count and when the child is bothered by allergies coincide with more challenging behavior by their child. The professional can develop a simple observation checklist for the family to collect information on wakefulness, high pollen count as reported by the newspaper, and the level of challenging behavior that the child exhibits. After a week or two of data, patterns may be revealed that support or dispute the relationship of challenging behavior to those events.

Families may have concerns about behavior that the interventionist would not typically define as challenging behavior such as echolalia or age-appropriate intolerance for long shopping trips. It is important to use these opportunities to assist families in understanding the nature of their child's disability, skill development, and developmentally appropriate expectations. The professional should guide the family in the identification of the challenging behaviors that are frequent, intense, or disruptive to the child's ability to engage in other activities.

It is our experience that parents of children with autism who have challenging behavior often feel as though they are ineffective. Families have reported that they feel scrutinized and judged by people who witness their child display challenging behavior (Turnbull & Ruef, 1996). Therefore, families may stop engaging in the public activities and routines in which their child may have challenging behavior (e.g., shopping, attending religious services, eating out, going to the park). When functional assessment information is gathered, the provider should examine the activity patterns of the family and be sensitive to the likelihood that a restricted family lifestyle may be a result of the child's challenging behavior.

When children have challenging behavior, their behavior may shape the behavior of adults (Carr et al., 1991; Taylor & Carr, 1992). Taylor and Carr (1992) examined adults' reactions to the challenging behavior of children that was controlled by adult attention. In their study, adults who were in a teaching role responded to children with autism whose challenging behavior was attention seeking by increasing their attention and physical contact with the children. Adults responded to children with autism whose challenging behavior was to escape social interaction by decreasing their attention and physical contact with the children.

Many parents may respond to their child's challenging behavior by decreasing demands and providing the child access to desirable events and objects without restriction. As a result, it may be difficult to observe challenging behavior unless demands are placed on a child or unless the child is restricted in some manner. For example, Jimmy was a child with autism who had tantrums that consisted of screaming, dropping to the floor, and on occasion hitting his parents. Jimmy would not sit at the table for meals and wanted to fast-forward videos on television during dinnertime. His parents responded to his tantrums by feeding him (although he was capable of feeding himself) while he stood on the couch and fast-forwarded videos. An observation of mealtimes would not reveal challenging behavior because the family had developed accommodations so that challenging behavior would not occur. To get an accurate assessment of the challenging behavior that may occur if the developmentally appropriate demand of eating at the table were placed on Jimmy, the observer asked the family to ask Jimmy to sit at the table with the television off.

Behavioral Hypotheses

The final step of a functional assessment is to develop hypotheses about the challenging behavior. These behavioral hypotheses are summary statements of what was learned through the functional assessment information. Hypothesis statements represent the best informed guess about the relationship of environmental features to challenging behavior and the purposes of challenging behavior given the functional assessment information.

Often the behavioral hypotheses can be developed from the functional assessment interview or other informant methods and validated by direct observation information. For example, during the interview the parent may report that the child is more likely to have challenging behavior during mealtimes, when at restaurants, and when asked to do self-care tasks and is less likely to have challenging behavior when playing alone or watching videotapes. An observation of mealtime showed that one child immediately began having a tantrum after being seated in his chair and was allowed to get out of the chair after several minutes of crying. The parent then placed the child's meal on the coffee table so the child could watch a videotape and eat. The observation confirmed the interview information and provided the observer with insight on the purpose and maintaining consequence of the behavior. Sometimes the observer will see events and challenging behavior that were not mentioned in the interview, and additional hypotheses will be developed based on those observations.

Hypothesis Development

Hypothesis statements should include information on the following: 1) the predictors of challenging behavior; 2) what the behaviors look like (i.e., intensity, duration, topography); 3) the responses that maintain or reinforce the behavior; and 4) a proposed function of the behavior (O'Neill et al., 1997). The following are two examples of hypothesis statements:

1. When informed that it is bathtime, Jordan will drop to the floor, cry, and then hit his head with his hand to escape taking a bath. Often his parents

will respond to the behavior by delaying the bath or deciding to give him a bath the next day.

2. Kara will bang her head lightly and repetitively on the floor to escape play activities with adults when adults try to direct her play or to place demands (i.e., instructions) on her. When Kara bangs her head, adults will cease their demands, provide her with comforting attention, or leave her alone. When Kara plays alone, head banging does not occur.

It is important that the professional who works with the family in the analysis of functional assessment information and the development of the hypotheses statements maintain sensitivity to how the family may react to the information presented. Discussions about how behaviors are maintained must be carefully presented so the parents do not feel that they have "done something wrong." It is important not only that the parents understand that challenging behaviors are communicatively based and that their response may maintain behavior but also that their child's development of conventional communication skills can be shaped with purposeful intervention.

Functional Analysis

When there is ambiguity about the purpose of behavior, functional analysis may be used to confirm a hypothesis or to identify clear patterns regarding the predictors and consequences associated with challenging behavior (O'Neill et al., 1997). In functional analysis, hypotheses are tested by creating controlled situations in which challenging behavior is examined. For example, if the hypothesis was that a child was using challenging behavior to escape difficult tasks or to gain an adult's attention, then a functional analysis could illuminate those relationships. The child could be provided with difficult tasks and then observed for challenging behavior. That situation could then be compared with times when the child was provided with easy tasks. To understand whether the challenging behavior was to request attention, the child could be provided with desired play materials and unconditional attention contrasted with a situation where the child was provided with desired play materials and no adult attention. Functional analysis procedures are most commonly used within research studies because they provide an experimental demonstration of a causal relationship. Researchers who conduct functional analyses typically use single-subject research designs and conduct the analyses within controlled environments. It has been our experience that formal functional analyses are rarely necessary with younger children because their behaviors are less complex and their histories with behavior are relatively brief (in comparison to adults with challenging behavior). Most often it is a straightforward process to develop a useful understanding of young children's challenging behavior through interviews and observations.

The hypothesis statements are the foundation for building the behavioral support plan. An examination of the hypotheses reveals what skills the child will need to learn to replace the challenging behavior. The goal of the support plan will be to create conditions that make the challenging behavior not necessary (irrelevant) and ineffective (not resulting in reinforcement) for the child (Dunlap et al., 1998; O'Neill et al., 1997). This is done by teaching the child a skill that is the functional equivalent of the challenging behavior (i.e., results in achieving the same outcome) while removing the reinforcer for the challenging behavior. In addition, prevention or antecedent strategies are developed to provide the child with adjustments in the environment, activities, and events that reduce the need for the child to use challenging behavior to achieve a goal (Dunlap et al., 1998; O'Neill et al., 1997).

Developing a Support Plan

The development of a behavioral support plan with the family to address the child's challenging behavior is a vital step in the provision of comprehensive, communication-based intervention. The support plan should begin with the identification of behavioral hypotheses that are consistent with the functional assessment information and caregivers' interpretations and observation of the child's behavior.

Once hypotheses are developed, replacement skills are identified that match the identified purpose of the challenging behavior or will result in the same effect as the challenging behavior. For example, if the child currently throws toys to signal that he wishes to escape an activity, then the child may be taught to signal *finished* as a replacement skill. In selecting the replacement skill or functional equivalent to the challenging behavior, it is critical that the skill be easy for the child to perform and readily interpretable (and responded to) by others in the environment. Instruction in the replacement skills should occur throughout the day and within a variety of situations using systematic instructional techniques and effective reinforcement strategies.

In addition to teaching new skills, strategies and modifications in the environment are identified that may reduce the likelihood that the child will use challenging behavior. For example, a visual schedule and transition warnings may be used for a child who has challenging behaviors each time he is requested to transition because he does not understand what is coming next. Environmental modifications may also address the sensory issues of the child. For example, Nicky is a child who is avoidant of certain auditory events. He avoids going in the garage where the fluorescent lights make a humming noise, has tantrums to escape the bathroom when the bathtub is being filled, and screams to leave the porch when it is raining. Environmental modifications for Nicky may include replacing the garage lights, filling the bathtub before he enters the bathroom, or softening the splattering by placing a towel under the faucet, and guiding him to anticipate the beginning of a storm and to signal to leave the porch using a gesture or picture card.

When setting events that may have an impact on challenging behavior (e.g., child is more disruptive following a night without sleep) have been identified, strategies should be developed to address those issues. For example, if a child has more challenging behavior at school when he or she has skipped eating breakfast, then he or she may be offered breakfast on arrival at school. Or, if a child is more difficult following a night without sleep, strategies that will help the child settle down for sleep (e.g., decreasing caffeine in the evening, establishing a consistent bedtime routine) may be included in the support plan. Often there may be questions about the impact of setting events that are more difficult to identify, such as allergies or illnesses. Discovering the impact of those setting events and developing solutions or strategies may require collaboration with medical professionals or other providers (e.g., occupational therapists, speech-language pathologists).

Support plans should also include procedures for ensuring that children receive adequate positive reinforcement and attention. Adults may respond to the challenging behavior of children with autism by decreasing their interactions with and social attention to the child. In addition, the support plan must also provide instructions for how adults will react to challenging behavior when it occurs. It is important that strategies are outlined that guide adults in responding to challenging behavior in ways that make the behavior ineffective (O'Neill et al., 1997). If the challenging behavior is not severe, the occurrence of challenging behavior may be treated as an instructional opportunity in which the child may be guided to use the replacement skill (Dunlap et al., 1998), although instructional situations in which a child is upset are not the most effective.

The final component of the behavioral support plan is to develop long-term support strategies that address lifestyle considerations. Although it may seem unusual to think about a child's lifestyle, children with autism and challenging behavior and their families often have very restricted lives (Turnbull & Ruef, 1996). When children have significant challenging behavior, they are often excluded from activities that peers without disabilities and their families engage in. It is important that families of children with autism be supported in building the kind of lifestyle they would envision if their children did not have a disability.

Providing Intervention

The development of a technically sound behavioral support plan with contextual fit provides a framework for the delivery of comprehensive, communication-based intervention. The behavioral support plan will include many ways in which adults will change what they do to support and respond to the child with challenging behavior. Once a plan is developed, the interventionist will need to work closely with the family and other caregivers to facilitate their use of the support plan strategies and modification of their interactions with the child. It is critical that all of the people who interact with the child become fluent in the use of the support plan within all of the child's activities.

Children with autism often have difficulties with establishing joint attention, communicating conventionally, social interaction and social comfort, responding to multiple stimuli, and interpreting language (Klinger & Dawson, 1992; Prizant & Duchan, 1981; Wetherby, 1986; Wetherby & Prutting, 1984; see also Chapter 6). They may appear to be rigid in their play and to need excessive predictability in routine. These behaviors may be evident in all of their routines and activities. Thus, strategies designed to support the child should be ones that may be applied within all of the child's routines and activities.

Activity-based instruction (Bricker, 1999) offers a framework for embedding the instruction of new skills and the application of support strategies within the context of the child's daily activities. In activity-based instruction, systematic instructional techniques are used within teaching opportunities that are embedded within the routine and planned activities of the child and family. Thus, instructional trials are provided across the day and within meaningful contexts. For example, Emma is learning to use a visual schedule to understand the activities of the day and is being taught to signal *finished* to end an activity. These skills are taught during her morning routine with her mother, in her play and group activities at preschool, and within her after-school activities of having a snack and playing with her siblings.

The goal of comprehensive intervention is to achieve rapid, durable, and generalized changes in the child's challenging and communication behavior that are evident in all environments (Horner & Carr, 1997). To achieve those ambitious outcomes, it is essential that intervention focus on the support of the family and other caregivers to understand and implement the behavioral support plan. Moreover, it is vital that the interventionist respond to other family support needs and issues. Families are the most vital and enduring influence on the child (Dunlap & Fox, 1996; Fox, Dunlap, et al., 1997). Intervention efforts must recognize the critical need to provide supports that strengthen and sustain the family system. The following case study description demonstrates how comprehensive, communication-based intervention addresses the challenging behavior of a young child with autism and the critical needs of the family as they nurture the development of their child.

AARON'S STORY

The following case study describes how comprehensive, positive behavioral support was provided to Aaron Chan and his family through the Individualized Support Project (Fox, Dunlap, et al., 1997). Aaron was 32 months old and diagnosed as having pervasive developmental disorder and overall moderate delay in development including significant deficiencies in social and communication skills. Aaron vocalized frequently but did not verbally communicate with language.

He attended community child care two mornings a week and received speech-language and occupational therapy from private service providers. Aaron's caregivers reported intense tantrums throughout the day. His preschool teacher was very concerned about his challenging behavior, difficulties with transition, and inability to interact with peers. The preschool was concerned about meeting Aaron's needs and wished to reevaluate his enrollment in their program.

Aaron lived with his mother and father. His father was a systems analyst, and his mother was a homemaker. When project staff met Aaron and his family, his parents reported that they were experiencing increased frustration and anxiety propelled by Aaron's challenging behavior. Daily routines such as mealtimes, dressing, and bedtime were difficult because of Aaron's noncompliance. His parents reported that he would not sit at a table to eat. Aaron refused to remain clothed and insisted on sleeping in his parents' bed at night. Aaron had very limited play skills and spent most of his time watching videotapes.

A functional assessment of Aaron's challenging behavior revealed that Aaron used tantrums to escape demand situations. When a developmentally and age-appropriate demand was presented (e.g., "Play with this toy," "Come to the table"), Aaron responded by crying, screaming, dropping to the floor, and banging his head. If the demand situation persisted, Aaron would seek adult comfort by clinging to the adult to escape the demand situation or to inhibit the adult from making additional demands. Aaron would become calm after removal of the demand. He also used tantrums to escape transitions. For example, when Aaron was prompted to leave an activity or environment, he responded by crying, screaming, and dropping to the floor. In response to the tantrum, Aaron was often comforted and the transition was delayed.

Following the functional assessment, a comprehensive behavioral support plan was developed for Aaron with his family. For Aaron, increased predictability was crucial. The assessment process revealed that Aaron could not understand which activity was coming next. A photograph activity schedule was implemented to inform Aaron of the activities of the day and choices that he may make. Caregivers (e.g., parents, child care teachers, therapists) were instructed in ways to prepare Aaron for transitions using the picture schedule and safety signals. In addition to following a predictable schedule, Aaron's daily care providers set a uniform group of expectations and limits for him. Caregivers learned strategies to facilitate Aaron's communication and social development within play sequences. Adaptive communication behaviors that matched the communicative function of his challenging behavior were identified and included in skill instruction. Aaron was taught to use word approximations and natural gestures to signal *no, help, up,* and *want.* There was also a focus on increasing Aaron's action schemes and play level through the use of naturalistic instruction. The entire team believed that ongoing communication was essential for consistency. Therefore, the team developed a notebook to accompany Aaron to different environments (e.g., speech-language therapy, preschool, occupational therapy). In addition, the interventionist coached all care providers on the strategies outlined in the behavioral support plan and how to understand and intervene with challenging behavior from a communication-based perspective.

Although Aaron was in a preschool class with typically developing children, there were low levels of social interaction between Aaron and the other children. Outside of school, Aaron would occasionally see his classmates, either at a birthday party or at the park. These visits were also accompanied by relatively low levels of social interaction between Aaron and his peers.

Intervention was focused on increasing Aaron's play and communication skills, with an emphasis on developing these skills within meaningful social contexts. Naturalistic teaching strategies were used to teach Aaron how to play with his peers. As other children made play initiations to Aaron, his responses were interpreted for the children without disabilities. In addition, Aaron's teacher and family were taught how to adapt activities so Aaron could participate.

On days when Aaron did not go to school, he and his mother began participating in a play group with some children from his classroom. This participation increased Aaron's mother's sense of connection and support and gave Aaron and his peers the opportunity to strengthen their friendships.

A major component of Aaron's comprehensive behavioral support plan was to provide family support. An important family need was to increase the extended family's comfort level regarding Aaron's disability. Another critical need was to increase Aaron's family's network of informal supports. Family members, friends, and other caregivers were gathered for a Personal Futures Planning (Mount & Zwernik, 1988) meeting at the beginning of intervention. One outcome from the planning meeting was the identification of more informal support networks for Aaron's parents. For example, Aaron's mother decided to form a coffee and playgroup with the mothers from the preschool class. A second outcome was the heightened awareness of the extended family regarding Aaron's disabilities and abilities. The maternal grandparents reported after the meeting that they were encouraged and optimistic about Aaron's future.

Other support activities including helping Aaron's parents with environmental arrangement. The project interventionist worked with Aaron's parents to help them to understand the play value of different toys and how to arrange toys to promote play. Although Aaron's parents negotiated the system of doctors and therapists well, they requested support in developing appropriate educational goals for Aaron. Project staff helped them to articulate learning objectives and provided them with explicit information regarding legal rights.

Intervention support was provided to Aaron's family and caregivers that amounted to more than 12 hours a week for 6 months. Intervention support occurred in all of the contexts in which Aaron had difficulties and included time for family support. After 6 months of focused intervention, Aaron's recurrent and intense challenging behavior had completely diminished and there were notable gains in his communication development. He used sophisticated gestures and word approximations to indicate *no, want, more, yes,* and *help* and became proficient at selecting choices of activities and objects. Aaron also began showing pride in his achievements by smiling and vocalizing and then gazing at the adult for recognition. His play schemes increased from single actions to three or four actions within a play sequence. At school, Aaron joined the other children to play with them in a variety of play centers.

At home, Aaron began to follow age-appropriate routines and expectations. Aaron's parents reported that they felt confident in understanding and resolving Aaron's challenging behavior from a communication-based perspective. They learned new ways to support Aaron in play and routines and, as a result, Aaron's engagement in social interactions and reciprocal play dramatically increased. Aaron's parents were able to develop consistent and predictable home routines and implement strategies from his behavioral support plan that resulted in his sitting at the table for meals, sleeping in his own bed at night, remaining clothed, and participating in self-care activities.

CLINICAL AND EDUCATIONAL IMPLICATIONS

Aaron's case study presents an example of how comprehensive support can result in important outcomes for the child and family. Not all programs have the resources to provide this type of knowledgeable and focused support. Aaron's case study also presents a child whose challenging behaviors were not complicated by underlying medical conditions or confounded by many previous behavioral intervention efforts. Intervention efforts for children who present more complex challenging behavior or have underlying biomedical issues (e.g., allergies, seizures) are often more difficult to implement. Many complex factors and service system issues may compromise any intervention effort. What we have endeavored to present is a thorough discussion of an approach that offers great promise to children with autism and their families.

In this chapter we stress the importance of some core elements when working with families of young children with autism and related disabilities. Although our experience has been focused on the importance of these elements within early intervention programs, we believe that these elements provide a level of comprehensiveness that is essential for children with autism and their families. First, we emphasize the importance of family-centered intervention. In this context, we refer to *family centeredness* as a manner of interacting with families that is fully respectful of each family as an individual system characterized by idiosyncratic values, ambitions, interests, strengths, and challenges. In addition, each family that includes a child with autism experiences significant needs and, although there are commonalities, these needs differ from family to family and usually include identifiable concerns that span the areas of informational, instrumental, social, and emotional support (Turnbull & Turnbull, 1996). Because families are by far the most essential resource available for their children, the ultimate effectiveness of intervention corresponds directly with the extent that families can be supported in their efforts to maintain a cohesive, nurturing, and positive familial context. Therefore, it behooves support providers to adopt a comprehensive and individually responsive approach to family support so that the different kinds of needs that a family experiences can be addressed in a sensitive and meaningful manner.

Another implication that is important to reiterate is the central importance of functional communication in the repertoires of children with autism. Research has shown very clearly that challenging behavior is directly related to insufficient and ineffective communicative development. It follows, then, that early instructional efforts that enable a child to communicate important functions with conventional topographies are vital. From a technical perspective, there is no more important goal than rapidly establishing a successful, functional replacement for a child's serious challenging behavior (Carr & Durand, 1985). As discussed throughout the chapter, it is essential that such communicative interventions involve family members and be provided in the actual contexts in which the behavior problems occur.

DIRECTIONS FOR FUTURE RESEARCH

Although an impressive and important body of knowledge has accumulated, and children similar to Aaron have a much brighter outlook than in any previous time period, there is still much that we have to learn. Research in the coming years needs to address vital questions, and it can be anticipated that the answers will contribute even further to the development and implementation of optimal support programs. One set of important questions, for example, pertains to the long-term outcomes that can be realized from family-centered and communication-based intervention strategies. In this chapter and in other sources (Dunlap & Fox, 1996; Dunlap, Johnson, & Robbins, 1990; Fox, Dunlap, et al., 1997) we have proposed a model of supports that is designed to resolve challenging behaviors so that durable response reduction is promoted. Although the available evaluation data (e.g., Dunlap & Fox, 1996; Dunlap et al., 1990) are encouraging, there are no rigorously controlled experimental data that can attest to the effects of the approach as children pass through childhood and grow into adolescents and adults. The ultimate establishment of a powerful prevention agenda will require such experimental analyses as well as longitudinal correlational studies designed to identify risk factors and broad, multidimensional variables associated with the most favorable outcomes.

Another crucial focus for future research involves the need to deliver comprehensive and responsive programs of positive behavioral support to families who represent the range of economic and cultural diversity. Very little research has been conducted with families from minority cultures or with families who live in poverty. It is quite possible that families from different backgrounds have values, beliefs, lifestyles, and priority contingencies that could mitigate against full acceptance of positive behavioral support approaches. Although positive behavioral support is a broad approach that corresponds to a family's circumstances with considerable flexibility, systematic research needs to examine issues of contextual fit with diverse families and to examine the process by which efficacious support plans can be developed when there is a potential for conflict between cultural values or economic circumstances and communication-based positive behavioral support.

CONCLUSIONS

More than a decade of research has provided empirical evidence of the effectiveness of positive behavioral support. In this chapter, the use of positive behavioral support within the provision of early intervention supports for young children with autism has been described. Positive behavioral support offers a framework for the development of comprehensive, communication-based interventions that support the child with autism across environments. Through positive behavioral support, interventionists develop a plan within a partnership with families and other care providers that will result in challenging behavior reduction, communication skill development, and the achievement of meaningful outcomes.

REFERENCES

Albin, R.W., Lucyshyn, J.M., Horner, R.H., & Flannery, K.B. (1996). Contextual fit for behavioral support plans. In L.K. Koegel, R.L. Koegel, & G. Dunlap (Eds.), *Positive behavioral support: Including people with difficult behavior in the community* (pp. 81–98). Baltimore: Paul H. Brookes Publishing Co.

Bailey, D.B., Simeonsson, R.J., Huntington, G.S., Comfort, M., Isbell, P., O'Donnell, K.J., & Helm, J.M. (1990). Family-focused intervention: A functional model for planning, implementing, and evaluating individualized family services in early intervention. *Topics in Early Childhood Special Education, 10,* 156–171.

Bailey, D.B., & Wolery, M. (1992). *Teaching infants and preschoolers with disabilities* (2nd ed.). New York: Macmillan.

Beckman, P.J. (1996). Theoretical, philosophical, and empirical bases of effective work with families. In P.J. Beckman (Ed.), *Strategies for working with families of young children with disabilities* (pp. 1–16). Baltimore: Paul H. Brookes Publishing Co.

Bijou, S.W., & Baer, D.M. (1961). *Child development I: A systematic and empirical theory.* Upper Saddle River, NJ: Prentice Hall.

Billingsley, F.F., & Neel, R.S. (1985). Competing behaviors and their effects on skill generalization and maintenance. *Analysis and Intervention in Developmental Disabilities, 5,* 357–372.

Bird, F., Dores, P.A., Moniz, D., & Robinson, J. (1989). Reducing severe aggressive and self-injurious behaviors with functional communication training. *American Journal on Mental Retardation, 94,* 37–48.

Bricker, D. (with Pretti-Frontczak, K., & McComas, N.). (1999). *An activity-based approach to early intervention* (2nd ed.). Baltimore: Paul H. Brookes Publishing Co.

Bristol, M.M., & Schopler, E. (1983). Stress and coping in families of autistic adolescents. In E. Schopler & G.B. Mesibov (Eds.), *Autism in adolescents and adults* (pp. 251–278). New York: Plenum.

Bronfenbrenner, U. (1979). *The ecology of human development: Experiences by nature and design.* Cambridge, MA: Harvard University Press.

Carr, E.G., & Carlson, J.I. (1993). Reduction of severe behavior problems in the community through a multi-component treatment approach. *Journal of Applied Behavior Analysis, 26,* 157–172.

Carr, E.G., & Durand, V.M. (1985). Reducing behavioral problems through functional communication training. *Journal of Applied Behavior Analysis, 18,* 111–126.

Carr, E.G., Horner, R.H., Turnbull, A., Marquis, J., McLaughlin, D.M., McAtee, M., Smith, C.E., Ryan, K.A., Ruef, M., & Doolabh, A. (1999). *Positive behavior support for people with developmental disabilities: A research synthesis.* Washington, DC: American Association on Mental Retardation.

Carr, E.G., Levin, L., McConnachie, G., Carlson, J.I., Kemp, D.C., & Smith, C.E. (1994). *Communication-based interventions for problem behavior: A user's guide for producing behavior change.* Baltimore: Paul H. Brookes Publishing Co.

Carr, E.G., & McDowell, J.J. (1980). Social control of self-injurious behavior of organic etiology. *Behavior Therapy, 11,* 402–409.

Carr, E.G., & Newsom, C.D. (1985). Demand-related tantrums: Conceptualization and treatment. *Behavior Modification, 9,* 403–426.

Carr, E.G., Taylor, J.C., & Robinson, S. (1991). The effects of severe behavior problems in children on the teaching behavior of adults. *Journal of Applied Behavior Analysis, 24,* 523–535.

Colarusso, R.P., & Kana, T.G. (1991). Public Law 99-457, Part H, infant and toddler programs: Status and implications. *Focus on Exceptional Children, 28,* 1–12.

Dawson, G., & Osterling, J. (1997). Early intervention in autism. In M.J. Guralnick (Ed.), *The effectiveness of early intervention* (pp. 307–326). Baltimore: Paul H. Brookes Publishing Co.

Day, H.M., Horner, R.H., & O'Neill, R.E. (1994). Multiple functions of problem behaviors: Assessment and interventions. *Journal of Applied Behavior Analysis, 27,* 279–289.

Donnellan, A.M., Mirenda, P.L., Mesaros, R.A., & Fassbender, L.L. (1984). Analyzing the communicative functions of aberrant behavior. *Journal of The Association for Persons with Severe Handicaps, 9,* 201–212.

Dunlap, G., & Fox, L. (1996). Early intervention and serious problem behaviors: A comprehensive approach. In L.K. Koegel, R.L. Koegel, & G. Dunlap (Eds.), *Positive behavioral support: Including people with difficult behavior in the community* (pp. 31–50). Baltimore: Paul H. Brookes Publishing Co.

Dunlap, G., Johnson, L.F., & Robbins, F.R. (1990). Preventing serious behavior problems through skill development and early interventions. In A.C. Repp & N.N. Singh

(Eds.), *Perspectives on the use of nonaversive and aversive interventions for persons with developmental disabilities* (pp. 273–286). Sycamore, IL: Sycamore Publishing Co.

Dunlap, G., & Robbins, F.R. (1991). Current perspectives in service delivery for young children with autism. *Comprehensive Mental Health Care, 1,* 177–219.

Dunlap, G., Robbins, F.R., Morelli, M.A., & Dollman, C. (1988). Team training for young children with autism: A regional model for service delivery. *Journal of the Division for Early Childhood, 12,* 147–160.

Dunlap, G., Vaughn, B.J., & O'Neill, R. (1998). Comprehensive behavioral support: Application and intervention. In S.F. Warren & J. Reichle (Series Eds.) & A.M. Wetherby, S.F. Warren, & J. Reichle (Vol. Eds.), *Communication and language intervention series: Vol. 7. Transitions in prelinguistic communication* (pp. 343–364). Baltimore: Paul H. Brookes Publishing Co.

Dunst, C.J., & Trivette, C.M. (1987). Enabling and empowering families: Conceptual and intervention issues. *School Psychology Review, 16,* 443–456.

Dunst, C.J., Trivette, C.M., & Deal, A.G. (1988). *Enabling and empowering families: Principles and guidelines for practice.* Cambridge, MA: Brookline Books.

Durand, V.M. (1982). Analysis and intervention of self-injurious behavior. *Journal of The Association for Persons with Severe Handicaps, 7,* 44–53.

Durand, V.M. (1990). *Functional communication training: An intervention program for severe behavior problems.* New York: Guilford Press.

Durand, V.M., & Carr, E.G. (1991). Functional communication training to reduce challenging behavior: Maintenance and application in new settings. *Journal of Applied Behavior Analysis, 24,* 251–256.

Durand, V.M., & Carr, E.G. (1992). An analysis of maintenance following functional communication training. *Journal of Applied Behavior Analysis, 25,* 777–794.

Durand, V.M., & Crimmins, D.B. (1988). Identifying the variables maintaining self-injurious behavior. *Journal of Autism and Developmental Disorders, 19,* 99–117.

Featherstone, H. (1980). *A difference in the family.* New York: Viking Press.

Fox, L., Dunlap, G., & Philbrick, L.A. (1997). Providing individualized supports to young children with autism and their families. *Journal of Early Intervention, 21,* 1–14.

Fox, L., Vaughn, B.J., Dunlap, G., & Bucy, M. (1997). Parent–professional partnership in behavioral support: A qualitative analysis of one family's experience. *Journal of The Association for Persons with Severe Handicaps, 22,* 198–207.

Garland, C.W. (1993). Beyond chronic sorrow. In A.P. Turnbull, J.M. Patterson, S.K. Behr, D.L. Murray, J.G. Marquis, & M.J. Blue-Banning (Eds.), *Cognitive coping, families, and disability* (pp. 67–80). Baltimore: Paul H. Brookes Publishing Co.

Griffer, M.R. (1997). A competency-based approach to conducting family-centered assessments: Family perceptions of the speech-language clinical process in early intervention service delivery. *Infant–Toddler Intervention, 7,* 45–61.

Hagopian, L.P., Fisher, W.W., & Legacy, S.M. (1994). Schedule effects of noncontingent reinforcement on attention-maintained destructive behavior in identical quadruplets. *Journal of Applied Behavior Analysis, 27,* 317–326.

Hart, C. (1995). Teaching children what parents want. In K.A. Quill (Ed.), *Teaching children with autism* (pp. 53–69). New York: Delmar Publishers.

Horner, R.H., & Budd, C.M. (1985). Teaching manual sign language to a nonverbal student: Generalization of sign use and collateral reduction of maladaptive behavior. *Education and Training of the Mentally Retarded, 20,* 39–47.

Horner, R.H., & Carr, E.G. (1997). Behavioral support for students with severe disabilities: Functional assessment and comprehensive intervention. *Journal of Special Education, 31,* 84–104.

Horner, R.H., & Day, H.M. (1991). The effects of response efficiency on functionally equivalent competing behaviors. *Journal of Applied Behavior Analysis, 24,* 719–732.

Horner, R.H., Dunlap, G., Koegel, R.L., Carr, E.G., Sailor, W., Anderson, J., Albin, R.W., & O'Neill, R.E. (1990). In support of integration for people with severe problem behaviors: A response to four commentaries. *Journal of The Association for Persons with Severe Handicaps, 15,* 145–147.

Horner, R.H., O'Neill, R.E., & Flannery, K.B. (1993). Building effective behavior support plans from functional assessment information. In M.E. Snell (Ed.), *Systematic instruction for students with severe handicaps* (4th ed., pp. 184–214). Columbus, OH: Merrill.

Horner, R.H., Vaughn, B.J., Day, H.M., & Ard, W.R., Jr. (1996). The relationship between setting events and problem behavior: Expanding our understanding of behavioral support. In L.K. Koegel, R.L. Koegel, & G. Dunlap (Eds.), *Positive behavioral support: Including people with difficult behavior in the community* (pp. 381–402). Baltimore: Paul H. Brookes Publishing Co.

Individuals with Disabilities Education Act Amendments of 1991, PL 102-119, 20 U.S.C. §§ 1400 *et seq.*

Individuals with Disabilities Education Act Amendments of 1997, PL 105-17, 20 U.S.C. §§ 1400 *et seq.*

Individuals with Disabilities Education Act of 1990 (IDEA), PL 101-476, 20 U.S.C. §§ 1400 *et seq.*

Klinger, L.G., & Dawson, G. (1992). Facilitating early social and communicative development in children with autism. In S.F. Warren & J. Reichle (Series & Vol. Eds.), *Communication and language intervention series: Vol. 1: Causes and effects in communication and language intervention* (pp. 157–186). Baltimore: Paul H. Brookes Publishing Co.

Koegel, L.K., Koegel, R.L., & Dunlap, G. (Eds.). (1996). *Positive behavioral support: Including people with difficult behavior in the community.* Baltimore: Paul H. Brookes Publishing Co.

Lalli, J.S., Casey, S., & Kates, K. (1995). Reducing escape behavior and increasing task completion with functional communication training, extinction, and response chaining. *Journal of Applied Behavior Analysis, 28,* 261–268.

Lucyshyn, J.M., Albin, R.W., & Nixon, C.D. (1997). Embedding comprehensive behavioral support in family ecology: An experimental, single-case analysis. *Journal of Consulting and Clinical Psychology, 65,* 241–251.

Mahoney, G., & Wheeden, C.A. (1997). Parent–child interaction: The foundation for family centered early intervention practice. A response to Baird and Peterson. *Topics in Early Childhood Special Education, 17,* 165–184.

McGonigel, M.J., Kaufmann, R.K., & Johnson, B.H. (1991). A family-centered process for the individualized family service plan. *Journal of Early Intervention, 15,* 46–56.

Meyer, L.H., & Evans, I.M. (1989). *Nonaversive intervention for behavior problems: A manual for home and community.* Baltimore: Paul H. Brookes Publishing Co.

Michael, J. (1982). Establishing operations and the mand. *Analysis of Verbal Behavior, 6,* 3–9.

Moes, D. (1995). Parent education and parent stress. In R.L. Koegel & L.K. Koegel (Eds.), *Teaching children with autism: Strategies for initiating positive interactions and improving learning opportunities* (pp. 79–93). Baltimore: Paul H. Brookes Publishing Co.

Mount, B., & Zwernik, K. (1988). *It's never too early; it's never too late: A booklet about Personal Futures Planning.* St. Paul, MN: Metropolitan Council.

O'Neill, R.E., Horner, R.H., Albin, R.W., Storey, K., Sprague, J.R., & Newton, J.S. (1997). *Functional assessment of problem behavior: A practical assessment guide.* Pacific Grove, CA: Brooks/Cole.

O'Neill, R.E., Vaughn, B.J., & Dunlap, G. (1998). Comprehensive behavioral support: Assessment issues and strategies. In S.F. Warren & J. Reichle (Series Eds.) & A.M. Wetherby, S.F. Warren, & J. Reichle (Vol. Eds.), *Communication and language intervention series: Vol. 7: Transitions in prelinguistic communication* (pp. 313–341). Baltimore: Paul H. Brookes Publishing Co.

Piazza, C., Moes, D.R., & Fisher, W.W. (1996). Differential reinforcement of alternative behavior and demand fading in the treatment of escape-maintained destructive behavior. *Journal of Applied Behavior Analysis, 29,* 569–572.

Prizant, B.M., & Duchan, J.F. (1981). The functions of immediate echolalia in autistic children. *Journal of Speech and Hearing Disorders, 46,* 241–249.

Reichle, J., & Wacker, D.P., (1993). *Communicative alternatives to challenging behavior: Integrating functional assessment and intervention strategies.* Baltimore: Paul H. Brookes Publishing Co.

Sameroff, A.J., & Chandler, M.J. (1975). Reproductive risk and the continuum of caretaking casualty. In F.D. Horowitz (Ed.), *Review of child development research* (Vol. 4, pp. 189–244). Chicago: University of Chicago Press.

Taylor, J.C., & Carr, E.G. (1992). Severe problem behavior related to social interaction: II. A systems analysis. *Behavior Modification, 16,* 305–335.

Touchette, P.E., MacDonald, R.F., & Langer, S.N. (1985). A scatter plot for identifying stimulus control of problem behavior. *Journal of Applied Behavior Analysis, 18,* 343–351.

Turnbull, A.P., & Ruef, M. (1996). Family perspectives on problem behavior. *Mental Retardation, 34,* 280–293.

Turnbull, A.P., & Ruef, M. (1997). Family perspectives on inclusive lifestyle issues for people with problem behavior. *Exceptional Children, 63,* 211–227.

Turnbull, A.P., & Turnbull, H.R., III. (1996). Group action planning as a strategy for providing comprehensive family support. In L.K. Koegel, R.L. Koegel, & G. Dunlap (Eds.), *Positive behavioral support: Including people with difficult behavior in the community* (pp. 99–114). Baltimore: Paul H. Brookes Publishing Co.

Vaughn, B.J., Dunlap, G., Fox, L., Clarke, S., & Bucy, M. (1997). Parent–professional partnership in behavioral support: A case study of community-based intervention. *Journal of The Association for Persons with Severe Handicaps, 22,* 186–197.

Wetherby, A.M. (1986). Ontogeny of communicative functions in autism. *Journal of Autism and Developmental Disorders, 16,* 295–316.

Wetherby, A.M., & Prutting, C.A. (1984). Profiles of communicative and cognitive-social abilities in autistic children. *Journal of Speech and Hearing Research, 27,* 364–377.

14

Augmentative Communication and Literacy

Pat Mirenda and Karen A. Erickson

The importance of communication skills for individuals with autism is undeniable. Some will develop speech that is adequate for efficient, effective communication, whereas others may require augmentative and alternative communication (AAC) supports. This chapter summarizes the literature related to the use of nonspeech communication supports with individuals with autism as well as the literature regarding supports for literacy development.

AUTISM AND AUGMENTATIVE COMMUNICATION

In 1988, a summary article about AAC interventions for students with autism appeared in a special issue of *Topics in Language Disorders* (Mirenda & Schuler, 1989). In that article, Mirenda and Schuler stated that "no firm conclusions about the . . . efficacy of these interventions can be drawn at this point, as the outcome for the population as a whole has been mixed" (p. 25). It is somewhat surprising to note that since 1989 no summary or review article on AAC and autism has appeared in any journal indexed by *Psychological Abstracts*—certainly, though, both the fields of AAC and autism have changed dramatically! Thus, this chapter can be used as a platform from which to examine the 1990s (and earlier) and as an up-to-date summary of the challenges, advances, and yet unanswered questions that have occurred in this area. In this chapter, the term *AAC* will be used to refer to communication techniques that an individual uses either *in addition to* (i.e., augmentative) or *instead of* (i.e., alternative) whatever naturally acquired speech, gestures, or vocalizations that he or she may have.

Functions Versus Forms

A common mistake in teaching communication skills to children with autism is neglecting to build a strong communicative foundation for these skills. Initial interventions often involve introducing a symbolic AAC system such as manual signing or pictures, even though the individual may not enjoy communicating and may not understand many basic elements, such as turn taking, joint attending, and the role of other people as facilitators. As noted by Mirenda and Schuler, "It is simply not sufficient to teach individuals with . . . limited interest in communication how to say or sign something, or how to point to or show a picture or another visual display. Instead, attempts should be made to extend the current nonverbal means and to diversify the existing communicative functions across contexts" (1989, p. 29).

In typical development, early forms of communication, such as gestures and vocalizations, are gradually augmented by new forms and eventually result in an integrated multimodal system. With a developmental model as the basis, interventions to promote the use of natural gestures and vocalizations in a variety of natural contexts are a good beginning point with individuals who may show little evidence of intentional communication. The goal of such interventions, of course, should be the development of natural speech and language. If this does not occur, however, a strong foundation for later AAC interventions still will have been built.

An excellent example of a multimodal approach to AAC intervention was provided in a case study describing the process a school team used to support a 6-year-old boy with autism (Light, Roberts, Dimarco, & Greiner, 1998). The authors used a modified version of the Participation Model (Beukelman & Mirenda, 1998) to assess both the forms and the functions in the child's communicative repertoire. For example, they utilized a series of "communicative temptations" designed to elicit specific behaviors related to functions such as protesting; sharing and confirming information; requesting objects, actions, information, and assistance; responding to various question forms; and greeting others (Light, McNaughton, & Parnes, 1994; Wetherby & Prutting, 1984). On the basis of this and other assessments, they designed a comprehensive AAC intervention to support concurrent development with regard to *both* language forms and functions. As this case study demonstrated, initial communication goals should include 1) building intentionality, turn taking, joint attention, and initiation skills using unaided AAC techniques such as natural gestures, vocalizations, and speech (if any) and 2) expanding the individual's repertoire of communicative functions beyond the instrumental.

A Brief History of Symbol Use in Autism

A *symbol* can be defined as "something that stands for or represents something else" (Vanderheiden & Yoder, 1986, p. 15); the "something else" is often called the *referent.* Symbols can be divided into two general types: *unaided symbols,* which require no external device for production; and *aided symbols,* which require some type of external device such as a communication book, board, or computer (see Beukelman & Mirenda, 1998 for more extensive information). Typically, unaided symbols such as gestures, vocalizations, facial expressions, and body language are used by beginning communicators who are often thought of as "preintentional." Both unaided symbols (including manual signs[1] in addition to those listed previously) and aided symbols such as photographs, line drawings, or letters are used for more formalized communication.

Historically, symbol selection has received intense attention in the AAC field with regard to people with autism because their relatively intact motor skills make complex interventions involving alternative physical access unnecessary in most cases. The primary question in this regard is and has always been, "What type(s) of symbols are most readily acquired and used by people with autism?"

Chimps, Chips, Signs, and Lexigrams

One of the earliest descriptions of what was originally referred to as *nonspeech communication* with people with autism can be found in a 1974 book chapter by Premack and Premack. The Premacks had taught Sarah, a female chimpanzee, to associate varicolored pieces of plastic of various shapes with more than 130 words in semantic categories that included nouns, verbs, adjectives, and prepositions, among others. Sarah not only understood the meanings of the plastic chips, she could also use them both to produce and to comprehend a variety of simple sentences and questions (Premack, 1971). On the basis of this research, they then taught an 8-year-old boy with autism who could not speak and had a severe visual impairment to use the same plastic chips to communicate, noting that, "the plastic visual system is clearly preferable to no language at all, and it may also prove helpful in speeding the acquisition of natural language" (Premack & Premack, 1974, p. 375). The success of this intervention was followed by a number of additional research projects documenting the efficacy of the plastic chip system (which was later published and marketed as the Non-Speech Language Initiation Program; Carrier & Peak, 1975) with children with autism (e.g., de Villiers & Naughton, 1974; McLean & McLean, 1974).

Simultaneous with these efforts, another pair of language researchers was teaching a chimp named Washoe (and her friends) to communicate using sign language (Gardner & Gardner, 1969, 1975). Similar to the work of the Premacks, this successful research also was applied to children with autism. These early sign language intervention studies showed considerable promise (e.g., Fulwiler & Fouts, 1976; Schaeffer, Kollinzas, Musil, & McDowell, 1978; Webster, McPherson, Sloman, Evans, & Kuchar, 1973). Meanwhile, yet

---

[1]The terms *manual signs, manual signing,* and *sign language* are used interchangeably in this chapter to refer to unaided symbols that include both natural sign languages (e.g., American Sign Language) and codes for spoken language, such as Signed English (Bornstein, Saulnier, & Hamilton, 1983) or Signing Exact English (Gustason, Pfetzing, & Zawolkow, 1980).

a third pair of researchers initiated a longitudinal project ("the LANA Project," named after its first subject) designed to teach chimps to communicate using abstract lexigrams composed of nine geometric forms (Rumbaugh, 1977; Savage-Rumbaugh, Rumbaugh, & Boysen, 1978). The lexigrams were accessed through computer-linked, touch-sensitive display panels that produced (in the early phases of the project) illuminated symbols or (in later phases) synthetic speech. The lessons learned in the LANA Project were successfully applied to 13 boys with severe cognitive impairments—2 of whom had autism—in a project initiated in the mid-1980s (Romski & Sevcik, 1996).

Letters and Words

Orthographic symbols (i.e., alphabet letters) were also used with people with autism in the early days of AAC. Structured operant conditioning interventions were initiated by several researchers to demonstrate that at least some individuals with autism could learn to associate printed words with their referents (e.g., Hewett, 1964; LaVigna, 1977; Marshall & Hegrenes, 1972; Ratusnik & Ratusnik, 1974). Interestingly, although these interventions proved at least as efficacious as the early demonstrations using other types of symbols, letters and words were not widely used for communication with this population, even after a flurry of interest in the mid-1980s related to hyperlexia (i.e., the precocious, self-taught ability to read printed words that is seen in many individuals with autism) (e.g., Frith & Snowling, 1983; Snowling & Frith, 1986; Whitehouse & Harris, 1984). At least in North America, it was not until the introduction of facilitated communication (FC) in the 1990s (Biklen, 1990) that attention refocused on the potential for using orthographic symbols to help individuals with autism communicate.

Visuospatial Symbols

Schuler and Baldwin, in a seminal paper on nonspeech communication and childhood autism published in 1981, were among the first to suggest that the relatively strong visuospatial strengths of individuals with autism were a natural "match" for visuospatial symbols such as photographs and line drawings. Subsequently, reports of the successful use of such visual-graphic symbol sets with people with autism began to appear in the literature and, by the late 1980s, their use was widespread, at least in North America (Mirenda & Mathy-Laikko, 1989; Mirenda & Schuler, 1989).

Manual Sign and Visual-Graphic Symbol Research

Plastic chips, manual signs, lexigrams, and line drawings—these were among the earliest types of symbols used in AAC interventions with individuals with autism. Today, the legacy of these early symbol interventions persists in the belief that *all people, regardless of the apparent extent of their disability,* can learn to communicate. In addition, the early research suggested that both manual signs and visual-graphic symbols hold particular promise for individuals with autism (Fay & Schuler, 1980). This section summarizes the research related to these two types of symbols.

By the mid-1980s, manual signing combined with speech (an approach often referred to as "total" or "simultaneous" communication) was the AAC technique most commonly used with people labeled "severely handicapped" (many of whom had autism) in the United States (Bryen & Joyce, 1985; Matas, Mathy-Laikko, Beukelman, & Legresley, 1985), the United Kingdom (Kiernan, 1983; Kiernan, Reid, & Jones, 1982), and Australia (Iacono & Parsons, 1986). Now, manual signing with individuals with autism has largely been supplanted in many places by the use of visual-graphic symbols (Schuler, Prizant, & Wetherby, 1997). This shift has occurred as a result of research findings in three main areas: imitation, iconicity, and intelligibility ("the three I's").

Imitation

Much of the early work in the area of simultaneous communication focused on using manual signs to facilitate the development of expressive speech in children with autism (Barrera & Sulzer-Azaroff, 1983; Konstantareas, Webster, & Oxman, 1979; Schaeffer et al., 1978). It was not long, however, before it became clear that this outcome was not always likely. In particular, Carr and his colleagues provided evidence to suggest that the success of simultaneous communication largely depended on whether the learner had mastered generalized imitation at the time of intervention (Carr & Dores, 1981; Carr, Pridal, & Dores, 1984). They described two groups of learners—good and poor verbal imitators—and noted that the use of manual signs plus speech with the good imitators often resulted in improved receptive *and* expressive language, whereas the same intervention with the poor imitators usually resulted in improved receptive language but not improved expressive output. In addition, poor imitators appeared to make fewer receptive gains than did their good imitator peers (Layton, 1988; Yoder & Layton, 1989). These results, coupled with research evidence of a generalized imitation deficit in autism (Dawson & Adams, 1984; see Smith & Bryson, 1994, for a review), somewhat tempered the initial enthusiasm for simultaneous communication as "the answer" for the communication problems of these individuals.

In addition, although the extent of co-occurrence of autism and fine motor problems (i.e., limb apraxia) is not clear, there is evidence to suggest that many individuals with autism do experience motor coordination difficulties (Hughes, 1996; Jones & Prior, 1985). Furthermore, a study demonstrated that manual sign vocabulary size and accuracy of sign formation were both highly correlated with measures of apraxia and fine motor skills in 14 individuals with autism (Seal & Bonvillian, 1997). This finding suggests that the problem with imitation might be due, at least in part, to underlying problems with motor planning and coordination (Rogers & Bennetto, 1996; see also Chapter 5). Cumulatively, the combined impact of the imitation and motor deficits in individuals with autism mitigates against the use of manual signing as an AAC symbol system in many cases, even though it may have other advantages such as portability and naturalness. In contrast, symbol systems such as those that are visual-graphic, which can be accessed simply by pointing, are motorically less demanding and may have this as an advantage.

Iconicity

The *iconicity hypothesis* states that "symbols having a strong resemblance to their referents [are] easier to learn and remember than those symbols having a weak visual relationship" (Fuller & Stratton, 1991, p. 52; see Fristoe & Lloyd, 1979, for the original discussion of this hypothesis). This hypothesis has largely been supported in studies examining manual sign learning in children with autism (Konstantareas, 1984; Konstantareas, Oxman, & Webster, 1978). Thus, the American Sign Language (ASL) signs for *eat, drink,* and *sleep,* which bear a close visual resemblance to their referents, are likely to be learned and used more readily than the signs for *help, stop,* and *toilet,* which do not (Sternberg, 1994). Yet, all of these words are highly functional and would usually be included in the initial sign lexicon taught to most children (Karlan, 1990). In fact, many of the most basic and functional signs fail the "iconicity test" implied by the hypothesis and thus are at least somewhat difficult for many individuals with autism to learn and use spontaneously (see Bryen & Joyce, 1985, for a more complete discussion of this issue).

In contrast to manual signs, visual-graphic symbols such as photographs and pictograms are usually quite iconic and thus capitalize on the visuospatial strengths commonly seen in people with autism (Mirenda & Schuler, 1989). The successful use of photographs as communication symbols has been reported in several studies involving both children (Krantz, MacDuff, & McClannahan, 1993; MacDuff, Krantz, & McClannahan, 1993; Pierce & Schreibman, 1994) and adults with autism (Vaughn & Horner, 1995). In these studies, photographs were used in addition to speech to provide augmented language input to the participants (this approach is discussed in more detail later in this chapter). Picture Communication Symbols (PCSs; Mayer-Johnson Co., 1994), perhaps the most widely used pictographic symbol set in North America, also have been used in both receptive (Peterson, Bondy, Vincent, & Finnegan, 1995) and expressive AAC interventions with these individuals (Bondy & Frost, 1994; Hamilton & Snell, 1993; Mirenda & Santogrossi, 1985; Rotholz, Berkowitz, & Burberry, 1989). In addition, the use of rebuses and Pictogram Ideogram Communication symbols (Maharaj, 1980) has been reported (Reichle & Brown, 1986).

This is not meant to imply that manual signing is not a viable symbol system for individuals with autism. Some would argue, in fact, that it should be the system of choice because it is more portable, more iconic, easier to teach, and easier to map onto speech (Shafer, 1993; Sundberg, 1993). It is also important to note that natural gestures, often considered less desirable than manual signs because they are not a formalized language system, are more likely to "pass" the iconicity test and thus have advantages with regard to spontaneous use. For example, Hamre-Nietupski and her colleagues (1977) catalogued 147 "generally understood gestures," which were later found to have a 77% recognition rate by adults who support individuals with severe disabilities (Fiocca, 1981). Although natural gestures may not develop in individuals with autism without support (Schuler, 1985), they should be incorporated as one component of a multimodal communication system in all cases.

Intelligibility

One of the primary reasons for the shift from manual signs to visual-graphic symbols has been more pragmatic than empirical, although there is some research to support it. The fact is that communication partners who are not familiar with manual signs are not likely to be successful when communicating with individuals with autism who have learned to sign and will probably require an interpreter to act as an intermediary. The learning demands placed on family members, teachers, classmates, and community members who support individuals with autism through manual signing are considerable, if independence from an interpreter is to be the goal. This demand, however, does not accompany visual-graphic systems, all of which present the printed word together with the symbol so that literate communication partners have two cues as to the meaning—the symbol itself (which may or may not be easily recognized) and the written word.

A study by Rotholz and colleagues (1989) illustrated quite clearly the intelligibility limitations of manual signing used with unfamiliar community members. Two adolescents with autism were taught to use both manual signs and PCSs to order food in a restaurant. On average, between 0% and 25% of the manual sign requests by one student and 0% of manual sign requests by the other student were successfully understood by the restaurant counterperson without assistance from the students' teacher. In contrast, the two students had average successful request rates of 80%–88% and 95%–100%, respectively, when they used PCSs in their communication books.

The preponderance of research evidence appears to support the use of visual-graphic symbols with individuals with autism who require AAC supports, although there is some disagreement in this regard (e.g., Shafer, 1993; Sundberg, 1993). Much of this disagreement is based on the argument that, because of its inherently linguistic nature, manual signing is more likely to support the development of speech—which is, after all, the ideal outcome of any communication intervention. Evidence suggests, however, that speech development secondary to AAC use is not necessarily an outcome that is confined to the use of manual signs (Bondy & Frost, 1995; Romski & Sevcik, 1996). In the next section, we review the evidence for and against the "symbol-to-speech" controversy in more detail.

What Is the Relationship Between AAC and Speech Development?

One of the most common concerns expressed by parents and teachers regarding the use of AAC techniques with individuals with autism is how the techniques are likely to affect speech development. Research has demonstrated quite clearly that "learning to communicate initially by sign transfers to the spoken word after the child learns approximately 200 signs and starts to chain two or more signs together" (Layton & Watson, 1995, p. 81; see also Carr & Dores, 1981; Konstantareas et al., 1979; Layton, 1988; Layton & Baker, 1981; Schaeffer et al., 1978; and Yoder & Layton, 1989). There is also ample evidence, however, that even after intensive manual sign instruction, a significant number of individuals continue to be mute and acquire only a few useful signs (Layton, 1988). Nonetheless, it appears that the use of manual signing does not inhibit the development of speech in individuals with autism and that there is *potential* for speech development in conjunction with manual signing.

The evidence for the impact of aided AAC on speech development is less clear, but two bodies of research evidence are promising in this regard. The first is from the work of Frost and Bondy (1994), who have developed and used a structured behavioral program entitled the Picture Exchange Communication System (PECS) with individuals with autism. PECS uses aided symbols (usually PCSs, although photographs and other visual-graphic symbols can be used as well) to teach the individual to exchange a symbol for a desired item (e.g., food, drink, toy). Once the individual can initiate this exchange under a variety of conditions and with a wide range of people, the system is gradually expanded to teach additional communicative functions such as labeling and information gathering. Bondy and Frost (1995) reported on the use of PECS with 66 young children with autism (5 years of age or younger) with no functional speech or previous experience with AAC systems. Over a 5-year period, 34 of the 66 children (52%) developed functional speech and no longer required AAC supports, and an additional 14 (21%) used a combination of speech and visual-graphic symbols or written words. Thus, a total of 73% of the children had developed at least some functional speech after 1–5 years of PECS instruction. Another group of 26 preschoolers with autism were taught to use PECS and were followed over a 3-year period; 7 of these children (27%) developed such sufficient speech that they were no longer educationally identified as having autism (Frost & Bondy, 1994). In both groups, the overall communicative development of the children was strongly related to their overall level of intellectual functioning. Frost and Bondy noted that speech tended to develop once the children were able to use 30–100 symbols to communicate.

Additional support for speech development with aided AAC use was provided through a research project conducted with 13 individuals with severe disabilities, 2 of whom had autism. All of the participants had 10 or fewer spoken word approximations at the start of the project. They were provided with an AAC intervention called the System for Augmenting Language (SAL) over a 2-year period (Romski & Sevcik, 1996). Communication displays using abstract lexigrams accompanied by printed words (similar to those used in the LANA Project discussed previously) were constructed for each participant. The displays were placed on voice-output communication aids (VOCAs) that produced synthetic speech output when the symbols were touch activated (e.g., if the lexigram JUICE was activated, the VOCA said, "juice"). Communication partners were taught to activate the symbols on the VOCAs to augment their speech input in naturally occurring communication interactions. For example, a teacher might say to a child, "Tami, let's go outside and play," while activating the symbols OUTSIDE and PLAY on Tami's VOCA. Thus, the child would see the teacher model use of the symbols OUTSIDE and PLAY and at the same time hear both the teacher and the VOCA say the words out loud. The participants were encouraged though not required to use the device throughout the day. Thus, SAL differed dramatically from PECS in that instruction was provided through a "model and encourage" approach rather than through structured training and response elicitation. Because the communication partners (e.g., parents, teachers, peers) were so critical to the integrity of SAL, a variety of strategies were included to ensure that their perceptions and experiences with the technique remained positive.

Romski and Sevcik (1996) reported multiple aspects of the project results, including those related to the issue at hand, speech development. Seven of the participants, including the two with autism, increased the proportion of spoken words in their vocabularies that were rated intelligible over the course of the project. The participants' speech improvements did not appear to be related to either their vocal imitation abilities or their rate of symbol use with SAL. Although the extent to which VOCA output contributed to the participants' speech development is not clear, the researchers speculated that the consistent models of spoken words provided by the VOCAs immediately following each symbol usage might have had a positive impact in this regard.

Together, the PECS and SAL results suggest that, as is the case with manual signing, aided symbol use does not appear to hinder and may, in fact, enhance the development of speech in individuals with autism, including those who are older than the age of 5 (Romski & Sevcik, 1996). The results also raise an additional issue regarding the role of VOCAs and other computer-based supports in communication interventions for people with autism.

The Role Of Voice-Output Communication Aids and Computers

Unlike the late 1980s, numerous VOCAs and computer software applications are now available to meet the needs of a wide range of individuals with autism. These include VOCAs in three categories: single-level devices, multilevel devices, and comprehensive devices. They also include computer software programs that provide writing and/or spelling assistance, support various aspects of literacy learning, or facilitate classroom participation in general.

Three Types of Voice-Output Communication Aids

Single-level VOCAs are designed to deliver a limited number of messages, usually not more than 20, and are very simple to program and operate. For example, the BIGmack (AbleNet, Inc.) is a small device with a built-in microswitch that, when activated, plays a single recorded message up to 20 seconds long. Recording a human voice message into the BIGmack takes only seconds, and new messages can be recorded over old ones throughout the day. Thus, with the assistance of an aide responsible for recording the messages, a kindergarten-age student with autism could use a BIGmack to 1) greet his or her teacher and classmates on arrival at school ("Hi, how are you today?"); 2) recite the class poem with his classmates; 3) participate in a language arts lesson by "reciting" the repeating line of a story the teacher is reading ("He huffed, and he puffed, and he blew the house down"); and 4) call out, "Duck, duck, duck, duck, goose!" when the group plays this common children's game. Additional examples of single-level devices (and the number of messages they can store) include the Talk Back (6) and Messenger (1), both by the Crestwood Company; Hawk (9) by ADAMLAB; MessageMate (8–20) by Words +, Inc.; Parrot (16) by ZYGO Industries, Inc.; SpeakEasy (12) by AbleNet, Inc.; and Voicemate (4–8) by Tash, Inc.

Multilevel VOCAs are capable of delivering more than 20 messages (in some cases, thousands!) and are more difficult both to program and to use because they are more complex. Of course, the advantage of multilevel devices is that they can contain a greater number of programmed messages (i.e., words, phrases, or sentences). Usually, multiple symbol displays are placed on the device to allow access to messages programmed on two or more "levels." Either the user or an assistant must manually change these displays in most cases. Some of the best-known examples include the Black Hawk, Whisper Wolf, and Wolf (ADAMLAB); Macaw (ZYGO Industries, Inc.); and Say-It-Simply Plus (Innocomp). Alternatively, some multilevel devices use various electronic techniques that allow users to access multiple message levels without having to change the symbol displays manually. These include the AlphaTalker and Walker Talker (Prentke Romich Co.) and the Digivox (Sentient Systems Technology, Inc.).

Finally, *comprehensive VOCAs* are designed to deliver multiple messages using a variety of rate enhancement techniques to increase efficiency and speed. Many of these devices have additional features, including printers, calculators, large memory capacities for storing lengthy text and speeches, and the ability to interface with standard computers. Some examples include the DeltaTalker, Liberator, and Vanguard (Prentke Romich Company); DynaVox (Sentient Systems Technology, Inc.); LightWRITER (Toby Churchill, Ltd.); Speaking Dynamically (Mayer-Johnson Co.); and Talking Screen (Words +, Inc.).

Computer Software

In addition to VOCAs that are designed for the specific purpose of communication, a proliferation of software is also used to support communication and literacy development via orthography for people with autism. In the early 1980s, research was undertaken to investigate the effects of computer-aided instruction on students with autism. The software used in these studies was designed to teach specific vocabulary and skills rather than to influence communication, literacy learning, and/or interaction. Nonetheless, computer use was found to have a positive effect on peer interactions and verbalizations (Panyan, 1984), problem-solving strategies (Jordan & Powell, 1990a, 1990b), motivation and behavior (Chen & Bernard-Opitz, 1993), and reading of individual words (Heimann, Nelson, Tjus, & Gillberg, 1995). Unfortunately, the efficacy of much of the software that is currently available to support communication and literacy development has only been investigated in students with disabilities other than autism (e.g., MacArthur, 1988, 1996; Staples, Heying, & McLellan, 1995; Williams, 1998).

The most common types of software are word processing programs that are operated in conventional computers equipped with speech synthesizers. Examples include IntelliTalk (IntelliTools, Inc.) and Write Out:Loud (Don Johnston, Inc.). These word processors can "read" individual letters, words, sentences, or paragraphs as they are entered with the keyboard. In addition, either selected words or entire text files can be reread by the speech synthesizer as individual words are visually highlighted on the computer screen. Such software provides consistent and immediate feedback that can be very useful to individuals who are learning to read, write, and communicate.

Word processing software with synthetic speech output and the additional feature of word prediction can also be used by many individuals. Word prediction software allows a user to enter the initial letter of a word to produce an on-screen list of common words that begin with the selected letter. Those who cannot read can use a mouse or arrow keys to select words that are recited out loud by the speech synthesizer. If a desired word appears in the list, the user can select it either by clicking on it with the mouse or by typing a corresponding number. If the word is not in the list, additional letters may be typed to produce a refined list. The most commonly available word prediction programs are EZ Keys (Words +, Inc.) and Co:Writer (Don Johnston, Inc.).

Although the availability of VOCA and computer technology has increased dramatically since the late 1980s, research related to their use with individuals with autism has not. There is some evidence, however that computer technology appears to enhance motivation, increase attention, and/or reduce challenging behavior in individuals with autism across the ability range, perhaps because of the highly visual nature of computer technology and the high degree of predictability it provides (Frost, 1984; Hedbring, 1985; Pleinis & Romanczyk, 1985). Thus, it is appropriate to at least *consider* providing technological supports on a trial basis to individuals with autism who experience communication and/or learning difficulties, based on comprehensive assessments. An example was provided in the case study cited previously (Light et al., 1998), in which a child's multimodal communication system consisted of natural speech, pointing and other conventional gestures, a communication book and dictionary, and a Macintosh Powerbook with a high-quality speech synthesizer and Write Out:Loud software (Don Johnston, Inc.). The extensive assessment conducted prior to implementing this intervention is an excellent example of state-of-the-art planning and decision making in this area; however, in reality, it remains the exception rather than the rule.

AAC Interventions for Challenging Behavior

As much as research related to autism and technology has been somewhat lacking over the past decade, research in another area—the interface between AAC and challenging behavior—has made great strides forward. AAC interventions have been used successfully in many empirical studies to provide both receptive and expressive communication supports to individuals with challenging behavior, as summarized in the next section.

Augmented Input Strategies

AAC interventions include a wide range of strategies and procedures whose common goal is to facilitate an individual's ability either 1) to *communicate* more effectively *with* others (i.e., expressive communication strategies) or 2) to *understand* communication *from* others (i.e., augmented input strategies; Wood, Lasker, Siegel-Causey, Beukelman, & Ball, 1998). Although the latter set of strategies has received relatively little attention until recently, there is increasing evidence that many individuals with autism who engage in problem behaviors benefit greatly when language input is augmented, particularly through the visual modality (Hodgdon, 1995, 1996; Quill, 1995). In this section, we describe the most common forms of augmented input used with these individuals.

Pictorial or Written Schedules One of the most common augmented input strategies involves the use of pictorial or written schedules to assist an individual to understand and follow predictable activity sequences in school and home settings (Wood et al., 1998). In some research studies investigating this approach, children with autism were taught to use *within-task* pictorial schedules to complete specific activities such as hanging up a coat or putting away a favorite toy (e.g., Krantz et al., 1993; MacDuff et al., 1993). In other studies, the participants used *between-task* schedules to predict what would happen next as they moved from one activity to the other (e.g., Flannery & Horner, 1994; Mirenda, Kandborg, & MacGregor, 1994). For example, Flannery and Horner (1994) used a written schedule to support Aviv, an adolescent with autism who engaged in aggression, self-injury, and property destruction. Aviv was known to exhibit challenging behavior when the sequence and duration of activities at school were unpredictable. Because he was able to read, Aviv was provided with a printed, sequential list of upcoming activities and their duration at the beginning of each school period and was prompted to consult the list regularly to predict, "Which activity is next?" When the schedule was not available, he engaged in moderately high rates of challenging behavior, compared with no such behaviors when the schedule was provided. Results such as this suggest that individuals with autism can learn to use pictorial or written schedules quite easily and that their challenging behavior may be reduced or eliminated dramatically when these supports are provided.

Within-Task Schedules (Symbol Scripts) Within-task schedules (or symbol scripts) can be particularly useful for individuals who experience difficulty *during* specific activities that do not appear to be unpleasant, painful, frightening, or otherwise aversive. In such cases, it may be that the individual simply does not understand the sequence of steps that compose the activity and thus attempts to escape from or avoid it. Augmented input is designed to clarify the activity through the use of symbols such as photographs, PCSs, or written words that correspond to the key steps of the task. *Key steps* means those steps in which the individual is expected to actively participate or that have an impact on him or her in some way. The symbols are sequences from the first to the last step of the activity, for example, on the pages of a photo album, a slide protector page, or a Velcro strip. Then, *prior* to the problem activity, the individual is assisted to preview the activity on a step-by-step basis, using the symbols for each step. For example, Mirenda, MacGregor, and Kelly-Keough (in press) described an intervention with Kerry, a child with pervasive developmental disorder and deafness. Every evening, Kerry had a tantrum in the bathtub when it was time to wash her hair; the tantrum consisted of kicking, self-injurious behavior, attempts to bite and hit her mother, and loud screaming. Her mother used a simple, four-symbol PCS sequence depicting the key steps in the hair washing routine: 1) get out the shampoo, 2) put shampoo on the hair, 3) wash the hair to the count of eight (the upper limit of Kerry's counting ability at that time), and 4) rinse off the shampoo. Use of the script resulted in immediate and long-term elimination of the tantrums after only a few exposures. This example illustrates the potential positive impact of this type of augmented input.

Rule Scripts A variation of the standard within-activity script is one that is used to clarify the "rules" related to an activity rather than the sequence of steps that compose it. For example, the rules for dinnertime might be 1) eat what is on your plate and don't eat what is on other people's plates; 2) use your knife, fork, and spoon to eat and don't eat with your fingers; and 3) eat slowly, take small bites, and don't eat quickly or take large bites. For some individuals, challenging behaviors may occur because they are unaware of or uncertain about the rules they are expected to follow; rule scripts can be useful in providing augmented input in this regard.

As with standard within-task scripts, symbols must first be compiled to represent the rules of concern (e.g., eat slowly, eat what's on your plate). The symbols and rules are then reviewed with the individual both *prior to* and *during* the activity, and positive feedback for following the rules is provided when appropriate (e.g., "You're doing a nice job of *eating slowly* and *eating what's on your plate*"). In addition, the symbols are used to provide corrective feedback if a rule violation occurs (e.g., "Remember, *no eating with your fingers.* You need to *eat with your fork*"). In effect, the symbols are used as visual prompts to teach the individual appropriate behaviors and expectations in specific situations. In this sense, rule scripts are similar to social stories (Gray, 1995) and cognitive picture rehearsal strategies (Groden & LeVasseur, 1995), which may also be useful as augmented input.

From this brief overview, it should be evident that augmented visual input strategies are likely to be essential components to the communication systems for many (if not most) individuals with autism who engage in challenging behaviors. Similarly, specific expressive AAC supports may be provided through approaches such as functional communication training (FCT).

Functional Communication Training Using AAC

One of the first empirical demonstrations of the potential for the expressive use of AAC in the remediation of the behavior problems of individuals with autism was offered in a 1985 study by Horner and Budd. The study involved an 11-year-old boy with autism who had extremely limited expressive language and displayed frequent grabbing and yelling behaviors during the school day. After informal assessment of the conditions in which the behaviors occurred, a decision was made to teach him five manual signs for items that appeared to be related to the grabbing/yelling. In other words, he was taught to request the items for which he usually grabbed/yelled. The data indicated quite clearly that after he had learned to use the signs in the natural environment of the classroom, his sign use increased as his grabbing and yelling behaviors decreased dramatically. The strategy of teaching individuals to use manual signs or other AAC techniques as "substitutes" for the "messages" underlying their challenging behavior is now known as *FCT.*

In a review of FCT studies published between 1985 and 1996 in which one or more AAC techniques were used (Mirenda, 1997), 8 of the 52 participants (15%) had autism (Bird, Dores, Moniz, & Robinson, 1989; Campbell & Lutzker, 1993; Day, Horner, & O'Neill, 1994; Horner & Budd, 1985; Horner & Day, 1991; Sigafoos & Meikle, 1996; Wacker et al., 1990). They ranged in age from 7 to 36 and engaged in one or more challenging behaviors, including self-injurious behavior, aggression, crying, screaming, property destruction, tantrums, noncompliance, and self-stimulatory behavior, as well as the aforementioned grabbing and yelling. The "messages" or functions of their behaviors included "Pay attention to me" (attention), "I want *x*" (tangibles), and "I don't want to do this" (escape), with the majority (63%) in the latter group. A variety of AAC techniques were taught as alternatives to the challenging behavior, including tangible symbols (one participant), manual signs and/or gestures (six participants), a card with printed words (e.g., *I want a BREAK*) (one participant), and line drawing symbols (one participant). There was an immediate and substantial reduction in the frequency of challenging behavior for all eight participants who had autism after the FCT interventions were initiated, which was maintained for as long as 1 year (follow-up data were not provided for all participants). FCT interventions have the clear advantage of "killing two birds with one stone"—they teach the individual to communicate one or more functional messages, while at the same time they provide a positive alternative to his or her challenging behavior(s).

Clinical and Educational Implications: AAC Interventions and Autism

From this brief overview, it should be clear that planning AAC interventions for individuals with autism is a complex and challenging task! Attention should be paid not only to providing appropriate communicative forms but (even more important) also to expanding communication functions. Selection of one or more types of symbols requires careful assessment and individualization. Instructional and facilitator supports may be provided in a variety of ways, ranging from direct instruction (e.g., PECS, FCT) to modeling and encouragement (e.g., SAL). Use of electronic devices and/or augmented input strategies may be appropriate for all or part of an intervention, depending on the individual. Finally, numerous communication opportunities in natural settings with responsive communication partners must be made available, to provide appropriate contexts for communication to occur.

The Participation Model, described in detail by Beukelman and Mirenda (1998), has been proposed as a multielement process for AAC assessment and intervention planning that incorporates many of the aforementioned elements.

The model consists of two strands for assessment and decision making, the Opportunity Strand and the Access Strand, and has six main components: 1) identification of communication needs in a variety of environments and activities; 2) assessment of partner interaction strategies and environmental barriers that may impede communication; 3) assessment of the individual's capabilities in areas such as positioning and motor skills, receptive language, expressive communication, symbol representation skills, literacy skills, cognitive organization, and sensory/perceptual skills; 4) implementation of strategies to remediate opportunity barriers; 5) intervention planning with regard to AAC techniques and instructional approaches; and 6) evaluation of AAC effectiveness in natural contexts. The Participation Model has been used successfully to plan school-based AAC interventions for individuals with autism and other severe disabilities (Light et al., 1998; Schlosser, Mirenda, McGhie-Richmond, Blackstein-Adler, & Janzen, 1998).

Directions for Future Research: AAC Interventions and Autism

It is probably clear by now that many questions remain when it comes to autism and AAC in general. Before turning to a discussion of literacy and people with autism, we offer the "Top Five Questions" in this area for which empirical research is urgently needed (with apologies to David Letterman!):

1. What strategies are most successful for encouraging development of natural gestures and vocalizations in preintentional communicators? How can parents and teachers best promote the development of intentionality and expanded communicative functions?
2. How much incidental modeling is needed for efficient symbol learning, whether of manual signs or visual-graphic symbols? For example, should everyone in an individual's environment use manual signs to communicate all messages? Or is key word signing (Windsor & Fristoe, 1989, 1991) the best approach?
3. What are the comparative outcomes of the PECS and SAL approaches when both are implemented with *young children* with autism?
4. How does use of augmented input strategies for behavioral support affect communication and social development?
5. How much does the availability of voice-output technology contribute to symbol learning, speech development, and receptive language development, compared with visual-graphic symbol use without voice output?

In the next section, we turn to a brief discussion of autism and literacy, which is related to our previous discussion regarding the use of orthographic symbols (i.e., letters and words) as an AAC approach for at least some individuals.

AUTISM AND LITERACY

As mentioned previously, it was not until the introduction of FC in the 1990s (Biklen, 1990) that the potential for using orthographic symbols to help individuals with autism communicate was widely considered. FC involves the use of a keyboard communication device of some type (e.g., a Canon Communicator; a small, portable typewriter) on which messages are typed on a letter-by-letter basis. The typist's forearm, wrist, and, if necessary, index finger are physically supported by a facilitator, who provides emotional, physical, and instructional support. Gradually, the supports provided by the facilitator are faded, with the goal of independent typing. FC has been used widely with individuals with autism as well as other developmental disabilities.

Briefly, the debate around FC has centered on the source of the messages being typed: Who is authoring the messages, the typist or the facilitator? The question has been raised largely because of the unexpected quantity and quality of the messages produced by many facilitated typists (often, children or adults with autism) who have never received literacy instruction and were presumed to be unable to read or write. Numerous books, chapters, articles, and dissertations have attempted to answer the authorship question through various research approaches (e.g., Biklen, 1993; Biklen & Cardinal, 1997; Shane, 1994). The vast majority of this research has indicated that facilitated typists frequently are influenced by their facilitators in typing the messages (e.g., Eberlin, McConnachie, Ibel, & Volpe, 1993; Moore, Donovan & Hudson, 1993; for a complete discussion see Green & Shane, 1994). A few studies have found, however, that under certain conditions some typists appear to be able to compose messages without facilitator influence (see Cardinal, Hanson, & Wakeham, 1996; Sheehan & Matuozzi, 1996; Weiss, Wagner, & Bauman, 1996). Although the use of FC remains controversial, there is no doubt that the flurry of research and debate surrounding it created renewed interest in the literacy learning potential of people with autism in general.

Hyperlexia

Hyperlexia, the precocious self-taught ability to read words with an apparent lack of comprehension, has also played a role in the recently renewed interest in the literacy learning potential of people with autism. Although hyperlexia appears in children with a wide range of disabilities, it appears to occur most often in children with autism (Cobrinik, 1974, 1982; Elliot & Needleman, 1976; Goldberg & Rothermel, 1984). In one study of 5,400 children with autism, 9.8% were found to have some sort of exceptional or savant abilities in reading or some other area (Rimland, 1978).

Specific characteristics of hyperlexia include 1) word reading skills that exceed what is predicted or expected based on cognitive and language abilities; 2) compulsive or indiscriminate reading of words; 3) onset of ability when the child is 2–5 years old; and 4) onset of ability in the absence of direct instruction (Silberberg & Silberberg, 1967). In addition, hyperlexia is characterized by a discrepancy between reading comprehension and word reading abilities (Cobrinik, 1974).

Snowling and Frith (1986) compared the reading abilities of three groups of adolescents: those with autism and cognitive impairments, those with autism and no cognitive impairments, and those with no disabilities at all. The latter two groups were matched for mental age. Snowling and Frith concluded that deficits in reading comprehension were related to the participants' verbal abilities rather than to their autism per se. The participants without disabilities and those with autism but no cognitive impairments were all able to extract meaning from sentences and passages. The participants with autism and cognitive impairments performed these tasks at a lower level.

In general, receptive language ability has a strong influence on an individual's ability to read with comprehension. When word reading ability is controlled for, individuals with poor receptive language skills find it much more difficult to read with comprehension than do individuals with strong receptive language skills (see Cunningham, 1993, for a complete discussion of the relationship). The ability to read (i.e., decode) words, however, is linked to visual skills, the application of phonological rules, and the detection of patterns in words (Cunningham, 1992). Individuals who are skilled in these areas may develop extensive sight word vocabularies in the absence of comprehension. As reported in Aram (1997), at least seven studies suggest that people with autism and hyperlexia correctly utilize regular phonological rules in reading words (Aram, Rose, & Horwitz, 1984; Frith & Snowling, 1983; Glosser, Friedman, & Roeltgen, 1996; Goldberg & Rothermel, 1984; Seymour & Evans, 1992; Siegel, 1984; Temple, 1990). Therefore, it is not surprising that some young children with autism are able to combine their strong visual skills with the phonological skills needed to read words prior to understanding their meaning.

In short, empirical evidence supports the assertion that hyperlexia stems not from a problem with reading comprehension but from a problem with general receptive language comprehension coupled with strong word recognition skills. Of 13 participants reported across two studies (Aram, 1997; Patti & Lupinetti, 1993), 6 were able to comprehend text at levels as least as high as would be expected based on their chronological ages or their performance on language tests. All but one of the remaining participants (ages 10–12, IQ scores ranging from 71 to 82) were able to read with comprehension at the third grade level or higher. Thus, in terms of reading, children with autism and hyperlexia are not dramatically different from readers without disabilities. All readers require background knowledge and general language understanding in order to comprehend text. Even the very best readers encounter texts that can be decoded but not comprehended due to the complexity or unfamiliarity of the topic. Children with hyperlexia and autism should not be viewed as incapable of learning to comprehend what they read, nor should they be expected to comprehend all of the words they can decode. As discussed in the next section, reading is not simply a behavioral task that involves decoding individual words. It is a complex, interactive task that requires readers to call on background experience, knowledge, and language understandings.

What Is Literacy?

Literacy is a skill that usually is acquired by individuals who have numerous opportunities to interact with print in meaningful ways and receive appropriate instruction (for a complete discussion see Koppenhaver, Pierce, & Yoder, 1995). Literacy is not a unitary behavior that can be defined in terms of the number of words a person can read or spell correctly. Rather, literacy involves the interaction of many processes and skills. For the purposes of this chapter, *literacy* is defined as the *combination of reading and writing. Reading* is more precisely defined as *silent reading comprehension* (i.e., the ability to read a text for a personally or externally imposed purpose and gain understanding from it). The importance of subskills, such as identifying words in isolation or sounding out unknown words, is determined directly by how much they ultimately assist the reader to understand a larger text. That is, all things done in the name of reading instruction should work toward the long-term goal of improving learners' ability to read silently with comprehension. *Writing* refers to written composition or the translation of thoughts and words into written text. Again, the importance of subskills such as spelling and punctuation is determined directly by how much they ultimately assist a writer to compose a larger text (Cunningham & Erickson, 1996). Similar to reading, all things done in the name of writing instruction should lead to the long-term goal of improving learners' ability to compose written text.

Emergent Literacy and Readiness Perspectives

The *emergent literacy* perspective has had a significant impact on our understanding of how individuals with disabilities learn to read and write (Erickson, 1995; Koppenhaver, Coleman, Kalman, & Yoder, 1991; Musselwhite & King-DeBaun, 1997; Pierce & McWilliam, 1993). Emergent literacy theory holds that the ability to read and write is acquired in much the same way as spoken language (Teale & Sulzby, 1986). Thus, reading and writing are not learned through direct instruction of discrete skills that are accumulated over time. Rather, reading and writing skills begin to develop during the thousands of hours of meaningful interactions with others that most individuals receive before they enter school (Adams, 1990). During these experiences, young children learn first about the functions of print and then the forms (e.g., children learn that writing conveys meaning long before they learn to write the letters of the alphabet). These skills are refined and become conventional when those thousands of hours are followed by instruction that systematically combines sight word instruction with phonics or decoding instruction, reading comprehension instruction with opportunities to select and read easy texts, and writing instruction with opportunities to write for real purposes and audiences (Cunningham & Allington, 1994). Although literacy instruction programs emphasize these subprocesses in different ways, successful readers and writers develop skills within each of these areas.

Individuals with autism are most often provided with literacy instruction that is based on a readiness rather than an emergent literacy model. *Readiness* is typically thought of as a within-child characteristic. As a child grows and develops across the cognitive, psychomotor, and socioemotional domains, he or she achieves "readiness" by attaining certain core skills that are predetermined by policy makers and educators (Graue, 1993). From this perspective, children are "ready" for reading and writing instruction once they have mastered a set of skills that typically include: 1) shape, number, and color recognition; 2) letter identification; and 3) a pincer grasp and other fine motor skills associated with handwriting.

As demonstrated through the aforementioned research on orthography as a possible form of communication, individuals with autism and the most severe cognitive impairments can learn readiness skills including sight word identification (Duran, 1985; LaVigna, 1977; McGee, Krantz, & McClannahan, 1986). In addition, they can learn to recognize and use isolated words or phrases (Lanquetot, 1984; Marshall & Hegrenes, 1972; Rosenbaum & Breiling, 1976). There does not appear to be any research, however, regarding the ability of people with autism to comprehend paragraph-length or longer text, and only one study has addressed text composition at this level (Rousseau, Krantz, Poulson, Kitson, & McClannahan, 1994). In this study, Rousseau and colleagues (1994) investigated sentence combining as a strategy for increasing adjective use and writing quality in three adolescents with autism and moderate cognitive impairments and language delays. In the intervention, the students learned to combine two short sentences into one long sentence (e.g., *The horse is brown. + The horse is fast. = The brown horse is fast.*). Immediately after completing the sentence combining activities, the students wrote in response to picture prompts. There was a significant increase in adjective use in their writing, and the overall writing quality was judged to be better in the intervention phase than in the baseline phase. This research is important because it provides evidence that an intervention that was used effectively to increase clause length, phrase length, and the frequency of adjective and gerund use in students without disabilities (Evans, Venetozzi, Bundrick, & McWilliams, 1988; O'Hare, 1973; Weaver, 1979) was also effective with students with autism.

Center for Literacy and Disability Studies Preschool Project

A more comprehensive example of the potential for an emergent literacy perspective was provided by reading researchers at the Center for Literacy and

Disability Studies (CLDS) at the University of North Carolina. They provided a unique program in a self-contained preschool for children with autism in which seven children were provided with a literacy-rich classroom setting over a 5-month period (Koppenhaver & Erickson, 1998). The children were all 4 or 5 years old. One child achieved an age-equivalent score of only 4 months on the Bayley Scales of Infant Development (Bayley, 1993). The remaining children, who were all able to complete the PsychoEducational Profile–Revised (Schopler, Reichler, Dashford, Lansing, & Marcus, 1990), achieved age-equivalent scores between 9 and 37 months on this instrument (mean = 20 months).

In the first phase of intervention, the children were provided with a variety of independent writing activities. While they were engaged in the writing activities, researchers interacted with the children and modeled how to complete the writing activities in a conventional manner. For example, one daily activity was a sign-in routine. The children were asked to sign their names on a lined sheet of paper on entering the preschool classroom. After attempting to write their names, they were told, "You signed your name. That says _____. This is how I write _____." The researcher then wrote each child's name conventionally in a hand-over-hand manner with the child when possible. Only generative writing activities such as the sign-in sheet were used during the project, with no structured copying or tracing tasks. The children had numerous opportunities to select writing materials when they were not involved in small-group or one-to-one instructional activities. Some of the materials included letter stamps, talking word processors, pencils, crayons, markers, whiteboards, paintbrushes, and letter-shaped cookie cutters with Play-Doh.

Over the 3 months of this first phase, one child learned to write his name independently, and several others began to write in letter-like scribbles, with some of the letters from their names appearing regularly in the writing samples. Children also demonstrated knowledge of the difference between drawing and writing through distinctly different movements of their pens and pencils when doing each. They also demonstrated knowledge that text moves from left to right across a page, that letters are supposed to be written on lines, and that words are made up of several letters written next to each other and separated by a space. On the computer, they began typing letters in patterns, and the letters in their own names appeared more regularly in their typing. All of these behaviors are considered to be precursors to conventional writing in children who do not have disabilities (Strickland & Morrow, 1989).

In the second phase of the intervention, books and other print materials were added to the classroom, and the teacher incorporated print in her calendar activities. The children used the library, and the librarian came into the classroom to read aloud on a weekly basis. The teacher read aloud daily and involved the children in this activity by having them turn pages, point to pictures, and manipulate interactive features of the books. As the project progressed, she supplemented these book readings by making her own books that featured the children in various "true stories" and that included visual-graphic symbols (e.g., photographs, PCSs) representing the nouns in the stories. The children participated either by matching the symbols to printed words or by selecting names and symbols to fill in blanks in sentences.

In the play corner, where children played independently when not engaged in one-to-one instruction, other reading materials were added. These included the following: books with sound effect strips, ABC books, touch-and-feel books, repeated line storybooks, product boxes and cans in the play kitchen, and words added to existing PCSs used for communication. Other writing materials were also added, including a Magna Doodle, Glo-Doodler, Etch-a-Sketch, Video-Painter, portable chalkboards, peel/erase pads, and a manual typewriter.

Across all seven children, measurable growth in emergent reading and writing skills was observed during the 3-month period that composed the second phase. They all learned to recognize their own names in print, and three children learned to recognize the names of all of their classmates. In addition, five of the seven children learned to recognize 9 or more uppercase letters of the alphabet without any direct instruction in letter recognition; one of these children identified 23 uppercase letters and another child identified 19 uppercase plus 13 lowercase letters. There was also evidence of phonemic awareness in at least two children as shown through clapping syllables while the librarian was reading/singing a book and matching consonants with phonemes (e.g., when the researcher displayed three or four letters at a time and pronounced an individual phoneme such as /t/, the child selected the *t*). When given a test that measured concepts about print (Clay, 1985), all of the children were able to identify the front of a book, orient the book properly, and turn the pages appropriately. Five of the children also correctly reoriented an upside-down picture, three of the children verbally labeled pictures, and one child pointed to words when asked. These skills were not evidenced prior to the intervention.

This project suggests that children with autism develop emergent reading and writing skills in much the same way as their peers without disabilities. Given hours of meaningful and varied opportunities to explore print, see models of print use, and interact around reading and writing experiences, children with autism can develop the emergent literacy skills expected in the early years.

A Sociocultural Model of Literacy Learning

The CLDS preschool project supports the belief that multiple contexts influence literacy learning. A sociocultural model of literacy and language learning (Pappas, Kiefer, & Levstik, 1990) with modifications to account for the differences in communication and access found in people with developmental disabilities (Koppenhaver et al., 1991) describes these multiple contexts. A sociocultural perspective recognizes that an individual's abilities and disabilities are but one of the factors that contribute to literacy learning (Bos & Fletcher, 1997; Englert, 1992; Erickson, 1995; Koppenhaver, Pierce, Steelman, & Yoder, 1994; Koppenhaver & Yoder, 1992). Numerous sociocultural factors are also responsible for determining whether literacy success will occur for most individuals with developmental disabilities, including autism. Such factors include the attitudes and expectations of those in an individual's immediate environment, the availability of accessible reading and writing materials, and the nature of the interactions between the individual and his or her literacy instructors.

The implications of the sociocultural model for literacy learning in individuals with autism are far reaching and help to explain how some children who appear to have much more severe forms of autism may learn to read, write, and use print to communicate, whereas others with less severe forms may not. According to this model, the *sociocultural context* includes the attitudes and expectations of the individuals in a person's immediate environment as well as in the community at large. With the exception of the minority who are considered to be highly capable, most people with autism are faced with the assumption that they require routine, rote learning, and that they are unable to develop high-level comprehension skills in either written or oral language. The effect is that they are provided with reading programs that emphasize sight word learning in the context of controlled, carefully sequenced instructional activities aimed at teaching isolated skills. Such a repetitive, drill-based approach is not in line with recommended practices in reading and writing instruction (see Cunningham & Allington, 1994).

In addition, the *situational context* reflects the quantity and quality of the print materials available to people with autism in school and home environments. Many teachers of children with autism do not provide these children open access to print materials because the materials are easy to destroy or because of assumptions related to reading readiness (Koppenhaver, Yoder, et al., 1995). For example, the CLDS preschool class described previously (Koppenhaver & Erickson, 1998) was relatively devoid of print materials for independent exploration and use prior to the model project because of the assumption that the children were not yet ready for reading and writing. Yet, when the children were given access to books and print materials during their free time, they self-selected literacy activities from 32% to 98% of the time!

The *communication context* is influenced by the types of communication support provided to individuals with autism. It is here that the goals of AAC and literacy most closely overlap, in that literacy is a social process that involves interactions between readers and writers (Bloome, 1985; Cook-Gumperz, 1986; Rowe, 1989). Young children without disabilities negotiate their early understandings about print through interactions with adults and, once they enter school, with peers. Clearly, children with autism are faced with multiple challenges in achieving the communicative give-and-take that is a part of emergent literacy learning. The challenge for parents and professionals is to utilize a range of instructional supports in this regard, including those related to AAC and technology, to make such interactions possible. Communication or literacy instruction that does not allow the child to negotiate meaning but that instead demands only single, rote responses is not likely to be fruitful.

Clinical and Educational Implications: Autism and Literacy

The only conclusion that can be drawn definitively from the extant research regarding autism and literacy is that no one yet knows what type of intervention is best! Researchers have evidence that children with autism can learn sight words without teacher-directed rote drill and practice (McGee et al., 1986). Researchers have evidence that approaches borrowed from recommended practices in writing instruction for children without disabilities can promote learning for students with autism (Rousseau et al., 1994). There is evidence to suggest that literacy-rich and interactive preschool environments promote emergent literacy learning (Koppenhaver & Erickson, 1998). There also is evidence to suggest that people with other developmental disabilities can learn to read and write when provided with access to the types of instruction that are characteristic of recommended-practice instruction for children without disabilities (e.g., Cousin, Weekley, & Gerard, 1993; Erickson, Koppenhaver, Yoder, & Nance, 1997; Gipe, Duffy, & Richards, 1993; Katims & Pierce, 1995). No one knows, however, how all of these practices interact, nor what their relative impact is on successful literacy learning. Given this lack of definitive knowledge, we propose that reading and writing instruction utilize a balanced approach that incorporates all of the processes that are known to be involved in successful literacy learning. One such approach is the Four Block model of literacy instruction.

The Four Block model was initially named *Multimethod, Multilevel Literacy Instruction* to reflect that the approach incorporates more than one instructional method and addresses the needs of students at different levels of competence simultaneously (Cunningham, Hall, & Defee, 1991). The model has proven successful in general education classrooms in both urban and rural schools, with both high-achieving and low-achieving students (Cunningham, Hall, & Defee, 1998). The model is intended to incorporate several different instructional approaches in a systematic fashion that can be individualized across students. The Four Block model includes instruction in four areas: guided reading (comprehension), word study (sight words and decoding), writing (written composition), and self-selected reading. The most important features of each block are highlighted in Table 14.1 (for a more complete description, see Cunningham et al., 1998).

The Four Block model provides a framework in which direct instruction at the word level, in reading comprehension, and in writing is systematically

Table 14.1. The components of the Four Block balanced literacy instructional program

The Four Blocks	Brief description of the Block
Guided reading	Children learn that reading involves thinking. A variety of texts and reading materials are used. Comprehension strategies are taught. Children learn to read increasingly difficult materials.
Self-selected reading	Children select own reading materials. Children respond to parts of reading materials they select. Teacher reads aloud. Teacher guides children in selecting materials at their level.
Writing	Teachers use minilessons to teach through examples and nonexamples. Children participate in group editing of texts written by the teacher in the minilesson. Children write on topics they select. Children write three to five first drafts before selecting one to revise and publish.
Working with words	Children learn to read and spell high-frequency words. Children learn the patterns that are used to decode and spell. Several instructional activities allow children to apply their developing knowledge of patterns and decoding.

incorporated in literacy instruction, with regular opportunities to self-select reading materials and writing topics. Sight words, a relative strength for most people with autism because of their visual strengths, are taught, but not to the exclusion of decoding skills; effective reading comprehension requires both (Cunningham, 1993). Reading comprehension is taught in conjunction with language comprehension rather than as a separate, unique process because effective silent reading comprehension requires language comprehension. Writing skills are modeled and taught with a focus on meaning not mechanics because writing is learned by writing and seeing models of good writing, not through grammar, mechanics, and handwriting instruction (Hillocks, 1987).

This balanced approach provides a temporary solution to the fact that what does and does not work in teaching reading and writing to children with autism is simply not known. A balanced approach can ensure that practitioners are not "missing the boat" while developing a research base to understand what instructional strategies and programs are most effective for teaching silent reading comprehension and written composition to people with autism.

Directions for Future Research: Autism and Literacy

Addressing the questions of how, what, and under what conditions to teach literacy skills to individuals with autism is daunting, given the limited extant research base in this area. Thus, here are a second set of "Top Five Questions" that warrant further investigation:

1. Do the explanations of early literacy development provided by emergent literacy apply in whole, in part, or not at all to people with autism?

2. Is there a relationship between literacy learning and the development of communication and speech in people with autism?
3. To what extent can recommended-practice principles of literacy instruction from general education be applied to people with autism?
4. Can people with autism who have had limited success learning literacy "readiness skills" be taught to decode and read with comprehension using a comprehensive approach such as the Four Block model?
5. How does the use of graphic symbols for AAC influence the literacy learning of people with autism?

CONCLUSIONS

The predominant theme that has emerged from this chapter is the importance of social context for communication and learning. Both AAC and literacy instruction for individuals with autism must be embedded in relevant, motivating social contexts because of the very nature of autism itself as a social impairment. It may be relatively easy to teach specific communication forms and simple literacy-related skills in isolation, but the likelihood that such skills will generalize and will be used spontaneously in natural settings is tenuous at best. Thus, it is vastly preferable to "begin at the beginning" by ensuring that AAC interventions provide both expressive and receptive communication supports that are individualized and meaningful to the individual. Similarly, literacy supports should be constructed to incorporate both decoding and comprehension skills in developmentally appropriate and balanced reading and writing activities. As research in AAC, challenging behavior, and literacy endeavors to define the elements that are most essential to success, it is important to base assessment and intervention planning on comprehensive models for support.

REFERENCES

Adams, M.J. (1990). *Beginning to read: Thinking and learning about print.* Cambridge, MA: MIT Press.

Aram, D.M. (1997). Hyperlexia: Reading without meaning in young children. *Topics in Language Disorders, 17*(3), 1–13.

Aram, D.M., Rose, D.F., & Horwitz, S.J. (1984). Hyperlexia: Developmental reading without meaning. In R.N. Malatesha & H.A. Whitaker (Eds.), *Dyslexia: A global issue* (pp. 517–531). The Hague, the Netherlands: Martinus Nijhoff.

Barrera, R., & Sulzer-Azaroff, B. (1983). An alternating treatment comparison of oral and total communication training programs with echolalic autistic children. *Journal of Applied Behavior Analysis, 16,* 379–394.

Bayley, N. (1993). *The Bayley Scales of Infant Development* (2nd ed.). San Antonio, TX: The Psychological Corporation.

Beukelman, D.R., & Mirenda, P. (1998). *Augmentative and alternative communication: Management of severe communication disorders in children and adults* (2nd ed.). Baltimore: Paul H. Brookes Publishing Co.

Biklen, D. (1990). Communication unbound: Autism and praxis. *Harvard Educational Review, 60,* 291–314.

Biklen, D. (1993). *Communication unbound.* New York: Teachers College Press.

Biklen, D., & Cardinal, D. (1997). *Contested words, contested science: Unraveling the facilitated communication controversy.* New York: Teachers College Press.

Bird, F., Dores, P., Moniz, D., & Robinson, J. (1989). Reducing severe aggressive and self-injurious behaviors with functional communication training. *American Journal on Mental Retardation, 94,* 37–48.

Bloome, D. (1985). Reading as a social process. *Language Arts, 62*(2), 134–142.

Bondy, A., & Frost, L. (1994). The Picture Exchange Communication System. *Focus on Autistic Behavior, 9,* 1–19.

Bondy, A., & Frost, L. (1995). Educational approaches in preschool: Behavior techniques in a public school setting. In E. Schopler & G. Mesibov (Eds.), *Learning and cognition in autism* (pp. 311–333). New York: Plenum.

Bornstein, H., Saulnier, L., & Hamilton, L. (1983). *The comprehensive Signed English dictionary.* Washington, DC: Gallaudet University Press.

Bos, C.S., & Fletcher, T.V. (1997). Sociocultural considerations in learning disabilities inclusion research: Knowledge gaps and future directions. *Learning Disabilities Research and Practice, 12*(2), 92–99.

Bryen, D., & Joyce, D. (1985). Language intervention with the severely handicapped: A decade of research. *Journal of Special Education, 19,* 7–39.

Campbell, R., & Lutzker, J. (1993). Using functional equivalence training to reduce severe challenging behavior: A case study. *Journal of Developmental and Physical Disabilities, 5,* 203–216.

Cardinal, D., Hanson, D., & Wakeham, J. (1996). Investigation of authorship in facilitated communication. *Mental Retardation, 34*(4), 231–342.

Carr, E., & Dores, P. (1981). Patterns of language acquisition following simultaneous communication with autistic children. *Analysis and Intervention in Developmental Disabilities, 1,* 1–15.

Carr, E., Pridal, C., & Dores, P. (1984). Speech versus sign comprehension in autistic children. Analysis and prediction. *Journal of Experimental Child Psychology, 37,* 587–597.

Carrier, J., Jr., & Peak, T. (1975). *Non-SLIP (Non-Speech Language Initiation Program).* Lawrence, KS: H & H Enterprises.

Chen, S.H.A., & Bernard-Opitz, V. (1993). Comparison of personal and computer-assisted instruction for children with autism. *Mental Retardation, 31*(6), 368–376.

Clay, M. (1985). *Early detection of reading difficulties: A diagnostic survey with recovery procedures* (2nd ed.). Portsmouth, NH: Heinemann.

Cobrinik, L. (1974). Unusual reading ability in severely disturbed children. *Journal of Autism and Childhood Schizophrenia, 4,* 163–175.

Cobrinik, L. (1982). The performance of hyperlexic children on an incomplete words task. *Neuropsychologia, 20,* 569–577.

Cook-Gumperz, J. (1986). *The social construction of literacy.* Cambridge, England: Cambridge University Press.

Cousin, P.T., Weekley, T., & Gerard, J. (1993). The functional uses of language and literacy by students with severe language and learning problems. *Language Arts, 70,* 548–556.

Cunningham, J.W. (1993). Whole-to-part reading diagnosis. *Reading and writing quarterly: Overcoming learning difficulties, 9*(1), 31–49.

Cunningham, J.W., & Erickson, K.A. (1996). *Assessment to help them all read and write.* Keynote address at the fifth annual Symposium on Literacy and Developmental Disabilities, Durham, NC.

Cunningham, P.M. (1992). What kind of phonics instruction will we have? In C.K. Kinzer & D.J. Leu (Eds.), *Literacy research, theory, and practice: Views from many perspectives* (pp. 17–31). Chicago: National Reading Conference.

Cunningham, P.M., & Allington, R. (1994). *Classrooms that work: They can all read and write.* Reading, MA: Addison Wesley Longman.

Cunningham, P., Hall, D., & DeFee, M. (1991). Non–ability-grouped, multilevel instruction: A year in a first-grade classroom. *The Reading Teacher, 44,* 566–571.

Cunningham, P., Hall, D., & DeFee, M. (1998). Non–ability-grouped, multilevel instruction: Eight years later. *The Reading Teacher, 51,* 652–664.

Dawson, G., & Adams, A. (1984). Imitation and social responsiveness in autistic children. *Journal of Abnormal Child Psychology, 12,* 209–225.

Day, H.M., Horner, R., & O'Neill, R. (1994). Multiple functions of problem behaviors: Assessment and intervention. *Journal of Applied Behavior Analysis, 27,* 279–290.

de Villiers, J., & Naughton, J. (1974). Teaching a symbol language to autistic children. *Journal of Consultation in Clinical Psychology, 42,* 111–117.

Duran, E. (1985). Teaching functional reading in context to severely retarded autistic adolescents of limited English proficiency. *Adolescence, 20,* 433–440.

Eberlin, M., McConnachie, G., Ibel, S., & Volpe, L. (1993). Facilitated communication: A failure to replicate the phenomenon. *Journal of Autism and Developmental Disorders, 23,* 507–530.

Elliot, D.E., & Needleman, R.M. (1976). The syndrome of hyperlexia. *Brain and Language, 3,* 339–349.

Englert, C.S. (1992). Writing instruction from a sociocultural perspective: The holistic, dialogic, and social enterprise of writing. *Journal of Learning Disabilities, 25*(3), 153–172.

Erickson, K. (1995). *Literacy and inclusion for a child with severe speech and physical impairments.* Unpublished doctoral dissertation, University of North Carolina at Chapel Hill.

Erickson, K., Koppenhaver, D., Yoder, D., & Nance, J. (1997). Integrated communication and literacy instruction for a child with multiple disabilities. *Focus on Autism and Other Developmental Disabilities, 12*(3), 142–150.

Evans, R., Venetozzi, R., Bundrick, M., & McWilliams, E. (1988). The effects of sentence-combining instructions on writing and on standardized test scores. *Journal of Educational Research, 82*(1), 53–57.

Fay, W.H., & Schuler, A.L. (Vol. Eds.). (1980). *Emerging language in autistic children.* In R.L. Schiefelbusch (Series Ed.), *Language intervention series* (Vol. 5). Baltimore: University Park Press.

Fiocca, G. (1981). *Generally understood gestures: An approach to communication for persons with severe language impairments.* Unpublished master's thesis, University of Illinois at Urbana, Champaign.

Flannery, K.B., & Horner, R. (1994). The relationship between predictability and problem behavior for students with severe disabilities. *Journal of Behavioral Education, 4,* 157–176.

Fristoe, M., & Lloyd, L.L. (1979). Nonspeech communication. In N.R. Ellis (Ed.), *Handbook of mental deficiency: Psychological theory and research* (pp. 401–430). Mahwah, NJ: Lawrence Erlbaum Associates.

Frith, U., & Snowling, M., (1983). Reading for meaning and reading for sound in autistic and dyslexic children. *British Journal of Developmental Psychology, 1,* 329–342.

Frost, L., & Bondy, A.S. (1994). *PECS: The Picture Exchange Communication System training manual.* Cherry Hill, NJ: Pyramid Educational Consultants.

Frost, R.E. (1984). Computers and the autistic child. In D. Peterson (Ed.), *Intelligent schoolhouse* (pp. 246–250). Upper Saddle River, NJ: Prentice-Hall.

Fuller, D., & Stratton, M. (1991). Representativeness versus translucency: Different theoretical backgrounds, but are they really different concepts? *Augmentative and Alternative Communication, 7,* 51–58.

Fulwiler, R., & Fouts, R. (1976). Acquisition of American Sign Language by a noncommunicating autistic child. *Journal of Autism and Childhood Schizophrenia, 6,* 43–51.

Gardner, R., & Gardner, B. (1969). Teaching sign language to a chimpanzee. *Science, 165,* 664–672.

Gardner, R., & Gardner, B. (1975). Early signs of language in child and chimpanzee. *Science, 187,* 752–753.

Gipe, J., Duffy, C.A., & Richards, J.C., (1993). Helping a nonspeaking adult male with cerebral palsy achieve literacy. *Journal of Reading, 36*(5), 380–389.

Glosser, G., Friedman, R.B., & Roeltgen, D.P. (1996). Clues to the cognitive organization of reading and writing from developmental hyperlexia. *Neuropsychology, 10,* 168–175.

Goldberg, T.E., & Rothermel, R.D. (1984). Hyperlexic children reading. *Brain, 197,* 757–785.

Graue, E.M. (1993) *Ready for what? Constructing meanings of readiness for kindergarten.* Albany: State University of New York Press.

Gray, C. (1995). Teaching children with autism to "read" social situations. In K. Quill (Ed.), *Teaching children with autism: Strategies to enhance communication and socialization* (pp. 219–242). New York: Delmar Publishers.

Green, G., & Shane, H. (1994). Science, reason, and facilitated communication. *Journal of The Association for Persons with Severe Handicaps, 19*(3), 151–172.

Groden, J., & LeVasseur, P. (1995). Cognitive picture rehearsal: A system to teach self-control. In K. Quill (Ed.), *Teaching children with autism: Strategies to enhance communication and socialization* (pp. 287–306). New York: Delmar Publishers.

Gustason, G., Pfetzing, D., & Zawolkow, E. (1980). *Signing Exact English* (3rd ed.). Los Alamitos, CA: Modern Signs Press.

Hamilton, B., & Snell, M. (1993). Using the milieu approach to increase spontaneous communication book use across environments by an adolescent with autism. *Augmentative and Alternative Communication, 9,* 259–272.

Hamre-Nietupski, S., Stoll, A., Holtz, K., Fullerton, P., Ryan-Flottum, M., & Brown, L. (1977). Curricular strategies for teaching selected nonverbal communication skills to nonverbal and verbal severely handicapped students. In L. Brown, J. Nietupski, S. Lyon, S. Hamre-Nietupski, T. Crowner, & L. Gruenewald (Eds.), *Curricular strategies for teaching functional object use, nonverbal communication, problem solving, and mealtime skills to severely handicapped students* (Part I, Vol. 7, pp. 94–250). Madison: University of Wisconsin–Madison and Madison Metropolitan School District.

Hedbring, C. (1985). Computers and autistic learners: An evolving technology. *Australian Journal of Human Communication Disorders, 13,* 169–188.

Heimann, M., Nelson, K.E., Tjus, T., & Gillberg, C. (1995). Increasing reading and communication skills in children with autism through an interactive multimedia computer program. *Journal of Autism and Developmental Disorders, 25*(5), 459–480.

Hewett, F. (1964). Teaching reading to an autistic boy through operant conditioning. *Reading Teacher, 17,* 613–618.

Hillocks, G., Jr. (1987). Synthesis of research on teaching writing. *Educational Leadership, 44*(8), 71–76, 78, 80–82.

Hodgdon, L. (1995). Solving social-behavioral problems through the use of visually supported communication. In K. Quill (Ed.), *Teaching children with autism: Strategies to enhance communication and socialization* (pp. 265–286). New York: Delmar Publishers.

Hodgdon, L. (1996). *Visual strategies for improving communication.* Troy, MI: Quirk Roberts Publishing.

Horner, R., & Budd, C. (1985). Acquisition of manual sign use: Collateral reduction of maladaptive behavior and factors limiting generalization. *Education and Training of the Mentally Retarded, 20,* 39–47.

Horner, R., & Day, H.M. (1991). The effects of response efficiency on functionally equivalent competing behaviors. *Journal of Applied Behavior Analysis, 24,* 719–732.

Hughes, C. (1996). Brief report: Planning problems in autism at the level of motor control. *Journal of Autism and Developmental Disorders, 26,* 99–107.

Iacono, T., & Parsons, C. (1986). A survey of the use of signing with the intellectually disabled. *Australian Communication Quarterly, 2,* 21–25.

Jones, V., & Prior, M.R. (1985). Motor imitation abilities and neurological signs in autistic children. *Journal of Autism and Developmental Disorders, 15,* 37–46.

Jordan, R., & Powell, S. (1990a). Teaching autistic children to think more effectively. *Communication, 24,* 20–23.

Jordan, R., & Powell, S. (1990b). Improving thinking in autistic children using computer presented activities. *Communication, 24,* 23–25.

Karlan, G. (1990). Manual communication with those who can hear. In H. Bornstein (Ed.), *Manual communication: Implications for education* (pp. 151–185). Washington, DC: Gallaudet University Press.

Katims, D.S., & Pierce, P.L. (1995). Literacy-rich environments and the transition of young children with special needs. *Topics in Early Childhood Special Education, 15*(2), 219–234.

Kiernan, C. (1983). The use of nonvocal communication techniques with autistic individuals. *Journal of Child Psychology and Psychiatry and Allied Disciplines, 24,* 339–375.

Kiernan, C., Reid, B., & Jones, M. (1982). *Signs and symbols: Use of non-vocal communication systems.* London: Heinemann.

Konstantareas, M. (1984). Sign language as a communication prosthesis with language-impaired children. *Journal of Autism and Developmental Disorders, 14,* 9–23.

Konstantareas, M., Oxman, J., & Webster, C. (1978). Iconicity: Effects of the acquisition of sign language by autistic and other severely dysfunctional children. In P. Siple (Ed.), *Understanding language through sign language research* (pp. 213–237). San Diego: Academic Press.

Konstantareas, M., Webster, C., & Oxman, J. (1979). Manual language acquisition and its influence on other areas of functioning in four autistic and autistic-like children. *Journal of Child Psychology and Psychiatry and Allied Disciplines, 20,* 337–350.

Koppenhaver, D.A., Coleman, P., Kalman, S.L., & Yoder, D.E. (1991). The implications of emergent literacy research for children with developmental disabilities. *American Journal of Speech-Language Pathology, 1*(1), 38–44.

Koppenhaver, D., & Erickson, K. (1998). *Young children with autism and emergent literacy success.* Manuscript in preparation.

Koppenhaver, D.A., Pierce, P.L., Steelman, J.D., & Yoder, D.E. (1994). Contexts of early literacy intervention for children with developmental disabilities. In S.F. Warren & J. Reichle (Series Eds.) & M.E. Fey, J. Windsor, & S.F. Warren (Vol. Eds.), *Communication and language intervention series: Vol. 5. Language intervention: Preschool through the elementary years* (pp. 241–274). Baltimore: Paul H. Brookes Publishing Co.

Koppenhaver, D.A., Pierce, P.L., & Yoder, D.E. (1995). AAC, FC, and the ABCs: Issues and relationships. *American Journal of Speech-Language Pathology, 4*(4), 5–14.

Koppenhaver, D.A., & Yoder, D.E. (1992). Literacy issues in persons with severe speech and physical impairments. In R. Gaylord-Ross (Ed.), *Issues and research in special education* (Vol. 2, pp. 156–201). New York: Teachers College Press.

Koppenhaver, D.A., Yoder, D.E., Pierce, P.L., Staples, A., Stuart, C., & Erickson, K.A. (1995). *Project WRITE (Writing and Reading Interventions through Technology, Educational Media, and Materials): The preliminary phase.* Chapel Hill: University of North Carolina at Chapel Hill.

Krantz, P., MacDuff, M., & McClannahan, L. (1993). Programming participation in family activities for children with autism: Parents' use of photographic activity schedules. *Journal of Applied Behavior Analysis, 26,* 137–138.

Lanquetot, R. (1984). Autistic children and reading. *The Reading Teacher, 38,* 182–186.

LaVigna, G. (1977). Communication training in mute autistic adolescents using the written word. *Journal of Autism and Childhood Schizophrenia, 17,* 115–132.

Layton, T. (1988). Language training with autistic children using four different modes of presentation. *Journal of Communication Disorders, 21,* 333–350.

Layton, T., & Baker, P. (1981). Description of semantic-syntactic relations in an autistic child. *Journal of Autism and Developmental Disorders, 11,* 385–399.

Layton, T., & Watson, L. (1995). Enhancing communication in nonverbal children with autism. In K.A. Quill (Ed.), *Teaching children with autism: Strategies to enhance communication and socialization* (pp. 73–101). New York: Delmar Publishers.

Light, J., McNaughton, D., & Parnes, P. (1994). *A protocol for the assessment of the communicative interaction skills of nonspeaking severely handicapped adults and their facilitators.* Thornhill, Ontario, Canada: Sharing to Learn.

Light, J., Roberts, B., Dimarco, R., & Greiner, N. (1998). Augmentative and alternative communication to support receptive and expressive communication for people with autism. *Journal of Communication Disorders, 31,* 153–180.

MacArthur, C.A. (1988). The impact of computers on the writing process. *Exceptional Children, 54,* 536–542.

MacArthur, C.A. (1996). Using technology to enhance the writing process of students with learning disabilities. *Journal of Learning Disabilities, 29,* 344–354.

MacDuff, G., Krantz, P., & McClannahan, L. (1993). Teaching children with autism to use photographic activity schedules: Maintenance and generalization of complex response chains. *Journal of Applied Behavior Analysis, 26,* 89–98.

Maharaj, S. (1980). *Pictogram ideogram communication.* Regina, Saskatchewan, Canada: The George Reed Foundation for the Handicapped.

Marshall, N., & Hegrenes, J. (1972). The use of written language as a communication system for an autistic child. *Journal of Speech and Hearing Disorders, 2,* 258–261.

Matas, J., Mathy-Laikko, P., Beukelman, D., & Legresley, K. (1985). Identifying the nonspeaking population: A demographic study. *Augmentative and Alternative Communication, 1,* 17–31.

Mayer-Johnson Co. (1994). *The Picture Communication Symbols combination book.* Solana Beach, CA: Author.

McGee, G.C., Krantz, P.J., & McClannahan, L.E. (1986). An extension of incidental teaching procedures to reading instruction for autistic children. *Journal of Applied Behavior Analysis, 19*(2), 147–157.

McLean, L., & McLean, J. (1974). A language training program for nonverbal autistic children. *Journal of Speech and Hearing Disorders, 39,* 186–193.

Mirenda, P. (1997). Functional communication training and augmentative communication: A research review. *Augmentative and Alternative Communication, 13,* 207–225.

Mirenda, P., Kandborg, T., & MacGregor, T. (1994, October). *"What's next?": Activity schedule interventions for challenging behaviour.* Paper presented at the sixth biennial conference of the International Society for Augmentative and Alternative Communication, Maastricht, the Netherlands.

Mirenda, P., MacGregor, T., & Kelly-Keough, S. (in press). Teaching communication skills for behavior support in the context of family life. In J. Lucyshyn, G. Dunlap, & R. Albin (Eds.), *Families, family life, and positive behavioral support: Addressing the challenge of problem behaviors in family contexts.* Baltimore: Paul H. Brookes Publishing Co.

Mirenda, P., & Mathy-Laikko, P. (1989). Augmentative and alternative communication applications for persons with severe congenital communication disorders: An introduction. *Augmentative and Alternative Communication, 5,* 3–13.

Mirenda, P., & Santogrossi, J. (1985). A prompt-free strategy to teach pictorial communication system use. *Augmentative and Alternative Communication, 1,* 143–150.

Mirenda, P., & Schuler, A. (1989). Augmenting communication for persons with autism: Issues and strategies. *Topics in Language Disorders, 9,* 24–43.

Moore, S., Donovan, B., & Hudson, A. (1993). Facilitator-suggested conversational evaluation of facilitated communication. *Journal of Autism and Developmental Disorders, 23,* 541–551.

Musselwhite, C., & King-DeBaun, P. (1997). *Merging technology and whole language for students with disabilities.* Birmingham, AL: Southeast Augmentative Communication.

O'Hare, F. (1973). *Sentence combining: Improving student writing without formal grammar instruction* (Report Series No. 15). Urbana, IL: National Council of Teachers of English.

Panyan, M. (1984). Computer technology for autistic students. *Journal of Autism and Developmental Disorders, 14,* 375–382.

Pappas, C.C., Kiefer, B.Z., & Levstik, L.S. (1990). *An integrated language perspective in the elementary school.* Reading, MA: Addison Wesley Longman.

Patti, P.J., & Lupinetti, L. (1993). Brief report: Implications of hyperlexia in an autistic savant. *Journal of Autism and Developmental Disorders, 23*(2), 397–405.

Peterson, S., Bondy, A., Vincent, Y., & Finnegan, C. (1995). Effects of altering communicative input for students with autism and no speech: Two case studies. *Augmentative and Alternative Communication, 11,* 93–100.

Pierce, K., & Schreibman, L. (1994). Teaching daily living skills to children with autism in unsupervised settings through pictorial self-management. *Journal of Applied Behavior Analysis,* 27, 471–482.

Pierce, P.L., & McWilliam, P.J. (1993). Emerging literacy and children with SSPI: Issues and possible intervention strategies. *Topics in Language Disorders, 13*(2), 47–57.

Pleinis, A., & Romanczyk, R. (1985). Analyses of performance, behavior, and predictors for severely disturbed children: A comparison of adult vs. computer instruction. *Analysis and Intervention in Developmental Disabilities, 5,* 345–356.

Premack, D. (1971). Language in a chimpanzee? *Science, 172,* 808–822.

Premack, D., & Premack, A. (1974). Teaching visual language to apes and language-deficient persons. In R. Schiefelbusch & L.L. Lloyd (Eds.), *Language perspectives: Acquisition, retardation, and intervention* (pp. 347–376). Baltimore: University Park Press.

Quill, K. (Ed.). (1995). *Teaching children with autism: Strategies to enhance communication and socialization.* New York: Delmar Publishers.

Ratusnik, C., & Ratusnik, D. (1974). A comprehensive communication approach for a ten-year-old nonverbal autistic child. *American Journal of Orthopsychiatry, 43,* 396–403.

Reichle, J., & Brown, L. (1986). Teaching the use of a multipage direct selection communication board to an adult with autism. *Journal of The Association for Persons with Severe Handicaps, 11,* 68–73.

Rimland, B. (1978). Savant capabilities of autistic children and their cognitive implications. In G. Serban (Ed.), *Cognitive defects in the development of mental illness* (pp. 43–65). New York: Brunner/Mazel.

Rogers, S., & Bennetto, L. (1996). Imitation and pantomime in high functioning adolescents with autism spectrum disorders. *Child Development, 67,* 2060–2073.

Romski, M.A., & Sevcik, R.A. (1996). *Breaking the speech barrier: Language development through augmented means.* Baltimore: Paul H. Brookes Publishing Co.

Rosenbaum, M., & Breiling, J. (1976). The development and functional control of reading comprehension behavior. *Journal of Applied Behavioral Analysis, 9,* 323–333.

Rotholz, D., Berkowitz, S., & Burberry, J. (1989). Functionality of two modes of communication in the community by students with developmental disabilities: A comparison of signing and communication books. *Journal of The Association for Persons with Severe Handicaps, 14,* 227–233.

Rousseau, M., Krantz, P., Poulson, C., Kitson, M., & McClannahan, L. (1994). Sentence-combining as a technique for increasing adjective use by students with autism. *Research in Developmental Disabilities, 15*(1), 19–37.

Rowe, D.W. (1989). Author/audience interaction in the preschool: The role of social interaction in literacy learning. *Journal of Reading Behavior, 21*(4), 311–349.

Rumbaugh, D. (1977). *Language learning in the chimpanzee: The LANA Project.* San Diego: Academic Press.

Savage-Rumbaugh, S., Rumbaugh, D., & Boysen, S. (1978). Symbolic communication between two chimpanzees (Pan troglodytes). *Science, 201,* 641–644.

Schaeffer, B., Kollinzas, G., Musil, A., & McDowell, P. (1978). Spontaneous verbal language for autistic children through signed speech. *Sign Language Studies, 21,* 317–352.

Schlosser, R., Mirenda, P., McGhie-Richmond, D., Blackstein-Adler, S., & Janzen, P. (1998, August). Participation Model: Effects of teacher training on student participation. *Proceedings of the Biennial Conference of the International Society for Augmentative and Alternative Communication* (pp. 412–413). Dublin, Ireland: International Society for Augmentative and Alternative Communication.

Schopler, E., Reichler, R., Dashford, A., Lansing, M., & Marcus, L. (1990). *PsychoEducational Profile–Revised.* Austin: PRO-ED.

Schuler, A. (1985). Selecting augmentative communication systems on the basis of current communicative means and functions. *Australian Journal of Human Communication Disorders, 13,* 99–116.

Schuler, A., & Baldwin, M. (1981). Nonspeech communication and childhood autism. *Language, Speech, and Hearing Services in the Schools, 12,* 246–257.

Schuler, A., Prizant, B., & Wetherby, A. (1997). Enhancing language and communication development: Prelinguistic approaches. In D. Cohen & F. Volkmar (Eds.), *Handbook of autism and pervasive developmental disorders* (2nd ed., pp. 539–571). New York: John Wiley & Sons.

Seal, B., & Bonvillian, J. (1997). Sign language and motor functioning in students with autistic disorder. *Journal of Autism and Developmental Disorders, 27,* 437–466.

Siegel, L.S. (1984). A longitudinal study of hyperlexic children: Hyperlexia as a language disorder. *Neuropsychologia, 22,* 577–585.

Seymour, R.H.K., & Evans, H.M. (1992). Beginning reading without semantics: A cognitive study of hyperlexia. *Cognitive Neuropsychology, 9,* 89–122.

Shafer, E. (1993). Teaching topography-based and selection-based verbal behavior to developmentally disabled individuals: Some considerations. *The Analysis of Verbal Behavior, 11,* 117–133.

Shane, H. (1994). *Facilitated communication: The clinical and social phenomenon.* San Diego: Singular Publishing Group.

Sheehan, C., & Matuozzi, R. (1996). Validation of facilitated communication. *Mental Retardation, 34,* 94–107.

Sigafoos, J., & Meikle, B. (1996). Functional communication training for the treatment of multiply determined challenging behavior in two boys with autism. *Behavior Modification, 20,* 60–84.

Silberberg, N.E., & Silberberg, M.C. (1967). Hyperlexia: Specific word recognition skills in young children. *Exceptional Children, 34,* 41–42.

Smith, I., & Bryson, S. (1994). Imitation and action in autism: A critical review. *Psychological Bulletin, 116*(2), 259–273.

Snowling, M., & Frith, U. (1986). Comprehension in "hyperlexic" readers. *Journal of Experimental Child Psychology, 42,* 392–415.

Staples, A., Heying, K., & McLellan, J. (1995). *Project Co:Writer: A study of the effects of word prediction on writing achievements with learning disabilities.* Unpublished manuscript, Center for Literacy and Disability Studies, University of North Carolina at Chapel Hill.

Sternberg, M. (1994). *American Sign Language dictionary* (Rev. ed.). New York: HarperCollins.

Strickland, D.S., & Morrow, L.M. (Eds.). (1989). *Emerging literacy: Young children learn to read and write.* Newark, DE: International Reading Association.

Sundberg, M. (1993). Selecting a response form for nonverbal persons: Facilitated communication, pointing systems, or sign language? *The Analysis of Verbal Behavior, 11,* 99–116.

Teale, W.H., & Sulzby, E. (Eds.). (1986). *Emergent literacy: Writing and reading.* Greenwich, CT: Ablex Publishing Corp.

Temple, C.M. (1990). Auditory and reading comprehension in hyperlexia: Semantic and syntactic skills. *Reading and Writing: An Interdisciplinary Journal, 2,* 297–306.

Vanderheiden, G., & Yoder, D. (1986). Overview. In S. Blackstone (Ed.), *Augmentative communication: An introduction* (pp. 1–28). Rockville, MD: American Speech-Language-Hearing Association.

Vaughn, B., & Horner, R. (1995). Effects of concrete versus verbal choice systems on problem behavior. *Augmentative and Alternative Communication, 11,* 89–92.

Wacker, D., Steege, M., Northup, J., Sasso, G., Berg, W., Reimers, T., Cooper, L., Cigrand, K., & Donn, L. (1990). A component analysis of functional communication training across three topographies of severe behavior problems. *Journal of Applied Behavior Analysis, 23,* 417–429.

Weaver, C. (1979). *Grammar and what to do with it.* Paper presented at the annual meeting of the National Conference on Language Arts in the Elementary School, Indianapolis.

Webster, C., McPherson, H., Sloman, L., Evans, M., & Kuchar, E. (1973). Communicating with an autistic boy by gestures. *Journal of Autism and Childhood Schizophrenia, 3,* 337–346.

Weiss, M., Wagner, S., & Bauman, M. (1996). A case of validated facilitated communication. *Mental Retardation, 34,* 220–230.

Wetherby, A.M., & Prutting, C.A. (1984). Profiles of communicative and cognitive-social abilities in autistic children. *Journal of Speech and Hearing Research, 27,* 364–377.

Whitehouse, D., & Harris, J. (1984). Hyperlexia in infantile autism. *Journal of Autism and Developmental Disorders, 14,* 281–289.

Williams, S. (1998). *Effects of software equipped with speech feedback and word prediction on the writing of adolescents with learning disabilities.* Unpublished doctoral dissertation, University of North Carolina at Chapel Hill.

Windsor, J., & Fristoe, M. (1989). Key word signing: Listeners' classification of signed and spoken narratives. *Journal of Speech and Hearing Disorders, 54,* 374–382.

Windsor, J., & Fristoe, M. (1991). Key word signing: Perceived and acoustic differences between signed and spoken narratives. *Journal of Speech and Hearing Research, 34,* 260–268.

Wood, L., Lasker, J., Siegel-Causey, E., Beukelman, D., & Ball, L. (1998). An input framework for augmentative and alternative communication. *Augmentative and Alternative Communication, 14,* 261–267.

Yoder, P., & Layton, T. (1989). Speech following sign language training in autistic children with minimal verbal language. *Journal of Autism and Developmental Disorders, 18,* 217–229.

15

The Experience of Autism in the Lives of Families

Barbara Domingue, Barbara Cutler, and Janet McTarnaghan

Families of children with autism spectrum disorder (ASD) have much to share with professionals in understanding the differences and difficulties associated with ASD as well as the needs of families struggling to deal with the realities of both living with a child whose needs are complex and sometimes confounding and dealing with a service system that may not fully acknowledge or even comprehend the complexities of ASD.

In our more than 50 years of collective professional service, we have learned much from parents and indeed have shared their fear and frustration. Progress has occurred through the growth and refinement of services, but the search for greater understanding of the disability and family needs must continue.

Throughout this chapter we use the term *ASD* to describe this poorly understood and extremely variable disability. *ASD* is the term used to include autism (autistic disorder), pervasive developmental disorder-not otherwise specified (PDD-NOS), Asperger syndrome, Rett syndrome, and childhood disintegrative disorder. ASD is a syndrome that affects communication; social interaction, sensory and motor aspects of functioning; and, for some, cognitive processing (e.g., engagement, shifting of attention, perseveration, impulsivity, other aspects of executive functioning). We highlight throughout this chapter what we have learned from families, with the hope of allowing clinicians and educators to gain greater understanding and offer more meaningful support on what will prove for many to be a long journey.

THE EARLY FAMILY EXPERIENCE

Many parents report that in infancy, their children showed the promise of perfection. Parents stated that their children were attractive babies who were easy to care for. These babies were complacent and not very demanding of attention. For those parents, onset of ASD was insidious; awareness grew over time, typically during the second year of life. Other parents were suspicious from the very beginning that something was wrong. Their children were extremely difficult to comfort. Whatever the initial experience, parents report they had great difficulty finding information and support. Their children seemed to require more than the parents could understand, more than they could provide. Rejected by their communities and often rejected even by other family members, parents began their search for help, information, and guidance alone.

First Awareness

Bewilderment and confusion are often the first experiences faced by many parents. For others, there is guilt, grief, and even fear. In first seeking help from professionals, parents may hear that they are nervous parents or that their child is "perfectly normal." Time will prove for most families, however, that these children do in fact have a disability, one that affects multiple aspects of development. Social interaction and communication are usually the areas of development that first arouse parents' concern that something might be very different about their child.

It is important to note that each family is different. Experiences are varied, and unique family structure and dynamics define who the family is (Risley, 1997). A common theme, however, is a growing awareness and fear that the child is not progressing as he or she should. Given the fact that there is great variation in the rate at which children develop and certainly variation in personality and temperaments, it is often difficult for parents to know what is within usual limits and what is not. Parents go back and forth, wondering, even agonizing, "Is something wrong with our child, or does the problem lie with us? Is it something we're doing or failing to do?"

Our experience has been that for first children, parents tend to attribute their child's differences to their own parenting inadequacies. When there are older children, parents tend to recognize the differences in the child and are less likely to question their parenting skill or style as the source of the child's difficulties.

Although parents may doubt their ability, their intuition that something is different about their child is correct more often than not (Gillberg et al., 1990; Siegel, Pliner, Eschler, & Elliot, 1988), but it takes time and great effort before they are confirmed in their suspicions and gain the understanding of their child's disability that they so desperately seek. The search for information and services and the need for help and to gain understanding mark the beginning of the journey.

Finding a Reason (Diagnosis)

With no clear answers or direction, confused and often frightened parents turn first to medical professionals to shed some light on the puzzling aspects of their child's behavior, only to find that their search for answers often leads to greater confusion or to more questions. Parents therefore express tremendous frustration with the diagnostic process. Many report that their pediatrician, to whom they first turned when they suspected a problem, suggested a "wait-and-see" approach. Other advice typically included statements such as "Boys and girls develop at different rates," "You shouldn't compare your children," "You're just nervous," "You're overanxious," or "You're overly protective." So, parents, listening to this advice, wait, watch, and often continue to worry. All the while they are conscious of the passing of time. Parents, therefore, frequently report a feeling of resentment toward professionals for time that can never be recaptured. These experiences rob the family not only of possible opportunities but also of information or resources that could have been used to assist their son or daughter. For those parents who begin to see a series of specialists, there is often lack of agreement as to exactly what the problem is. Parents describe the tremendous drain on their time and energy, as well as the expense involved, in searching for the answers from the right people (Konstantareas, 1990).

Because of the complex and variable nature of the disability, as well as the age of the child, professionals often hesitate to "apply a label" or to make a diagnosis. Reasons shared with us by professionals include not wanting to stigmatize the child at a young age, not wishing to be the "bearer of bad news," or not wanting to overburden the family. Professionals who do not possess an up-to-date understanding of ASD typically consider the prognosis for children to be bleak at best, and some physicians may recommend private residential schools even for very young children.

Ambiguous professional communications as well as confusion concerning the diagnosis in general are often named as other obstacles faced by parents during the diagnostic process. One parent reported that after visits to several professionals in her search for diagnostic clarity, her child's neurologist said that he distinctly detected a "whiff" of PDD at the conclusion of the evaluation process—leading her to wonder if autism, in fact, was "aromatic!" Another professional thought that a "dash" of autism was detected in the child. Professionals' use of ambiguous or unclear language in describing a child's disability, as these examples illustrate, only serves to further complicate an already frightening and stressful experience. Furthermore, the lack of clarity concerning the diagnosis makes the challenge of understanding the child's needs and moving forward to meet those needs even more puzzling to the family (Konstantareas, 1990).

Parents who are not provided with the information they need to assist their sons or daughters often will continue their search. As a result of this, they are branded as "shoppers," or are accused of being in denial (Donnellan & Mirenda, 1984). There seems to be little recognition that professional behavior and the diagnostic process itself frequently perpetuate the "shopping" cycle.

Unfortunately, parents expect that once a diagnosis is given, the search for answers will end. Often, though, diagnosis is just the beginning (Cutler & Kozloff, 1987).

Decisions, Decisions

For some very young children, a formal diagnosis may not be given, but early intervention services will be recommended. With or without a formal diagnosis, parents are now faced with a confusing and sometimes conflicting array of choices with regard to the type of intervention warranted for their son or daughter. Parents, therefore, need information about what services and supports are available to make informed choices. Yet, parents report great frustration with professionals who choose to withhold information because the professionals fear that parents may not be capable of making good choices or because the professionals may have a personal/professional bias about the intervention. This "screening" of information usurps the parents' right to decide what is best for their child.

Though there are a number of different strategies for assisting young children with ASD (e.g., communication therapy, sensorimotor interventions, floor time, applied behavioral analysis, play, music therapies), some interventions may not be available to the family for a variety of reasons (e.g., funding, staffing, geographical restrictions, program philosophy). When parents know that help is available yet are not able to access it, they are in the position of having to compromise—to make do with what is available as opposed to what might be most beneficial for the child (Wolery, 1997). An example of this compromise is access to integrated programs. Despite documented evidence as to the efficacy of integrated programs for young children with autism (Strain, 1990), there is a lack of well-designed, adequately staffed, and community-based inclusive programs.

Conflicting information with regard to what constitutes recommended practice and the proliferation of numerous new interventions also mark the experience of autism in many families' lives. Parents simply do not have the luxury of waiting for science to validate the efficacy of new treatments (Lehr & Lehr, 1997). They fear that the treatment or intervention that they might not try may have in fact made all the difference in their child's life. Parents also feel the need to be aware constantly of all changes and new treatments in the field, leading them to expend time, energy, and financial resources to remain ever vigilant in their search for help for their son or daughter.

Unfulfilled Promises

Some professionals lead families to believe that a cure for their child's disability is available (Risley, 1997). These promises are very appealing to parents who may be emotionally vulnerable and anxious to do whatever they must to help their son or daughter.

The common practices of doing "too little, too late" or only intervening in crises are other illustrations of unfulfilled promises. Examples include the lack of availability of particular therapies in preschool programs or, when provided, therapies that are reduced or withdrawn once the child shows any progress; families who may have been well supported in early intervention programs find they are kept at a distance from the planning once their children leave the early intervention system and enter school. Finally, children may end up in crises in which a good match does not exist between the needs of the child and the supports offered. These experiences, again, cause families to feel the burden of lost time and missed opportunities.

How Parents See It

Adaptation to having a child with a disability is a lifelong process that occurs in a vastly different manner from family to family and even among members within the same family. Each parent or other family member responds to the needs of the child in his or her own unique way. In an effort to understand the experience of families who have a child with a disability, some professionals have applied the framework from the literature describing stages involved in the grieving process (Hanline, 1991). One of the problems in applying this model is the presumption that grief is the experience of all families; thus, each response made by a family member, therefore, results in the assignment of a particular stage within that process (e.g., "He's in denial," "She can't get past her anger"). An even greater problem with the use of this model is that it may lead the professional to give a stereotypical response to a parent, without engaging in a genuine dialogue about the parent's unique perspective and experience. Another significant problem is that this grief schema weakens the impact of social stressors such as exclusionary educational programs as well as the lack of needed family supports on the family's ability to cope (Cutler, 1993; Wikler, 1983).

Hanline noted that "current perspectives do not presume parental response to the birth of a child with a disability to always be that of a grieving process" (1991, p. 53). A growing body of research suggests that the presence of a family member with a disability may actually contribute to the strengthening of the family, thus enhancing the quality of life of the individual members. At an individualized education program (IEP) team meeting, one mother reported, "All they talked about was what my 6-year-old child could not do and how he did not fit in. They ignored all the progress he had made!" How disheartening it must be for parents who love, appreciate, and see possibilities for their child to have these perspectives interpreted either as unrealistic or as representative of aspects of denial.

Finding a Balance

One of the most difficult experiences faced by parents is the need to find a balance in family life. For those who have children in addition to their child with

ASD, meeting the needs of those other children while searching for information and services is exhausting. Many times, the demands placed on parents to be part of a child's intervention program or to coordinate necessary services leave little time for other family members. An additional concern to families is the extra cost of the therapies and services for the child with ASD that the schools do not or cannot provide. Balancing time, energy, attention, and finances within the family is a constant struggle.

Finding a Place within the Community

For many families the experience of autism in their lives is an isolating one (Cutler & Kozloff, 1987; Wolery, 1997). The public stares, the whispers, and the judgments—spoken and unspoken—constantly follow the family. Visits to restaurants and other family outings, once a source of joy, become experiences fraught with stress or embarrassment. People once considered friends no longer call as often or are too busy to stop by. One parent stated, "You really get to know who your true friends are." Another commented, "We just didn't attend family get-togethers any more—it was too stressful for our son and too stressful for me." Many have spoken about the pressure they feel to always have to explain their son's or daughter's behavior for fear that they might be misunderstood.

Parents who want their sons and daughters to be accepted and known within their communities accept the additional challenge of educating individuals everywhere they go, without understanding that they don't always have to assume the obligation to explain. Professionals must support families in their endeavors to have their children accepted and respected within their communities from the very beginning (Wolery, 1997).

What Lies Ahead

From the day their child receives a diagnosis of ASD, most parents wonder and worry about what the future might hold. The lives of their sons or daughters will be filled with change, opportunities for growth, and transitions from one stage of life to the next. This is true for all children but is particularly difficult for families of children with ASD because possibilities in their future might appear to be so limited. This perceived limitation is partially a result of the great variability among children with ASD and also a result of the lack of specificity regarding the best approach to intervention (Wolery, 1997).

Parents not only must manage the challenges inherent in raising a child with a disability but also must cope with recurring times when they cannot anticipate various milestones, transitions, or instances when younger siblings surpass the skills of the child with a disability (Hanline, 1991; Wikler, 1983). Although many of these experiences are prevalent in the first 5 years of the child's life, they are not limited to these early years. These moments, feelings, and perceptions represent themes that may be repeated over and over. These typical, familiar experiences will be interwoven throughout the remainder of this discussion as they relate to the provision of services to children with ASD.

SUPPORTING FAMILIES TO MAKE THE ASSESSMENT PROCESS EASIER

For many parents and professionals, the label of ASD is frightening. For some parents, who have been given little or no information and who have no previous knowledge of ASD, the label is meaningless and as a result they are still left adrift and without information. For others, the label provides an anchor—a starting point for gaining access to information and gathering resources.

Parents typically experience a kind of "screening process" for their child first, which flags problem areas and often results in a referral for a diagnosis or a more detailed picture of the strengths and challenges of the child. This multidisciplinary diagnostic *team* always includes the family and may include a neurologist, psychologist, developmental pediatrician, audiologist, speech-language pathologist, and occupational therapist with expertise in sensory integration. The team should focus on classification, which is critical for the purposes of intervention, prognosis, support, and broader areas including legal rights (Stone, 1997). One of the problems inherent in assigning a diagnostic label is that it might diminish the individuality of the child and cause others to have preconceived ideas about the child's abilities. For this reason, the assessment process can be a frightening and emotionally draining ordeal for parents. It can also be very time consuming. Sometimes assisting parents to think about this process as one of "ruling in or ruling out" a diagnosis of autism makes the experience a bit less intimidating. Guiding parents toward a screening or more detailed assessment process may require a high degree of professional sensitivity if the parents have not recognized any problems with their child or have recognized a problem but have not yet taken the first steps toward acknowledgment. This is a precarious position for families and also for early intervention staff who may be aware of the child's developmental challenges yet struggle with sharing this information with the families in a sensitive and respectful manner.

There is a growing trend away from the traditional standardized assessments toward more observational, functional, adaptive, and play-based strategies (Foley & Hochman, 1998). An additional dimension of assessment, consistent with this direction, includes observation of interactions between caregiver and child (Greenspan, 1992). Standardized assessments have been problematic because they do not always give an accurate picture of the child with ASD, often not crediting a child for skills he or she has but may not be able to demonstrate. Occasionally, evaluators may assume that the child has skills that do not exist as an artifact of the testing protocol (presuming that one skill is built on another and that skills are built in that sequence, which may or may not be the case for children with ASD) (Jordan & Powell, 1995). If the profile presented by assessment is too disparate from what the parents know and experience about their child, they might begin to mistrust the process or doubt their own instincts and lose confidence in the ability of the professionals involved with their child. Other areas of concern associated with standardized tests include the shortage of specific instruments for assessment of young children with ASD, especially those that solicit parental input, and the lack of staff who are trained in the administration of those tests.

Another problem with formal assessments revolves around the testing environment itself. For young children, assessments that take place in unfamiliar environments may automatically put them at a disadvantage. Evaluators may assess a child who is extremely anxious and unable to respond as he or she typically would, thus gaining a spurious picture of the child, which may be misrepresentative of the child's true abilities. This problem is true for older children as well, but for some older children the testing environment may be an ideal one—one that is free from social demands, usually with one-to-one attention and unambiguous instructions provided. This type of assessment may not yield information regarding the child's ability to function in a classroom situation in which the social and communication demands are more complex and sensory issues may interfere.

The lack of sufficient time allowed to complete some standardized tests is incompatible with the processing difficulties of many children with autism. The pacing of tests can also be problematic. Typically, the child visits one evaluator after another in a 1- or 2-day period. This pace is stressful for both the child and family. Such a "cookie-cutter" approach does not allow the evaluator to develop a relationship with the child or become attuned to the child and his or her family's unique needs (Eggbeer, Littman, & Jones, 1997). This combination of factors might lead the evaluator to conclude that the child is "untestable." Statements of this nature are not helpful and add to the burden and confusion that parents are already experiencing.

These difficulties lead us to conclude that assessments, particularly for very young children, must occur in an environment in which the children feel safe and comfortable and across settings with familiar caregivers. This level of comfort is essential because young children often command a range and complexity of behavior that is not displayed in unfamiliar or threatening clinical settings (Walizer & Leff, 1993). Despite the advantages of assessing the child in a comfortable environment such as his or her home, this approach may have drawbacks. Some family members may consider this approach to be intrusive and disruptive to the family's routine. Even though conducting assessments within natural environments is considered to be recommended practice, this option may not be readily available to families because of constraints in personnel or resources in their local service delivery systems.

Though we are not advocating the elimination of standardized testing with young children, the limitations of such testing need to be recognized and complemented through other means of gathering relevant information about the child. Assessment should never be considered a one-time or discrete event. Rather, it should be an ongoing process of gathering information over time about the child's strengths as well as challenges across situational contexts (Prizant & Wetherby, 1993). The limited snapshot presented through one-time formal assessments may result in recommendations that are not representative of the child's range of skills. Assessments need to yield useful and direct information for intervention that is compatible and consistent with the needs expressed by the family (Prizant & Wetherby, 1993).

Information presented throughout the assessment period, as well as subsequent recommendations, should be free from professional jargon. In conjunction with standardized testing, structured parental interviews and questionnaires, which document historical and developmental information, must be used. Formal assessments should always be supplemented by direct observation, checklists, and information provided by individuals familiar with the child in a variety of settings. The use of videotapes to pick up subtle information and capture familiar routines (Jordan & Powell, 1995; Klin et al., 1997; Prizant & Wetherby, 1993) may also yield valuable insights about the child that are not readily observable through other means. Assessments of this nature are particularly helpful for children suspected of having ASD because behavior may be idiosyncratic, situationally determined, or contextually specific and because the child's strengths and needs may be in danger of being overlooked or misread.

Primary to assessment and leveraged by laws pertaining to early intervention is the need for assessments to be family driven or family centered. Parents must be recognized and supported in understanding that they are truly the experts in knowing their child (Cutler, 1993). The first step in this process is to include parents in the discussion of what needs to be gleaned from the assessments and which areas present concerns for the family. Parents should feel free to share their observations of the child, both in terms of strengths and areas of greater challenge. Parents' active engagement in the evaluation procedures demystifies the process and also provides a common set of observations for subsequent discussion (Klin et al., 1997). By working in conjunction with parents during assessment, evaluators can understand the strategies parents have developed to assist their son or daughter. Assessment may also be seen as the first step in intervention in that additional strategies for interacting with the child may be modeled in the process (Klin et al., 1997; Prizant & Wetherby, 1993).

On completion of assessment, information should be presented to families in a clear, sensitive, and descriptive manner that addresses the unique learning patterns of their son or daughter (Marcus, Kunce, & Schopler, 1997). Walizer and Leff explained that "the manner in which the bad news is presented to caregivers has a profound effect on [parents'] views of themselves, their child, and their future contact with those helping their child" (1993, p. 21). Assessments must provide the family and others who interact with the child with practical recommendations that cannot be summarily dismissed by early intervention professionals or school systems (Stone, 1997).

Finally, in keeping with the idea of assessment as a fluid and ongoing process, clinicians must make themselves available to the families to provide ongoing information and support. Periodic discussion to gather information about the child's progress in relation to recommendations made is extremely helpful to families and provides a sense of continuity of information.

PLANNING SERVICES: HELPING PARENTS DEFINE THEIR NEEDS

"Families represent the most powerful and pervasive influence that a child will ever experience" (Fox, Dunlap, & Philbrick, 1997, p. 4). It is this primary role of the family as the "constant" in the child's life that defines the need for intervention to be both family driven and family centered. Family-centered practice is focused on the idea that each family is unique, should be involved in helping to define their own needs, and should ultimately control services that are provided. Family-centered practices should be consumer driven and should enhance competency (Dunst, Johanson, Trivette, & Hamby, 1991). In actuality, for services to be truly family centered, they must focus on the family's strengths and characteristics as a whole rather than solely addressing the needs of the child (Allen & Petr, 1997; Brotherson & Goldstein, 1992). When family dynamics are not considered, members may feel betrayed or alienated from one of the most important events in their child's life. If families are relegated to a secondary role so early in the intervention process, this could set the stage for them to presume that their continued involvement should be only minimal at best.

It is obvious that there exists tremendous variability among families. This variability includes but is not limited to the following factors: the presence of brothers and sisters; single-parent families; two working parents; socioeconomic conditions; cultural traditions; existence or absence of natural or extended support systems; and the family's perception of the child and the child's disability. These factors help define the unique characteristics within each family. Therefore, clinical practice needs to reflect sensitivity, flexibility, and creativity in addressing these differences. These qualities are the central components of family-centered services. This kind of service provision requires that the clinician suspend professional judgement of the family and resist the urge to superimpose a predetermined agenda on them. Families have been very clear and consistent over time about what does and does not help. They have stated it over and over again, only to have their statements studied and restudied in search of validity, as though this validity exists somewhere outside of the family's lived experiences.

Support that is family centered has the following characteristics (Allen & Petr, 1997; Fenichel, 1991; Mikus, Benn, & Weathertson, 1995; Wolery, 1997):

- Infants and toddlers must be provided support within the context of their families.
- Services should provide a foundation for building a trusting, respectful, and collaborative relationship with the family.
- Supports should be responsive to the idiosyncratic needs and strengths of the family, and services should be coordinated to ease the burden on families.
- Interventions must be specifically designed to be developmentally appropriate.

Although there is general agreement as to what family-centered services should encompass, in practice, implementation of these principles is somewhat challenging. Often, professional preparation focuses on working with the child and not with the family system. Professionals are often in the position of working with many families simultaneously, making it difficult for them to take the necessary time for building relationships. There can be conflict regarding what the family values and what the professional values. What a family might define as an important goal may be considered by the professional to be of lesser importance. Professionals who are unfamiliar with cultural norms and traditions within a family may be at a disadvantage when attempting to respond to the needs of the entire family in keeping with those cultural mores (Lynch & Hanson, 1998).

Shortages of resources or trained personnel are other formidable barriers. It is not enough to simply identify family needs; the team also has to be able to provide the actual service or offer the support necessary in a timely fashion. Research in early intervention for children with autism has shown that children make greater progress when services are provided early and are intensive in nature (Dawson & Osterling, 1997). For families of children with autism, this is often easier said than done. One parent, when speaking about her 4-year-old child, noted that "I was offered intensive family support services but was told there was no one available to provide the one piece we all felt was most important—respite! I had to find my own respite worker. It took 2 months."

Many families are aware that intensive early services are necessary and also recognize the neurological underpinnings of their child's autism. This results in an urgency to find the right services that begin early and will have the greatest impact on their child's development.

Another critical obstacle to family-centered services lies within the service delivery system itself. Often, these systems are not set up to allow for the flexibility and creativity needed for responsive planning, or for fluid communication among providers who offer different aspects of support.

A major obstacle perceived by professionals is the constant shifting of goals to meet the everchanging needs of the child and the family, compounded by the need to accomplish this with many different families. A professional in the field of family support stated the following:

> Sometimes, what you set out to accomplish with a family may not be what you end up doing with the family. For example, when called to assist a child with joining a YMCA swim class, I discovered that the mom had lost her job, had no public assistance, little food in the house, and another child who was also demanding much of her attention. After meeting with the mother, the goal of joining the YMCA, though important, became secondary to the more fundamental goal of putting food on the table.

There is ambiguity regarding how to implement the steps necessary for family-centered planning to take place. The role of the professional can be very confusing when trying to respond genuinely and respectfully to the needs of families.

The Role of the Family

Despite the present challenges, a family-centered approach to planning is essential. Parents spend more time with their child than anyone else. They know their child's nuances and responses and can lend a unique perspective with regard to intervention goals. Individuals will come and go in a child's life, but parents are the constant (Cutler, 1993). This makes the involvement of parents in the planning process critical and essential. There is a greater chance for the child to generalize skills from one environment to another and to maintain those skills when parents are involved.

Dawson and Osterling (1997) found that parents experienced a greater sense of relatedness with their child, an increase in their sense of competence and feeling of well being, and a decrease in emotional stress when they were involved in their child's program. When parents help prioritize the goals to be addressed and are genuinely engaged in the planning and intervention process, true change can occur (Berlin, O'Neal, & Brooks-Gunn, 1998). When parents are viewed as "key mediators" in interpreting the child's experiences (Klein & Wieder, 1995), they can be helped to fine-tune this role thereby creating greater opportunities for the child to learn within natural contexts throughout the day.

Families should be extended the opportunity to make decisions and choices regarding instructional activities and their degree of involvement in those activities. These opportunities for choice should be embedded within ongoing routines and activities (Brotherson & Goldstein, 1992; Wolery, 1997). When this does not take place, a situation similar to the following may occur. The staff of one child's day program, trying to be responsive to the family's needs, agreed to help in meeting the child's needs at home. The parents had hoped for assistance in helping their child learn some functional skills, development of a communication system, and assistance in creating some recreational opportunities within the community. The staff responded by suggesting a jogging program for the entire family. This program would begin at 5:00 A.M., would last for about 20 minutes, and was to take place 7 days a week. The family tried to comply with the program but soon discovered that this truly didn't meet their needs or reflect their goals for their son in their home.

It is unreasonable for professionals to expect all parents to assume a role that extends beyond the normal challenges of parenting (Robbins, Dunlap, & Pleinis, 1991). Professionals need to respect the roles that parents are comfortable in assuming regarding the degree of their involvement, as well as the amount of time a family can realistically make available. Professionals must be sensitive to time as a limited resource for families. Parents spend time traveling to and from various appointments, therapies, and so forth. Their time must be used efficiently and effectively. There is also the need to balance the time allotted for other family members to be involved in intervention along with the time needed to assure family well-being. Embedding activities within natural family routines provides another way of respecting how a family's time is spent. This structure, however, may also pose problems due to the need for clinicians to respect a family's privacy while being helpful (Able-Boone, Sandall, Loughry, & Frederick, 1990). Although parents think of time in terms of daily routine, they also see the care of their child as a lifelong, ever-evolving commitment, "not simply a short-term education or therapeutic contact" (Brotherson & Goldstein, 1992, p. 523). Professionals need to be aware of this significant difference in the way families view time as they support and work with families.

Another essential element in family-centered planning is the development of a collaborative relationship between parents and professionals. In addition to being viewed as unique in their experiences, parents should be considered as competent, contributing members of the team with knowledge to share. Some parents have emphasized that "struggling to be heard is time consuming and stressful!" (Brotherson & Goldstein, 1992, p. 523). Much time and energy could be saved if the team acknowledged parents as the experts on their child and as such, valued and respected their contributions.

According to state and federal law, the vehicle used to design and implement services for young children is the individualized family support plan (IFSP). The importance of family participation is the "bedrock" of Part C of the Individuals with Disabilities Education Act (IDEA; PL 105-17) Amendments of 1997, formerly Part H of the Education of the Handicapped Act Amendments of 1986 (PL 99-457) (Able-Boone et al., 1990). Parents, as part of a multidisciplinary team, should participate in defining the key elements of their child's IFSP. This includes providing information about the child; developing a profile of the family's strengths, needs, and priorities; delineating expected outcomes; setting criteria, procedures, and time lines to assure these outcomes; defining the frequency, intensity, setting (home, center, community, combination of all), and method of early intervention services; assignment of a services coordinator, or case manager (a term many families dislike), to coordinate needed elements; and the design of transition plans at age 3 if necessary (Fewell, Snyder, Sexton, & Hockless, 1991). Parents need to be well-informed, active participants in this process. That these intervention plans reflect family cultures and life experiences is extremely important (Berlin et al., 1998). A well-constructed IFSP helps to ensure that interventions will occur in a manner that is most helpful to the child and family.

MOVING TOWARD AN INDIVIDUALIZED EDUCATION PROGRAM: THE CHANGING ROLE OF THE FAMILY

For families of children with autism, time spent within the early intervention system may be very brief due to late diagnosis. Many families receive a diagnosis only to find themselves in the process of making the transition to a new system—with new sets of rules, new means of delivering services, and requests for additional assessments. In many cases the family just begins to develop relationships that may be abruptly severed, leaving the family once again in a tenuous and vulnerable position. For others, the ambiguity and length of the diagnostic process may have prevented their child from receiving services before the age of 3. Families may enter this process with no prior knowledge or experience of working with any system or receiving any services.

Moving into the Unknown

As stated previously, children younger than age 3 receive services through the IFSP. The IFSP defines the system in which evaluation, intervention planning, and implementation of services for infants and toddlers at risk take place. The cornerstone of this plan is the incorporation of the strengths and concerns of the entire family as well as those of the child.

On turning 3 years old, children receive services under Part B of IDEA. As mandated by this law, children receive an IEP that focuses on the development of goals and objectives for the child. Although the parents are participants in this process, the manner in which the parents participate is vastly different. The family needs as a whole are not addressed as part of the plan. Many families report that there is a diminished sense of partnership. Often it appears to the family as though the care and time involved in cultivating their participation is no longer seen as valuable. Many families will feel the impact of the difference between the philosophical approaches of these two systems. Though a child will move from receiving services from one type to another, the larger family support needs remain and there is no delineation as to how those needs will be met. In addition to the distinction regarding the recipient of services (family centered versus child centered), some face a loss of services entirely because of differing eligibility criteria.

The criterion of providing services to children who are "at risk," used for those younger than 3, is far broader than the federal criteria of "child with a disability" and "child with a developmental delay," set for children 3 years of age and older. This difference in scope creates a double-edged sword for children with autism. The "at risk" definition allows a child younger than 3 to receive services without a formal diagnosis of autism or PDD. Conversely, if a child does not have a diagnosis, and his or her symptoms have not been clearly understood or defined, he or she runs the risk of not being eligible for services at the age of 3. This leads some families to enter the transition process feeling resentful, confused, and angry.

With the changes in service focus and delivery, families report feeling a sense of loss. Something that had been given is now perceived as having been taken away. This also applies to the role filled by some early interventionists as advocates for the child and family. Families feel this loss acutely because it is viewed as an essential service that is no longer available.

BUILDING BRIDGES FOR WORKING TOGETHER: PARENT–PROFESSIONAL RELATIONSHIPS AND COLLABORATION

Though federal law (PL 105-17) stipulates the participation of parents, the law cannot mandate the quality or extent of that involvement. The need for continuity and consistency in program planning and intervention across individuals and environments, so vital for children with autism, further accentuates the importance of parents' and professionals' working together to ensure that these factors exist. The combination of social, cognitive, and communicative challenges present in autism, however, often results in complex relationships between parents and professionals (Donnellan & Mirenda, 1984). In addition, numerous sources have indicated that parent–professional relationships, in general, often reflect conflict, tension, and disharmony (Leyser, 1988). Therefore, it is important to consider some of the factors contributing to problems in parent and professional relationships and delineate elements of successful parent–professional relationships.

One source of conflict often cited by parents is the perception of continually having to "prove" that they are, in fact, the ones who know the child best. This speaks to the issue of parental credibility. Parents state that professionals need to realize that the "stakes are high" when the topic is their child's life. Although parents are emotionally involved, that does not diminish the quality of their contribution. As stated earlier, parents are the constants in their child's life. Professional involvement frequently changes, subsequently offering only time-limited glimpses of a child's skills and needs. Commenting on one of the major sources of stress in her life, one mother stated that "it isn't parenting the child with autism that's the problem, it's the constant struggle to have your voice heard and your opinions respected that is most stressful."

The fragmented input from and frequent turnover of professionals puts the onus on parents to be the "gatekeepers" of information regarding their child's progress and continued challenges. This requires that parents constantly reeducate the steady stream of professionals who move into and out of their son's or daughter's lives (Allen & Petr, 1997; Brotherson & Goldstein, 1992).

A number of factors relating to professional training and development have also been cited as obstacles to mutually satisfying parent–professional relationships. The ability of professionals to work not only with the child but also with the family as a system is paramount. For example, some studies show only a moderate level of perceived competence among early intervention staff when they were asked to rate themselves and their ability to work effectively with families (Bailey, Palsha, & Simeonsson, 1991). The skills that a team member needs to work specifically with a child will differ from those that he or she needs to work within a family system. Working within a family system requires the refinement of techniques for building solid relationships, communicating openly with families, and interviewing and collaborating in decision making, to name just a few, in addition to particular expertise in working with children with disabilities (Brotherson & Goldstein, 1992). Another major skill needed is the ability to find the balance among listening to families, discovering what the family can do realistically, and deciding where the professional may need to fill in the gaps (Bailey, 1987). The integration of these skills is not always easy. Many professionals have not had adequate training to meet these challenges.

Critical to the parent–professional relationship is the level of trust on the part of families that the professionals have the skills and understanding necessary to effectively meet the needs of their child with autism. It should not be assumed, however, that particular expertise for working with children with autism is a given. In fact, the lack of specific training in meeting the unique needs of children with ASD is another concern often raised by parents. Because of the range of characteristics presented within the spectrum of autism, strategies developed for one child may not be helpful for another. There is a tendency to apply the same template across all children within a given diagnosis. This creates a danger for both families and professionals. Professionals providing intervention to children with autism need a broad range of information and an eclectic array of strategies at their disposal. In addition, they need to apply these strategies flexibly and in a manner that is compatible with the families' style and priorities. When this is not done, parents and professionals may be at odds as to what intervention should be and the specifics regarding intervention (e.g., where, how much, at what point). Much energy is invested by both sides defending positions and determining whose position is most important, or essentially, who is in control. Parents claim that professionals have withheld information regarding possible interventions based on spurious judgments of the parents' ability to handle that information or on preconceived notions that the interventions have no credibility or relevance for their child. Specific programs that rely heavily on family participation for implementation also run the risk of scapegoating families if the intervention fails (Schopler, 1971; Snell, 1983).

Conversely, professionals cite frustration with parents for a number of reasons, including lack of parental attendance at meetings; lack of follow-through; parents who do not listen to or trust the skills of the professionals; and lack of motivation to execute the suggested programs (Bailey, 1987). Poor communication between parents and professionals, as well as limited resources for providing services, were also identified as common barriers to effective relationships (DeGangi, Wietlisbach, Poisson, & Stein, 1994). As noted previously, what professionals have termed "shopping behavior" (collecting information from various sources and attempting to implement that information into program planning) is another source of conflict frequently cited by professionals in their relationship with parents.

The nature and origin of parent–professional differences are based on more fundamental issues of differing values and priorities. Complicated family dynamics and structure and differences in cultural beliefs and socioeconomic status all challenge the quality of parent–professional collaboration. The wider the gap, the greater the challenge to working together on behalf of the child.

Despite these obstacles, parents and professionals have a fundamental need to develop good working relationships. A number of factors contribute to the cultivation of healthy parent–professional partnerships. To begin with, professionals need to have an awareness of and sensitivity to the uniqueness of the family situation and the family's changing needs. Flexibility and creativity regarding services available to families is critical (Brotherson & Goldstein, 1992). One parent acknowledged,

> It made such a positive impression on me when the kindergarten teacher came to my home to spend some time with our family the summer before my son was to enter her classroom. He had never attended a formal school program before, and this really helped us all to feel more comfortable and less anxious when he started school.

It is often easy to lose sight of the seemingly small gestures of kindness and genuine human understanding that can enrich and strengthen parent–professional partnerships.

An array of support services, including emotional support, should be readily available to families. Professionals, however, should not assume that all families need these services or the same intensity of services. Another primary factor in relationship building is a willingness of all to acknowledge that parents and professionals do not always share the same goals. This suggests the need to negotiate values and priorities to reach a joint solution. To do this effectively, both parties must be willing to listen respectfully to one another and resist the urge to pass judgment. Other factors that have an impact on the development of good relationships include a sensitivity to cultural values and traditions; recognition of the family's socioeconomic background; and acceptance of the family's reactions as normal and legitimate. Professionals need to make available to parents diagnostic and educational information that will assist them in making informed decisions about the best course of intervention for their child. As stated previously, dialogue with families should be free of jargon and confusing professional rhetoric. Professionals need to be able to share with families their concerns and experiences regarding specific interventions but ultimately respect the family's right to make whatever decisions they feel are necessary for their child. It is incumbent on professionals to subscribe to the *criterion of the least dangerous assumption;* that is, if an intervention fails, professionals should not assume that failure is the parent's fault (Donnellan & Cutler, 1990).

Parents should be aware that professionals possess varying degrees of expertise in understanding the dynamics of ASD. Limited resources or constraints of time may hamper professionals' ability to actualize goals and objectives that have been mutually developed. Parents need to be actively engaged in problem solving with professionals around these issues (Bailey, 1987; Donnellan & Cutler, 1990).

Sometimes, the best efforts at working together meet with failure. At this point, it may be helpful to engage another party in assisting parents and professionals to find some common ground. In this regard, programs providing family support might complement or support parents and professionals in their pursuit of specific goals. Parent and professional relationships will be ongoing and everchanging. Despite inherent challenges to working together, indeed, the success of the child's development depends on the quality of these relationships.

Though this period of time might be traumatic for families, there are certain elements that can make the transition easier to services after children turn 3. Parents need to be fully informed of the process. Parents cannot be expected to make informed choices without knowing that there are options available to them and what those options entail. They need to be aware of how the process works, including the steps involved and the role they play in actualizing the steps. This involves an understanding of the law and the rights accorded to their son or daughter. They also need to know what they might possibly gain or lose in terms of services and what can be done if they believe their child's needs are not being met. Knowledge is power, and once armed with knowledge, families are in a better position to obtain the needed supports for their child.

FUTURE DIRECTIONS: HOW RESEARCH CAN HELP

Families of children with ASD experience difficulty from the time of their first awareness because of the limited understanding of ASD held by professionals who will diagnose, assess, recommend, and deliver services to their children. Though much is known about ASD with more information continually emerging (Hart, 1993), many professionals hold to earlier images of children with ASD as atypical, asocial, noncompliant, and bewildering. These images are based on inferences derived from the children's more obvious behaviors and do not take into account the deficits and difficulties that are neurologically based (Rogers, 1992; Wing, 1976). No wonder some well-intentioned professionals are still reluctant to assign such a dismal and stigmatizing label to young children! A broader framework for learning about ASD is essential for a more comprehensive understanding of this developmental disability through those areas of research that currently have had a minimal impact on the service system.

Sensory Problems

There is sufficient evidence to indicate that children with ASD have serious sensorimotor difficulties (Ayres, 1995; Gillingham, 1995; see also Chapter 7). Practitioners have known for a long time of hypersensitive hearing in some children, for example, and parents have spoken of their children's being able to hear a candy unwrapped from the next room. Clinicians are becoming aware that differences such as toe walking or resistance to being picked up, once labeled "maladaptive behaviors," are likely evidence of extreme sensitivity to touch. Some children with ASD are obviously uncomfortable with bright light under certain conditions. What is needed is research to develop information about how children with ASD respond to noise, crowds, touch, and so forth and under what conditions their responses may vary. These behaviors are observable and measurable but will require more sophisticated research completed across environments rather than a simple behavioral or developmental checklist done in a single environment. Some focus on these difficulties may sensitize more professionals to recognizing early signs of ASD, perhaps as early as the first year. Although it may not be appropriate to label such young children as having ASD, practitioners may at least be able to recognize a child who is at risk and begin intervention.

Motor Difficulties

There are also motor aspects of autism that have been given some attention (Damasio & Maurer, 1978; Donnellan & Leary, 1995; Hill & Leary, 1993; Rapin, 1997) and are now becoming items of interest. An article in *The New York Times* (1999) highlighted the work of Teitlebaum in studying subtle abnormal movements of infants on videotapes who were later diagnosed as having ASD.

Many parents have told us that their babies, later diagnosed with ASD, failed to hold up their arms in anticipation of being picked up and that many at the age of 1 year did not or could not use a spoon (and some continued to have poor skills with utensils and later had poor handwriting). Motor difficulties and differences in ASD are an area that requires greater attention and more intensive research. More work in this promising area of research may enlighten clinicians' understanding of ASD and improve their abilities to serve these children.

Communication

The research on echolalia (see Prizant & Rydell, 1993, for a review) has helped to enlighten the field since the mid-1980s. Echolalia, once considered to be "nonsense" talk, is now understood by many, if not all, to represent a child's best efforts to communicate. Work on the communicative intent of aberrant or "challenging" behaviors has shown that children will use the means they have available (which may be shouting or throwing) to make a protest when they are unable to say, "No" (Donnellan, Mirenda, Mesaros, & Fassbender, 1984).

Children with ASD who are verbal have been accused of changing topics in conversation without regard for the listener. Here an inference is made about the children's social inadequacy, and rarely is it thought that the child may be trying to maintain a social connection with the limited verbal means available to him or her. We have seen and heard children with ASD who are being co-treated by speech-language and occupational/sensory therapists produce language that is qualitatively different from their usual utterances. Some children produce better language on computers, which have a low motor demand, than they do in their typical environments.

Much needed research in these areas (sensory, motor, and communication, including cross-disciplinary research) could provide a more comprehensive and clearer picture of ASD for earlier diagnosis and possibly for earlier and more substantial intervention. Information should be garnered from many groups. Researchers and practitioners are particularly blessed that an increasing number of people with ASD can talk about their experiences (Barron & Barron, 1992; Grandin, 1995; Williams, 1994). These individuals and others with ASD should be interviewed further to increase knowledge about ASD. In addition to better information about ASD, which should be provided at the undergraduate and graduate levels, new and improved models of partnering and supporting families should be developed.

IMPROVING SERVICES AND SUPPORTS

New models and supports need to be developed for working with families. People have been talking about parent–professional partnerships since the early 1980s (Cutler, 1981, 1996; Donnellan & Mirenda, 1984). Still we hear from parents who feel that they are expected to cooperate unquestioningly, that is, to follow professional advice often without understanding the full array of interventions or the impact on their children (Donnellan & Cutler, 1990; Donnellan & Mirenda, 1984).

The new models would require greater understanding of living with a child with ASD and how the community responds to these families (Cutler & Kozloff, 1987), more acceptance of cultural and life differences and family crises, more empathy for the difficulties that families face on all fronts, and the ability to assume some responsibility for developing a model parent–professional partnership that the parent can then use as a measure for future parent–professional relationships (Cutler, 1996). This model partnership shifts the burden from the parents who should "cooperate" to the professional who can support the skills, characteristics, and efforts that parents will need to be lifelong and effective advocates. This includes helping parents to be organized and assertive at meetings; supporting productive work with other professionals; and assisting parents in learning how to search for information, resources, and other allies. Not all professionals will or can assume such responsibility, but a cadre of professionals competent in partnering to serve as models for parents as well as for other professionals is needed.

For good partnership models to develop, training must happen at the preservice levels (undergraduate or graduate) when young professionals are learning without having to deal with the stressors of the service system and are more open to new ideas. The development of curriculum for such training would require more work and extended interviews with parents in nonthreatening environments by professionals who are not stakeholders in the system serving the child. Parents have the experiences, know their needs, and can articulate them with empathic and knowledgeable professionals.

CONCLUSIONS

If research prevails in discovering and disseminating more and better information on ASD, that is, developing a fuller, more sympathetic, and even more optimistic picture of the array of children who are eventually diagnosed with ASD, the children and their families could enjoy a number of benefits:

1. Earlier diagnosis of ASD or at least recognition of children at risk
2. A willingness on the part of the professional to make the diagnosis based on a future less bleak than past and current images present
3. A longer period of early intervention services given earlier diagnosis
4. Reduced emotional stress experienced by parents in daily living with their children at home, with their extended families, and in their communities
5. Better ability of parents to focus their energies on their children and their optimal development

If new models of partnering with parents can be designed, parents will be less "dragged down" by the difficulties they face in dealing with the service system. Their growing abilities, supported by their mentoring professional partners, may further enhance knowledge of ASD, and the parents may become stronger and more effective in gathering the services they and their children need.

We are constantly amazed by the strength, resilience, and commitment of many families as we have worked alongside them in their often frustrating and sometimes frightening journey through the complexities of a service system that itself is still struggling to understand and meet the needs of children with ASD. Families surely are bowed by their experiences but still stand committed to their children. Although collectively the service system now knows more about ASD and is more responsive, it has yet to provide the full array of understanding and support to families and their children with ASD. Accomplishing this is a challenge for the new century.

REFERENCES

Able-Boone, H., Sandall, S., Loughry, A., & Frederick, L. (1990). An informed, family-centered approach to Public Law 99-457: Parental views. *Topics in Early Childhood Special Education, 10*(1), 100–111.

Allen, R.I., & Petr, C.G. (1997, Summer). Family-centered service delivery: A cross-disciplinary literature review and conceptualization. *Families and Disability Newsletter,* 5.

Ayres, A.J. (1995). *Sensory integration and the child.* Los Angeles: Western Psychological Services.

Bailey, D.B. (1987). Collaborative goal-setting with families: Resolving differences in values and priorities for services. *Topics in Early Childhood Special Education, 7*(2), 59–71.

Bailey, D.B., Palsha, S.A., & Simeonsson, R.J. (1991). Professional skills, concerns, and perceived importance of work with families in early intervention. *Exceptional Children, 58*, 156–165.

Barron, J., & Barron, S. (1992). *There's a boy in here.* New York: Simon & Schuster.

Berlin, L.J., O'Neal, C.R., & Brooks-Gunn, J. (1998). What makes early intervention programs work? The program, its participants, and their interaction. *ZERO TO THREE Bulletin, 18*(4), 4–15.

Brotherson, M.J., & Goldstein, B.L. (1992). Time as a resource and constraint for parents of young children with disabilities: Implications for early intervention services. *Topics in Early Childhood Special Education, 12*(4), 508–527.

Cutler, B.C. (1981). *Unraveling the special education maze.* Champaign, IL.: Research Press.

Cutler, B.C. (1993). *You, your child, and "special" education: A guide to making the system work.* Baltimore: Paul H. Brookes Publishing Co.

Cutler, B.C. (1996). Parent professional partnership. In *Positive Behavioral Supports Project.* Durham, NH: Institute on Disability.

Cutler, B.C., & Kozloff, M.A. (1987). Living with autism: Effects on families and family needs. In D.J. Cohen & A.M. Donnellan (Eds.), *Handbook of autism and pervasive developmental disorders* (pp. 513–527). New York: John Wiley & Sons.

Damasio, A., & Maurer, R. (1978). A neurological model for childhood autism. *Archives of Neurology, 35,* 777–786.

Dawson, G., & Osterling, J. (1997). Early intervention in autism. In M.J. Guralnick (Ed.), *The effectiveness of early intervention* (pp. 307–326). Baltimore: Paul H. Brookes Publishing Co.

DeGangi, G.A., Wietlisbach, S., Poisson, S., & Stein, E. (1994). The impact of culture and socioeconomic status on family–professional collaboration: Challenges and solutions. *Topics in Early Childhood Special Education, 14*(4), 503–520.

Donnellan, A.M., & Cutler, B.C. (1990). A dialogue on power relationships and aversive control. In L.H. Meyer, C.A. Peck, & L. Brown (Eds.), *Critical issues in the lives of people with severe disabilities* (pp. 617–624). Baltimore: Paul H. Brookes Publishing Co.

Donnellan, A.M., & Leary, M.R. (1995). *Movement differences and diversity in autism/mental retardation.* Madison, WI: DRI Press.

Donnellan, A.M., & Mirenda, P.L. (1984). Issues related to professional involvement with families of individuals with autism and other severe handicaps. *Journal of The Association for the Severely Handicapped, 9*(1), 16–25.

Donnellan, A.M., Mirenda, P.L., Mesaros, R.A., & Fassbender, L.L. (1984). Analyzing the communicative functions of aberrant behavior. *Journal of The Association for the Severely Handicapped, 9*(3), 201–212.

Dunst, C.J., Johanson, C., Trivette, C.M., & Hamby, D. (1991). Family-oriented early intervention policies and practices: Family-centered or not? *Exceptional Children, 58,* 115–126.

Education of the Handicapped Act Amendments of 1986, PL 99-457, 20 U.S.C. §§ 1400 *et seq.*

Eggbeer, L., Littman, C.L., & Jones, M. (1997). ZERO TO THREE's Developmental Specialist in Pediatric Practice Project: An important support for parents and young children. *ZERO TO THREE Bulletin, 17*(6), 3–8.

Fenichel, E. (1991). Learning through supervision and mentorship to support the development of infants, toddlers, and their families. *ZERO TO THREE Bulletin, 12*(2), 1–9.

Fewell, R.R., Snyder, P., Sexton, D., & Hockless, M.F. (1991). Implementing IFSPs in Louisiana: Different formats for family-centered practices under Part H. *Topics in Early Childhood Education, 11*(3), 54–65.

Foley, G.M., & Hochman, J.D. (1998). Programs, parents, and practitioners: Perspectives on integrating early intervention and infant mental health. *ZERO TO THREE Bulletin, 18*(3), 13–18.

Fox, L., Dunlap, G., & Philbrick, L.A. (1997). Providing individual supports to young children with autism and their families. *Journal of Early Intervention, 21*(1), 1–14.

Gillberg, C., Ehlers, S., Schaumann, H., Jakobsson, G., Dahlgren, S.O., Lindblom, R., Bagenholm, A., Tjus, T., & Blidner, E. (1990). Autism under age 3 years: A clinical study of 28 cases referred for autistic symptoms in infancy. *Journal of Child Psychology and Psychiatry and Allied Disciplines, 31,* 921–934.

Gillingham, G. (1995). *Autism: Handle with care!* Edmonton, Alberta, Canada: Tacit Publishing, Inc.

Grandin, T. (1995). *Thinking in pictures.* New York: Bantam Doubleday Dell.

Greenspan, S.I. (1992). Reconsidering the diagnosis and treatment of very young children with autistic spectrum or pervasive developmental disorder. *ZERO TO THREE Bulletin, 13*(2), 1–9.

Hanline, M.F. (1991). Transitions and critical events in the family life cycle: Implications for providing support to families of children with disabilities. *Psychology in the Schools, 28,* 53–59.

Hart, C. (1993). *A parent's guide to autism.* New York: Pocket Books.

Hill, D.A., & Leary, M.R. (1993). *Movement disturbances: A clue to hidden competencies in persons diagnosed with autism and other developmental disabilities.* Madison, WI: DRI Press.

Individuals with Disabilities Education Act Amendments of 1997, PL 105-17, 20 U.S.C. §§ 1400 *et seq.*

Jordan, R., & Powell, S. (1995). *Understanding and teaching children with autism.* West Sussex, England: John Wiley & Sons.

Klein, P.S., & Wieder, S. (1995). Mediated learning, developmental level, and individual differences: Guides for observation and intervention. *ZERO TO THREE Bulletin, 15*(3), 16–20.

Klin, A., Carter, A., Volkmar, F.R., Cohen, D.J., Marans, W.D., & Sparrow, S.S. (1997). Developmentally based assessments. In D.J. Cohen & F.R. Volkmar (Eds.), *Handbook of autism and pervasive developmental disorders* (2nd ed., pp. 411–447). New York: John Wiley & Sons.

Konstantareas, M.M. (1990). A psychoeducational model for working with families of autistic children. *Journal of Marital and Family Therapy, 16*(1), 59–70.

Lehr, S., & Lehr, R. (1997). *Scientists and parents of children with autism: What do we know? How do we judge what is right?* Unpublished manuscript.

Leyser, Y. (1988). Let's listen to the consumer: The voice of parents of exceptional children. *The School Counselor, 35,* 363–369.

Lynch, E.W., & Hanson, M.J. (Eds.). (1998). *Developing cross-cultural competence: A guide for working with children and their families* (2nd ed.). Baltimore: Paul H. Brookes Publishing Co.

Marcus, L.M., Kunce, L.J., & Schopler, E. (1997). Working with families. In D.J. Cohen & F.R. Volkmar (Eds.), *Handbook of autism and pervasive developmental disorders* (2nd ed., pp. 631–649). New York: John Wiley & Sons.

Mikus, K.C., Benn, R., & Weatherston, D. (1995). Parallel processes, *ZERO TO THREE Bulletin, 15*(3), 35–40.

Movement may offer early clues to autism. (1999, January 26). *The New York Times,* p. D3.

Prizant, B.M., & Rydell, P.J. (1993). Assessment and intervention considerations for unconventional verbal behavior. In J. Reichle & D.P. Wacker (Eds.), *Communicative alternatives to challenging behavior: Integrating functional assessment and intervention strategies* (pp. 263–297). Baltimore: Paul H. Brookes Publishing Co.

Prizant, B.M., & Wetherby, A.M. (1993). Communication in preschool autistic children. In E. Schopler, M.E. Van Bourgondien, & M.M. Bristol (Eds.), *Preschool issues in autism* (pp. 95–128). New York: Plenum.

Rapin, I. (1997). Autism. *New England Journal of Medicine, 337*(2), 97–104.

Risley, T.R. (1997). Family preservation for children with autism. *Journal of Early Intervention, 21*(1), 15–16.

Robbins, F.R., Dunlap, G., & Pleinis, A.J. (1991). Family characteristics, family training, and the progress of young children with autism. *Journal of Early Intervention, 15*(2), 173–183.

Rogers, D. (1992). *Motor disorder in psychiatry.* New York John Wiley & Sons.

Schopler, E. (1971). Parents of psychotic children as scapegoats. *Journal of Contemporary Psychotherapy, 4,* 17–22.

Siegel, B., Pliner, C., Eschler, J., & Elliot, G.R. (1988). How children with autism are diagnosed: Difficulties in identification of children with multiple developmental delays. *Developmental and Behavioral Pediatrics, 9,* 199–204.

Snell, M. (1983). Forum: The view from a different angle. *Newsletter: The Association for the Severely Handicapped, 9*(11), 1–2.

Stone, W.L. (1997). Autism in early infancy and early childhood. In D.J. Cohen & F.R. Volkmar (Eds.), *Handbook of autism and pervasive developmental disorders* (2nd ed., pp. 266–282).

Strain, P.S. (1990). LRE for preschool children with handicaps: What we know, what we should be doing. *Journal of Early Intervention, 14,* 291–296.

Walizer, E.H., & Leff, P.T. (1993). Personal narratives and the process of educating for the healing partnership. *ZERO TO THREE Bulletin, 14*(1), 21–25.

Wikler, L. (1983). Chronic stresses of families of mentally retarded children. In L. Wikler & M. Keenan (Eds.), *Developmental disabilities: No longer a private tragedy.* Joint publication of the National Association of Social Workers and the American Association on Mental Deficiency.

Williams, D. (1994). *Somebody somewhere.* New York: Times Books.

Wing, L. (1976). Diagnosis, clinical description and prognosis. In L. Wing (Ed.), *Early childhood autism* (2nd ed.). Oxford, England: Pergamon.

Wolery, M. (1997). *Children with autism.* Paper presented at the National Early Childhood Technical Assistance System meeting on developing state and local services for young children with autism and their families, Denver.

Author Index

Page references followed by *t* and *n* indicate tables and footnotes, respectively.

Subject Index

Page references followed by *f* and *t* indicate figures and tables, respectively. Those followed by *n* indicate footnotes.